T0391168

Phosphorus Dendrimers in Biology and Nanomedicine

Phosphorus Dendrimers in Biology and Nanomedicine

Synthesis, Characterization, and Properties

edited by

Anne-Marie Caminade
Cédric-Olivier Turrin
Jean-Pierre Majoral

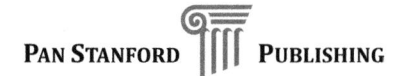

PAN STANFORD PUBLISHING

Published by

Pan Stanford Publishing Pte. Ltd.
Penthouse Level, Suntec Tower 3
8 Temasek Boulevard
Singapore 038988

Email: editorial@panstanford.com
Web: www.panstanford.com

British Library Cataloguing-in-Publication Data
A catalogue record for this book is available from the British Library.

ISBN 978-981-4774-33-8 (Hardcover)
ISBN 978-1-315-11085-1 (eBook)

Dedicated to
Prof. Donald A. Tomalia
on the occasion of his 80th birthday

Contents

Preface

Branched structures are widely found in Nature, at all scales, from the spiral galaxies to some types of cells. The best representatives at the macroscopic level are certainly the trees, with their branches and roots. Branched structures are also found in the blood vessel network, or in the structure of kidneys and lungs in mammals. On a smaller scale, some cells, such as dendritic cells of the immune system also have a branched structure. Surprisingly, at the molecular scale, Nature has not produced any branched structures, with the exception of glycogen (a protein surrounded by multibranched polysaccharide of glucose).

About 40 years ago, man began to produce branched structures at the molecular level, which were first called "cascade" molecules [1]. Then Prof. D. A. Tomalia synthesized the now well-known poly(amidoamines), or PAMAMs, and proposed the name "dendrimer" [2], which is created from two Greek words, "dendros" for tree and "meros" for part (also used for polymer) for naming these branched molecular objects. The term "dendrimer" is now widely accepted and used.

In these 40 years, creative chemists have proposed different types of dendrimers, which are well known to the whole scientific community. An exponential growth of the number of publications has been observed, leading to several tens of thousands of publications, and numerous patents and books [3] about dendrimers to date.

The synthesis of dendrimers consists in the repetition of generally two steps, which must be quantitative to ensure harmonious growth of each branch. Such necessity limits the number of methods suitable to obtain large dendrimers. Among them, the synthesis of

[1]Buhleier, E., Wehner, F., and Vögtle F. (1978). "Cascade-" and "Nonskid-chain-like" syntheses of molecular cavity topologies, *Synthesis*, **78**, pp. 155–158.

[2]Tomalia, D. A., Baker, H., Dewald, J., Hall, M., Kallos, G., Martin, S., Roeck, J., Ryder, J., and Smith, P. (1985). A new class of polymers: Starburst-dendritic macromolecules, *Polym. J.*, **17**, pp. 117–132.

[3]See in particular our previous book: Caminade, A. M., Turrin, C. O., Laurent, R., Ouali, A., and Delavaux-Nicot, B., Editors (2011). *Dendrimers: Towards Catalytic, Material and Biomedical Uses*, John Wiley & Sons Ltd., Chichester, UK.

PAMAM dendrimers was the first process in which large dendrimers were produced, and these dendrimers are undoubtedly the most widely used. Besides PAMAM dendrimers, several classes of dendrimers have emerged, in particular poly(propylenimine) (PPI), polycarbosilane, and phosphorus dendrimers. This book is devoted to phosphorus dendrimers, with emphasis on their properties for biology and nanomedicine. It comprises 14 chapters.

Chapter 1 describes the different types of phosphorus-containing dendrimers, in particular the (poly)phosphorhydrazone (PPH) dendrimers, which were the first ones synthesized in our group [4], and are still the most widely used type of phosphorus dendrimers. The modularity of this synthesis is unique among all types of dendrimers as it permits to easily modify the nature of not only the terminal functions (as for almost all types of dendrimers) but also of the core, and of the constituents of the branches. This method is compliant with other methods of synthesis of dendrimers, to include for instance P=N–P=S linkages at specific levels (for further internal functionalizations), or recently, viologen units (to include positive charges inside the structure). Very unusual types of dendrimeric structures have been obtained, such as new branches grown from within [5] or Janus dendrimers (two faces).

Chapter 2 presents the different types of techniques that have been used to characterize the phosphorus dendrimers, to ascertain their purity, and to measure their size and shape. These techniques originate on one side from molecular chemistry and on the other side from polymer chemistry. Most of these techniques are also usable (and have been used) for the characterization of other types of dendrimers, with the exception of ^{31}P nuclear magnetic resonance (NMR). This technique is especially useful and powerful for the characterization of phosphorus dendrimers, in particular, to ascertain the purity of dendrimers at each layer.

Chapter 3 emphasizes the utility of electron paramagnetic resonance (EPR), in particular, for studies in biologically relevant

[4]Launay, N., Caminade, A. M., Lahana, R., and Majoral, J. P. (1994). A general synthetic strategy for neutral phosphorus-containing dendrimers, *Angew. Chem. Int. Ed. Engl.*, **33**, pp. 1589–1592.
[5]Galliot, C., Larre, C., Caminade, A. M., and Majoral, J. P. (1997). Regioselective stepwise growth of dendrimer units in the internal voids of a main dendrimer, *Science*, **277**, pp. 1981–1984.

conditions. It is indeed a precious tool to investigate biological systems at a molecular level for obtaining *in situ* information about the interactions between molecules and biological entities and the chemical transformations occurring in the system under study. The method can use spin probes or take profit of the presence of paramagnetic atoms in the dendrimer such as Cu(II). The utility of this method is illustrated by the study of interactions of phosphorus dendrimers with amyloid prion peptides involved in Alzheimer and prion neurodegenerative diseases, and also with cancerous cells.

Chapter 4 concerns the fluorescence properties of phosphorus dendrimers. It shows the different types of fluorescent phosphorus dendrimers, with a description of the location of the fluorophores and of their types. Indeed, the classical fluorescent groups and the two-photon absorption fluorophores have both been incorporated either as terminal groups, or at the core, or off-center (linked to the core), or in the branches of phosphorus dendrimers. In all cases, emphasis is put on the use of these fluorescent dendrimers in a biological context, for transfection experiments, and for studying the interaction of dendrimers with cells or blood vessels of living animals, that is, for bioimaging in general.

Chapter 5 discusses the functionalization of solid surfaces by phosphorus dendrimers, in particular, in the context of biomaterials. This chapter is divided into two parts: functionalization of surfaces by non-covalent interactions and functionalization of surfaces by covalent interactions. The first part concerns either weak interactions such as π-stacking or strong interactions such as electrostatic interactions. Hybridization of DNA in this context could be detected up to quantities as small as 10^{-18} M. Different chemical functions of dendrimers have been used for covalent interactions with surfaces: thiols for gold, alcoxysilanes for silica, phosphonates for titanium oxide, or aldehydes for aminosilanized surfaces. Surfaces suitable for cell culturing and sensitive detection of dangerous nitrophenols and very robust DNA chips have been obtained.

Chapters 6 and 7 concern the use of dendrimers against human immunodeficiency virus (HIV), but with two different approaches. Chapter 6 is particularly focused on the strategies based on multivalent non-covalent HIV entry inhibitors and contains several short updates related to this context. GalCer, which is a glycosphingolipid connected to a ceramide group, has been identified as an alternative receptor of HIV, mediated by the V3 loop of gp120 of HIV. However, GalCer is not soluble in water. Water-soluble synthetic analogs of GalCer targeting the gp120 V3 loop are expected to prevent the infection of GalCer presenting cells. In particular, catanionic analogs of GalCer, based on the non-covalent association of carboxylic acids (from the phosphorus dendrimers) and amine (from GalCer) have been synthesized, and tested *in vitro*.

Chapter 7 focuses on the use of various types of positively charged dendrimers against HIV, and more precisely on the role of these dendrimers in the development of new immunotherapies based on dendritic cells against HIV-1 infection. Indeed, dendritic cells–based immunotherapies are being researched as therapeutic HIV-vaccine candidates. The role of dendrimers in this context is to be non-viral vectors to achieve a targeted delivery of specific antigens to dendritic cells, for improving their response to HIV-1 infection. The types of dendrimers tested are PAMAM, PPI, polycarbosilane, and PPH dendrimers.

Chapters 8 and 9 concern two different approaches against cancers. Chapter 8 displays other uses of positively charged dendrimers as vectors of biological entities, in the context of gene therapy against cancers. It discusses and summarizes the ability of phosphorus dendrimers, on one side to deliver therapeutic genes into nuclei of cells, to have these genes permanently expressing themselves, and on the other side to deliver small interfering RNAs into the cytoplasm for the (temporary) silencing of unwanted genes. Several low toxicity and efficient phosphorus dendrimers have been found as promising candidates for gene delivery against cancers.

Chapter 9 presents another approach against cancers that uses phosphorus dendrimers bearing potential ligands as terminal functions, either free or complexing copper. The anti-proliferative activities of both families against various human cancer cell lines were assessed, and their mechanisms of action were elucidated. The detailed mechanism of action was found to be different for the free dendrimers and their copper complexes. Their modes of action were found unusual in the nanomedicine field, occurring *via* activation of the pro-apoptotic protein Bax, a central death regulator.

Chapter 10 concerns a series of mannose derivatives grafted as terminal functions on phosphorus dendrimers and their use for targeting human C-type lectin receptors to prevent lung inflammation. The rationale of this work is based on the mannose-capped lipoarabinomannan, produced by the human pathogen *Mycobacterium tuberculosis*, which displays anti-inflammatory properties. The aim was to mimic the bioactive supramolecular structure of mannose-capped lipoarabinomannan, with the objective of developing innovative anti-inflammatory molecules. A dendrimer bearing trimannosides as terminal groups was found particularly efficient, including *in vivo*, to prevent lung inflammation in mice.

Chapter 11 proposes several approaches concerning the use of phosphorus dendrimers against diseases of the central nervous system. Positively charged dendrimers were found efficient against prion diseases such as the mad cow disease and the Creutzfeldt–Jakob disease, including *in vivo* (for mice). These dendrimers, bearing positive charges on the surface or inside the structure, were also found suitable to inhibit the aggregation of specific peptides responsible for the accumulation of fibrils and senile plaques in the brain, inducing Alzheimer's and Parkinson's diseases. A negatively charged phosphorus dendrimer ABP [amino-bis(methylene phosphonate)] was found to be efficient *in vivo* to treat mice developing a model of multiple sclerosis.

Chapter 12 tells the long story of ABP, which is a single (small) phosphorus dendrimer, and its 12 azabisphosphonate terminal functions. This compound has many properties to trigger the human immune system, as shown by numerous tests with peripheral blood mononuclear cells (PBMCs). The primary cellular target of dendrimer ABP is the monocytes after which it selectively amplifies the natural killer cells (essential against viral, bacterial, and parasitic infections), a change that can be observed after few weeks. The activation of monocytes by ABP occurs via an anti-inflammatory pathway, offering a promising solution against chronic inflammatory diseases. *In vivo* assays were successfully carried out on mice suffering from diseases, models of rheumatoid arthritis and multiple sclerosis, and rats with uveitis.

Chapter 13 is a reflection about dendrimers and their potential and future role in biology and nanomedicine. Indeed, dendrimer nanostructures represent outstanding nanocarriers in nanomedicine, and they have often been referred to as the "polymers of the 21st century". In this chapter, the "dendrimer space concept" has been proposed analogous to the space concepts of chemistry and biology, which are extensively used in the pharmaceutical industry to develop new drugs.

Chapter 14 is the last one. It emphasizes the first industrial use of phosphorus-containing dendrimers, proposed by a start-up Dendris [6]. It concerns the use of phosphorus dendrimers in a multiplexing technology based on DNA for the rapid and accurate diagnosis of pathogens. These DNA arrays (DendrisChips) have been tested in several French hospitals for the detection of pathogens pulmonary and sexual diseases and in food industries for detection of food bacteria.

In conclusion, we do believe that phosphorus-containing dendrimers, which already have a brilliant past as emphasized by all the biological properties reported in this book, will also have a brilliant future, particularly in the field of nanomedicine, as shown by the recent creation of IMD-Pharma S.A.S [7]. Phosphorus dendrimers are indeed just another type of dendrimers but they also have their own properties.

Anne-Marie Caminade
Cédric-Olivier Turrin
Jean-Pierre Majoral
Winter 2017

---

[6]www.dendris.fr
[7]www.IMD-Pharma.com

Chapter 1

Synthesis of Phosphorus-Containing Dendrimers

Jean-Pierre Majoral, Régis Laurent, and Anne-Marie Caminade
Laboratoire de Chimie de Coordination, CNRS, 205 Route de Narbonne,
BP 44099, 31077 Toulouse Cedex 4, France
jean-pierre.majoral@lcc-toulouse.fr, anne-marie.caminade@lcc-toulouse.fr

1.1 Introduction

Among the different types of dendrimers, those incorporating phosphorus in various positions in their structure present undoubtedly the largest variety of constitutive elements of the core, branching units, internal branches, backbones, and surfaces due to the fascinating versatility of the organophosphorus chemistry. The use of ^{31}P NMR, which is a highly valuable tool for the characterization of these dendrimers, explains why a large number of synthetic procedures were proposed. Reactions are generally easy to perform, in mild conditions, the by-products being removed without sophisticated techniques (water and nitrogen are often the only by-products of the sequence of reactions) and the

Phosphorus Dendrimers in Biology and Nanomedicine: Synthesis, Characterization, and Properties
Edited by Anne-Marie Caminade, Cédric-Olivier Turrin, and Jean-Pierre Majoral
Copyright © 2018 Pan Stanford Publishing Pte. Ltd.
ISBN 978-981-4774-33-8 (Hardcover), 978-1-315-11085-1 (eBook)
www.panstanford.com

final compounds being obtained in high yields. As a consequence, properties and applications of these nano-objects were intensively studied and successfully illustrated in different fields ranging from nanomaterials, biology, nanomedicine, catalysis, etc.

The aim of this chapter is not the full presentation of what was done in the field of the construction of phosphorus dendrimers but simply to give to the reader a flavor of what it is possible to do playing with phosphorus chemistry in this very important domain of nanoscience. Therefore, this non-exhaustive review will illustrate via selected examples the multiple possibilities to create such macromolecular species.

1.2 Synthesis and Selected Reactivity of Dendrimers Involving Phosphorhydrazone Linkages

Our first and main method of synthesis of phosphorus dendrimers [1] consists in the repetition of two quantitative reactions, the first step being the nucleophilic substitution of Cl by hydroxybenzaldehyde in basic conditions. The second step is the condensation of the aldehydes with the dichlorophosphothiohydrazide. This compound is also issued from the organic chemistry of phosphorus (substitution of one Cl of $P(S)Cl_3$ with methylhydrazine, at low temperature). The second step generates PCl_2 functions at the periphery of the dendrimer suitable to perform again substitutions with the 4-hydroxybenzaldehyde (Fig. 1.1). Remarkably, this method has been carried out up to generation 12 from $P(S)Cl_3$ [2] and to generation 8 starting from $P_3N_3Cl_6$ [3]. All the reactions are quantitative in most cases, using less than 5% excess of reagents.

The presence of $P(S)Cl_2$ end groups on the outer shell of the dendrimers allows the grafting of many types of functionalized phenols and, therefore, the incorporation of a variety of other functional groups bringing original properties. Several examples are shown in Fig. 1.2; the colors indicate for which type of use they were synthesized. Besides the aldehydes, which are obtained during the course of the synthesis of these dendrimers, and which are used for the elaboration of DNA chips (see Chapter 14) [4, 5], the main properties obtained with these functionalizations concern electrochemistry, catalysis, fluorescence, biology, or even as precursors for other types of functions. For the electrochemical properties, one can cite ferrocenes for studying the evolution of the properties depending on the generation [6], also the evolution of chirality [7], or catalysis [8], with an efficiency depending on the type of linker between ferrocene and phosphine [9], and the possibility to switch ON/OFF the catalysis [10]. Electropolymerization of thiophene derivative was carried out to obtain electroconductive polymers [11].

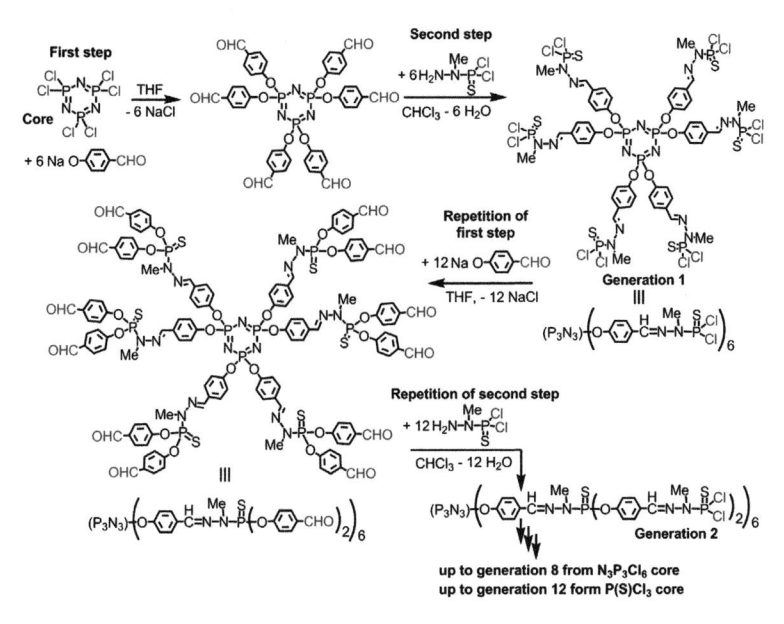

Figure 1.1 The most widely used method of synthesis of phosphorus dendrimers.

Many types of catalytic entities have been grafted on the surface of phosphorus dendrimers, which have been recently reviewed [12]. The examples shown in Fig. 1.2 concern derivatives of triphenylphosphine [13, 14], thiazolylphosphines [15], iminophosphines [16], diphosphines [17], azabis-oxazolines [18], diketones [19], pyridineimine [20], terpyridine [21], and cinchonine [22]. Diverse types of fluorophores (see Chapter 4) have been grafted to the surface of phosphorus dendrimers, in particular maleimide derivative obtained by reaction of tyramine with 2,4-diphenyl maleic anhydride

[23], dansyl [24], and also dabsyl [25] derivatives, or fluorophores having two-photon absorption (TPA) properties [26], with eventually interchromophoric interactions [27], or third-order nonlinear properties [28]. Some of these chromophores have been used as biological tools, in connection with other functions having biological properties. These functions comprise D-xylose derivatives [29], carboxylates, and phosphonates derivatives as precursors of anti-HIV compounds [30] (see Chapter 6), azabisphosphonates [31] (and isosteric carboxylic esters analogs [32]) precursors of symmetrical [33] or non-symmetrical [34] azabisphosphonic salts having important anti-inflammatory properties (see Chapter 12) [35]. In most cases, the methoxy derivatives are grafted, then the deprotection affords dendrimers with phosphonic or carboxylic acid salts as terminal functions. The importance of the number of terminal functions

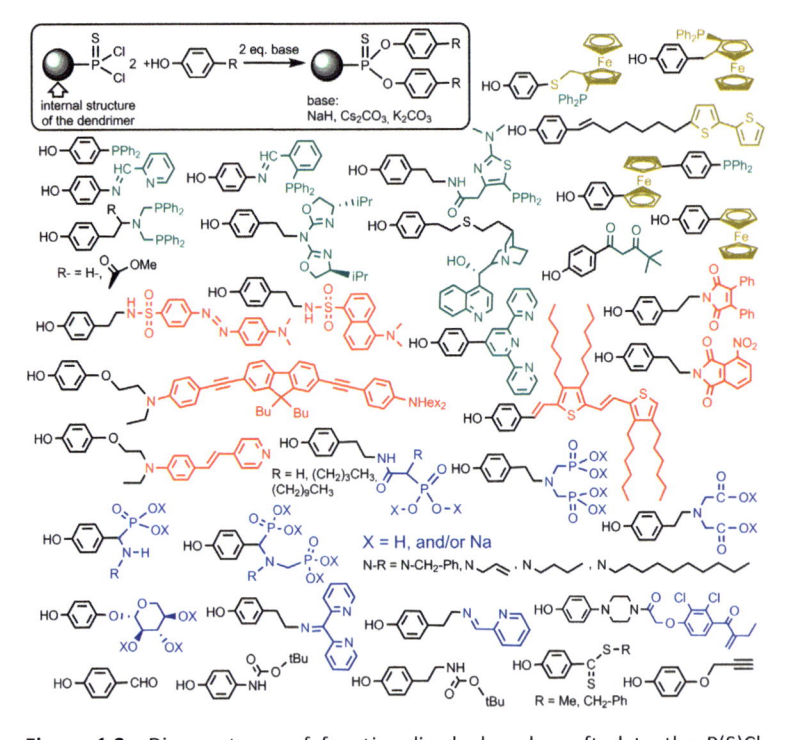

Figure 1.2 Diverse types of functionalized phenols grafted to the P(S)Cl$_2$ terminal functions of dendrimers; in yellow-gold for electrochemistry; in green for catalysis (after complexation of a metal); in red for fluorescence; in blue for biological purposes; and in black for precursor of other functions.

[36] and of the nature of the internal structure for the anti-inflammatory properties have been emphasized [37]. Recent results in the field of oncology have been obtained with dendrimers functionalized by copper complexes of pyridine derivatives [38] (see Chapter 9), and ethacrynic acid [39, 40] (Fig. 1.2).

A few functional phenols are precursors of other functions, after their grafting to dendrimers. The aldehydes have been used for condensation reactions with amino crown ether [41], hydrazine [42] or methylhydrazine [43], Girard P and T reagents [44], but also for Wittig [41, 42, 45], and Horner–Wadsworth–Emmons reactions [46]. The aldehydes can also be reduced to benzylalcohols, then modified to benzylchloride or bromide, for the grafting of catalytic entities such as PTA [47] or cinchoninium salts [48]. Dithioesters have been used for acylation reactions [49], and as precursors of star polymers obtained by reversible addition-fragmentation chain transfer (RAFT) [50]. The Boc-protected amines afford primary amines as terminal functions after deprotection, which have been used for the capture of CO_2 [51], or for the grafting of other functions such as diverse mannose derivatives [52], or gem-bisphosphonates [53]. Propargyl groups have been recently used for the click reaction with azidopoly(vinylidenefluoride) [54].

Besides phenols, diverse amines have been reacted with the $P(S)Cl_2$ terminal functions. Among them, one can cite allyl and propargyl amines [55], and also diethylethylenediamine, which affords in a single-step water-soluble dendrimers, HCl generated by the substitution reaction being trapped by the tertiary amine [56]. The latter family of compounds has many properties in the field of materials for the elaboration of nano-tubes [57, 58], microcapsules [59], and highly sensitive DNA chips [60] (see Chapters 5 and 14), and in the field of biology as transfection agents [56], anti-prion agents [61], anti-aggregation agents of Alzheimer peptides [62], and Parkinson peptides [63] (see Chapters 7, 8, and 11). Other types of diamines, such as morpholine or piperidine derivatives, have also been grafted in view of transfection experiments [64]. In other examples, both Cl linked to the same P can react with a single diamine, creating a diazaphospholane cycle. This cycle was obtained from various macrocycles [65], or was linked to a triazamacrocycle that is able to complex Pd^0 [66] or Pt^0 [67], to create nanoparticles of these metals, and even to organize them in dendritic networks [68], or to afford liquid crystal dendrimers [69]. Several examples of the reactivity of diverse amines are displayed in Fig. 1.3.

The reaction with amines is also suitable to perform specific monosubstitutions on each $P(X)Cl_2$ (X = S, O) end group. The reaction is regiospecific, but not enantioselective. The monosubstitution using sequentially two types of amines leads to dendrimers with two, three, or four functional groups on each chain end [42]. The second substitution can be performed also with phenols, in particular HOC_6H_4CHO (Fig. 1.3) [70]. A recent example concerned the possibility to graft both triethoxysilyl groups (for grafting to silica) together with a primary amine (free or Boc-protected), for the capture of CO_2 [71].

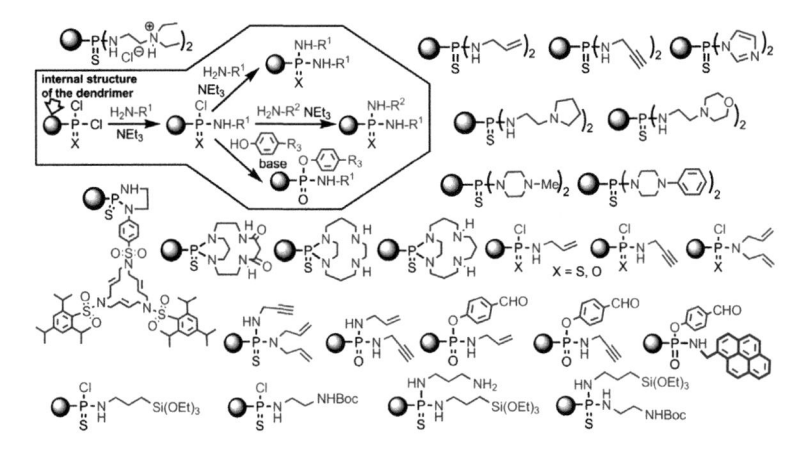

Figure 1.3 Examples of functionalization of the surface of dendrimers by amino derivatives on $P(X)Cl_2$ (X = O, S) terminal functions, with one or two amines, or one amine and one phenol, leading to multifunctionalized dendrimers. Only one function is shown, representative of all the terminal functions.

Most of the examples shown above concern phosphorus dendrimers issued from the reactivity of the core $P_3N_3(OC_6H_4CHO)_6$. Alternatively, the higher homolog $P_4N_4(OC_6H_4CHO)_8$ has been also synthesized [36]. Ways of preparation of phosphorus-containing dendrimers can be conducted from other cores, such as the modified phthalocyanine bearing eight external aldehyde groups [72]. This monomer, using the process shown in Fig. 1.1, permits the preparation of fluorescent dendrimers up to generation 5 bearing 256 terminal protonated amines (Fig. 1.4). This dendrimer was found as a nanotool, able to modify its environment and to be modified by it [73]. It has been used also for the visualization of transfection experiments [74].

An analogous sequence of reactions developed around a bisphenol derivative presenting remarkable TPA properties leads to the synthesis of blue organic nanodots useful for medical imaging [75]. Such a water-soluble polycationic highly fluorescent dendrimer allows, for example, the two-photon imaging (excitation at 710 nm) of the vascular network in the dorsal part of the rat olfactory bulb, after injecting intravenously the dendrimer of generation 2 in water. Similarly a "green" organic nanodot prepared from a green TPA monomer (Fig. 1.4) permits the visualization of the vascular system of the muscle tissue of tadpole [76]. Remarkably, these new brilliant nanodots were demonstrated to be nontoxic and represent, therefore, a new family of dendrimers for *in vivo* multiphotonic imaging.

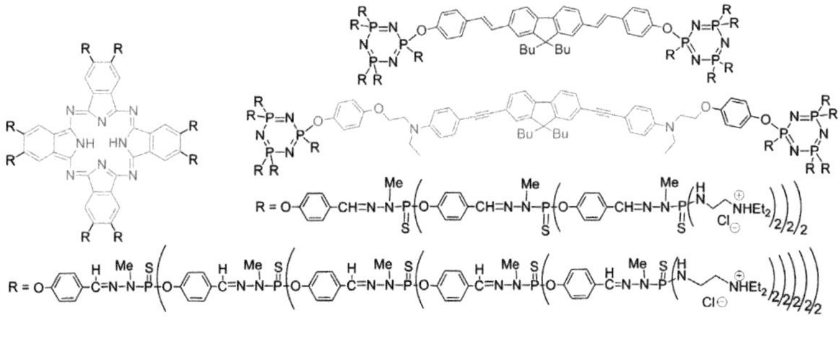

Figure 1.4 Examples of fluorescent cores of water-soluble dendrimers ended by ammonium groups and used for imaging.

The use of TPA fluorophores as cores of dendrimers was made possible by the specific reactivity of hexachlorocyclotriphosphazene [77]. Indeed, the reactivity of each Cl can be differentiated, and the desired products isolated by chromatography. This method was used in particular to afford dendrimers with one, two, three, four, or five branches ended by azabisphosphonate functions, and emanating from the cyclotriphosphazene core, for studying their anti-inflammatory properties [36]. However, in most cases, only one function different from all the others is linked to the core. These types of dendrimers are called "off-center" [78]. Such a process used with the N_3P_3 core is illustrated in Fig. 1.5. In many cases, the single function is a Boc-protected tyramine, used in combination with five aldehydes, to continue the growing of the branches [79], or with five phosphines in view of catalysis experiments [79], or with five dyes such as dabsyl [25] and dansyl in view of the synthesis of Janus dendrimers [24]. A single aldehyde has been used in combination with five methylesters [36], or with five fluorophores such as dansyl [24] or maleimide derivatives, used as sensors for the detection of nitrophenols [80]. One methyl ester (to be deprotected to afford the corresponding carboxylic acid) has been used in combination with either five aldehydes [71] or five Boc-protected tyramine to afford Janus dendrimers [24]. One thioctic acid has been used in combination with five aldehydes to continue the growing of the dendrimer, to afford finally either positively or negatively charged dendrimers. The thioctic function was used for the grafting of the dendrimers to gold surfaces and studying the influence of the charge on the behavior of osteoblast cells [81]. Combinations of one methylhydrazine with five phosphines on one side and of one azide with five aldehydes on the other side afforded two monomers based on N_3P_3 suitable for the rapid synthesis of dendrimers [82], as will be shown in Section 1.3.1. A single fluorescent entity has been grafted also in several cases to the N_3P_3 core, together with five aldehydes. This concerns, in particular, a maleimide derivative [23], used for biological experiments after grafting ammoniums as terminal functions [33, 36, 83], a pyrene derivative, used for catalysis experiments after grafting phosphine complexes as terminal functions [13], and a julolidine derivative used for bioimaging after grafting bisphosphonates as terminal functions [36] (Fig. 1.5).

Other families of dendrimers incorporating phosphorhydrazone linkages have been synthesized by replacing hydroxybenzaldehyde by other hydroxyaldehydes (Fig. 1.6). Among them, one can cite the possibility to have longer branches [84], various types of ferrocene derivatives for studying the influence of the burying of this function on electrochemical properties [6, 85, 86], azobenzenes for studying the possibility to induce trans-cis isomerizations [87], or fluorophores having TPA properties emitting in the blue-green for the fluorene linked to two triple bonds [88] and in the green for the fluorene linked to two double bonds [89], for bioimaging.

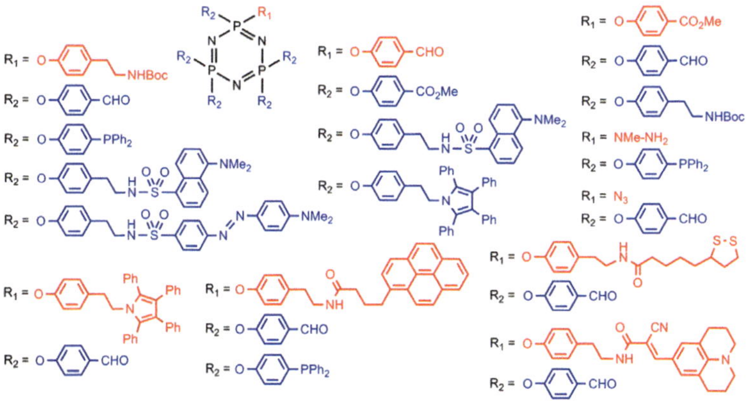

Figure 1.5 Examples of selective functionalization of N_3P_3 for the synthesis of off-center dendrimers. The function in red is used one time; the function in blue is used five times.

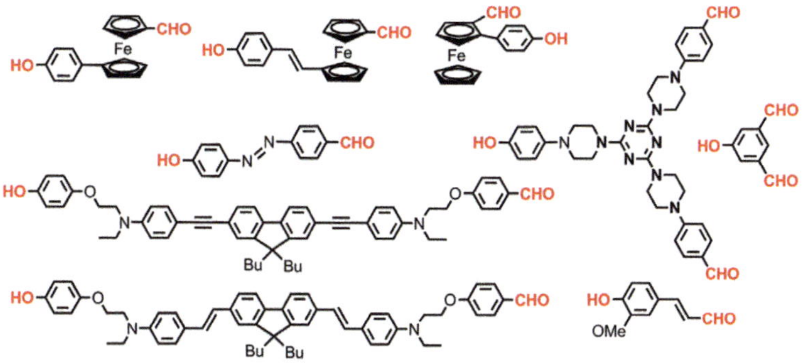

Figure 1.6 Examples of hydroxyl aldehydes used for replacing 4-hydroxyben-zaldehyde in the branches of phosphorus dendrimers.

The replacement of hydroxybenzaldehyde also offers the possibility to multiply more rapidly the number of terminal functions, using phenol dialdehydes. The first example was obtained using hydroxybenzene dicarboxaldehyde. The generation 4 dendrimer was obtained in only four steps instead of 8 when using the classical method of synthesis shown in Fig. 1.1 [90]. This concept was recently developed for the synthesis of dendrimers intrinsically composed in alternation of building blocks pertaining to two known families of dendrimers, namely the phosphorhydrazone dendrimers and the triazine-piperazine dendrimers [91, 92]. The synthesis is based on a monomer having one phenol and two benzaldehyde moieties linked to a triazine-trispiperazine entity (Fig. 1.6). The resulting "mixed" dendrimers with layered controlled architecture have inherited some properties from their "parents," but they have also their own and original characteristics. Both parent families are white powders, whereas the mixed dendrimers are yellow, orange, or red powders, depending on the generation, due to an increased electronic delocalization. These dendrimers incorporate redox active organic entities (triazine and piperazine) that allow for the first time the monitoring of the growth of an organic dendrimer by electrochemistry [93].

1.3 Synthesis Involving P=N–P=S Linkages

The Staudinger reaction of phosphines with azides creates P=N bonds, which are generally sensitive to hydrolysis. However, if the P=N function is conjugated, its stability is largely increased. Thus, instead of using organic azides, thiophosphoryl azides can be used to generate P=N–P=S linkages [94] (or eventually P=N–P=N when using azides linked to the cyclotriphosphazene), as shown in the following figures.

1.3.1 Accelerated Synthesis from Orthogonal Systems

Several types of AB_5 and CD_5 monomers were prepared and used alternatively, affording accelerated synthesis of very original dendrimers from the hexaaldehyde cyclotriphosphazene $P_3N_3(OC_6H_4 CHO)_6$ used as core [95]. This method allows to create a new generation at each step and a rapid multiplication by 5 of the number of terminal groups (and not by two as usual), with A = NMe–NH$_2$, B = ArPPh$_2$, C = N$_3$, and D = ArCHO. Only three steps (condensation D + A, then Staudinger B + C, then again condensation D + A) are necessary to build a phosphorus dendrimer of generation 3 bearing 750 end groups! (Fig. 1.7) [82].

An analogous accelerated strategy using AB_2 and CD_2 monomers, starting from $(S)P(OC_6H_4CHO)_3$, was also developed up to the synthesis of a dendrimer of generation 4 [96]. Other combinations based on another series of monomers (CA$_2$ and DB$_2$) have been used, as shown in Fig. 1.8 [97].

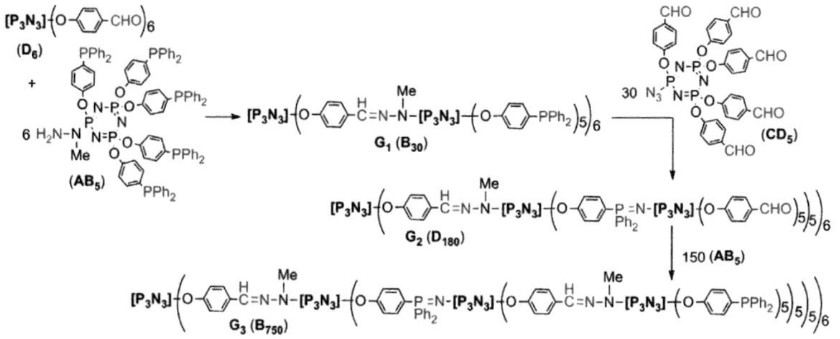

Figure 1.7 Accelerated synthesis of phosphorus-containing dendrimers, using two branched monomers for condensation and Staudinger reactions.

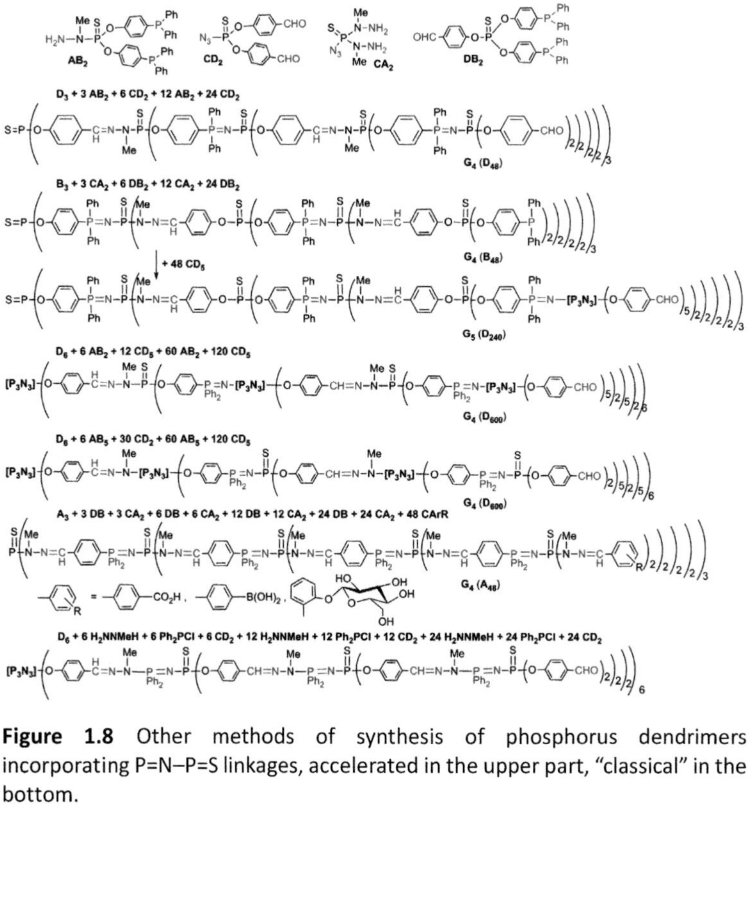

Figure 1.8 Other methods of synthesis of phosphorus dendrimers incorporating P=N–P=S linkages, accelerated in the upper part, "classical" in the bottom.

Other methodologies have used condensation reactions and Staudinger reactions for the synthesis of dendrimers, but necessitating two steps for the synthesis of one generation. The hydrazine terminal functions were used for condensation reactions with functionalized benzaldehydes, affording carboxylic acids, boronic acids, or carbohydrates terminal functions [98]. A three-step process was also used for the synthesis of dendrimers up to generation 3 [99] (Fig. 1.8).

Figure 1.8 displays the linear structure of two generation 4 dendrimers having the same number of terminal aldehyde groups (60) after the same number of steps, but using two different methods. For this reason, both compounds have a different internal structure, as shown by the full chemical structure of their second generations in Fig. 1.9 [82].

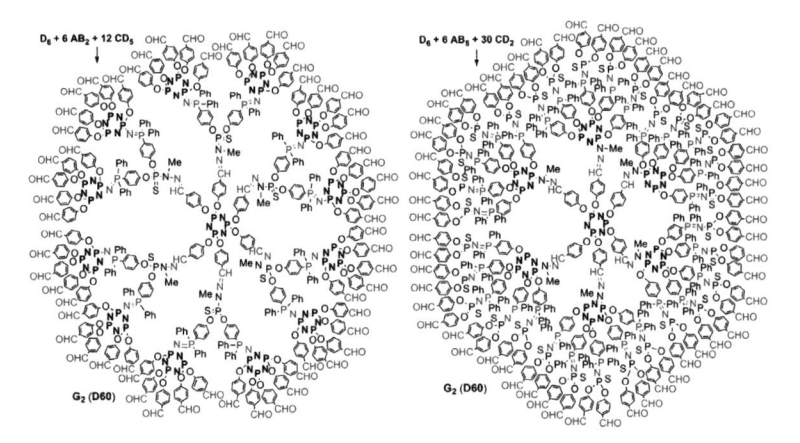

Figure 1.9 Two second-generation dendrimers having 60 aldehyde terminal functions, built from the hexaaldehyde core using two different accelerated methods of synthesis.

1.3.2 Growing Dendrimers inside a Dendrimer

The compatibility of the Staudinger reaction with the condensation reaction allows having P=N–P=S linkages selectively at one or several layers. The P=S groups linked to a P=N group have distinguishable properties compared to the other P=S groups, due to a delocalized form [100] $^+$P–N=P–S$^-$ with a negative charge on S, which renders it sensitive to alkylation reactions using methyltriflate [101], or allyl- and propargyl-triflates [102], whereas the other P=S groups do not react. The P=N–P=S linkages are also suitable for the complexation of gold [103] (see hereafter). Interestingly, the alkylation provokes a weakening of the P=S bond, which can be easily cleaved with nucleophilic phosphines and in particular $P(NMe_2)_3$. The formed tricoordinated phosphorus linkages at specific layers of the internal structure can be submitted to Staudinger reactions, in particular with the CD_2 monomer (see Fig. 1.8), thus affording P=N–P=N–P=S linkages [103]. The presence of aldehydes inside the dendrimers allows either the step-by-step growing of new branches [104] (Fig. 1.10) or the grafting of dendrons, leading to highly sophisticated phosphorus dendritic structures [105]. In addition, some other reactions can be undertook as, for example, the regioselective incorporation of macrocycles, metals [106], zwitter-ions [107], or fluorescent groups [108].

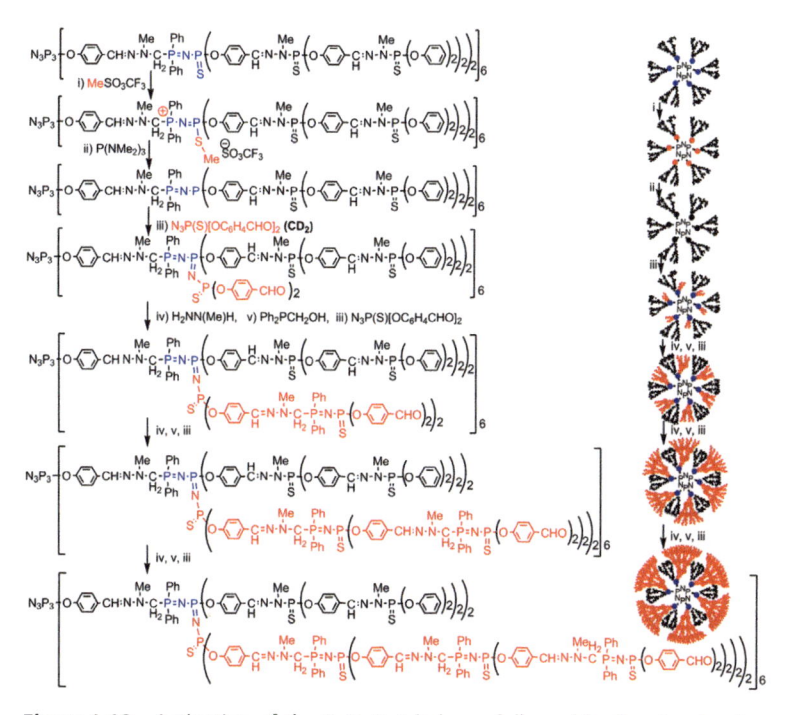

Figure 1.10 Activation of the P=N–P=S linkage, followed by the step-by-step growing of new branches inside the dendritic structure.

1.3.3 Dendritic Structures owing P=N–P=S at Each Generation

The synthetic strategy involves the reiteration of a sequence of two reactions: (i) a Staudinger-type reaction between species that have free phosphino groups and an azide, the latter bearing complexed phosphino groups with BH_3, and (ii) the deprotection of the resulting phosphino-boron adducts with a base such as DABCO. Such a methodology was applied to the preparation of dendrimers up to the fifth generation (Fig. 1.11) [109]. The same process has been applied starting from PPh_3 as core and has been carried out up to generation 4 [110].

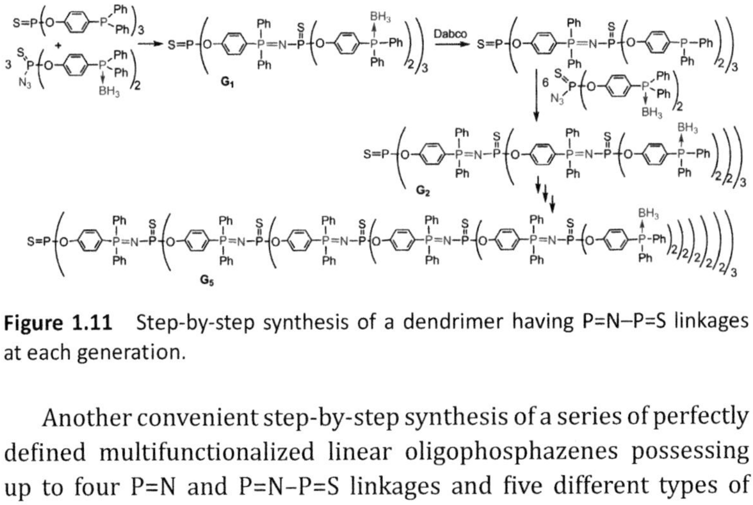

Figure 1.11   Step-by-step synthesis of a dendrimer having P=N–P=S linkages at each generation.

Another convenient step-by-step synthesis of a series of perfectly defined multifunctionalized linear oligophosphazenes possessing up to four P=N and P=N–P=S linkages and five different types of substituents on the phosphorus atoms was described affording a novel core for the design of original macromolecules combining linear oligomeric monomer and dendritic structures as it was illustrated with the grafting of dendrons diversely functionalized in a specific location of the oligophosphazene linkage (Fig. 1.12) [111].

1.3.4   P=N–P=S Linkages at the Core of Dendrons

The Staudinger reaction applied to thiophosphoryl azides (in particular the CD_2 monomer $(S)PN_3(OC_6H_4CHO)_2$ shown in Fig. 1.8) has been extremely useful for the synthesis of dendrimers, as shown in numerous previous figures. This reaction has been used also for the synthesis of dendrimers having special cores such as 1,6-diphosphine [101], bisdiphenylphosphino ferrocene [94], a triazamacrocycle [112], a cage diphosphine [113], or alkenylphosphines [114] and a phosphonate-phosphine [115], for the synthesis of dendrons (dendritic wedges) [116], and a triethoxysilyl phosphine for the grafting to silica [117]. The main types of cores used for Staudinger reactions are shown in Fig. 1.13.

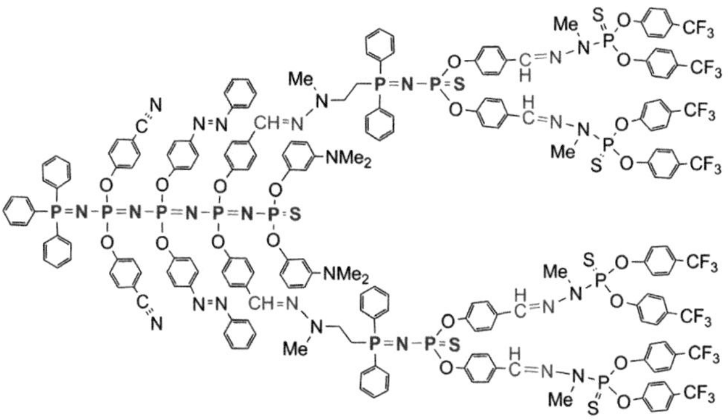

Figure 1.12 A linear oligophosphazene as core, synthesized step-by-step, bearing two dendritic branches.

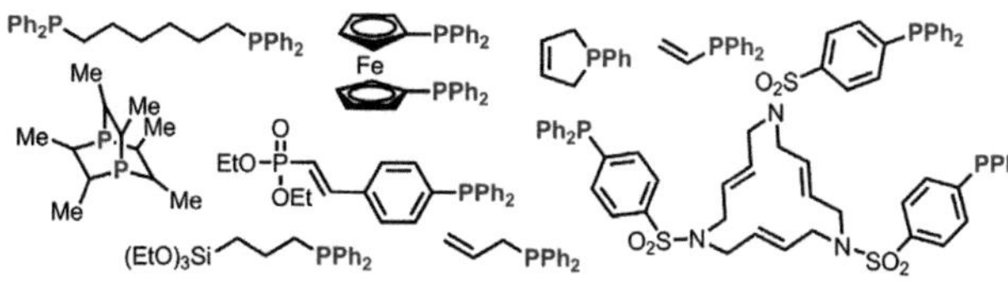

Figure 1.13 Types of cores used for Staudinger reactions with (S) $PN_3(OC_6H_4CHO)_2$.

The case of diphenylvinylphosphine is particularly interesting, as the presence of the P=N–P=S linkage activates the vinyl function, which reacts easily in Michael-type additions with amines and hydrazines. The main types of reactions are shown in Fig. 1.14; they have been carried out in most cases up to generation 3, having various types of terminal functions. The reactions comprise the addition of propargylamine, tyramine, diallylamine, thiomorpholine, and trans-diaminocyclohexane [105], as well as aminopropyl triethoxysilane [117]. Methylhydrazine and ethylenediamine, which can be further functionalized to afford phosphine or azide derivatives, suitable for the synthesis of highly sophisticated dendritic architectures having different types of terminal functions in a single dendritic object [118] and also for catalysis experiments [119], have been also added to the vinyl group. These reactions are also suitable for the synthesis of Janus dendrimers (see Section 1.6). A cyclam derivative linked to a cross-linked polystyrene nanoparticle was functionalized by polycationic dendrons (Fig. 1.14). The colloidal and thermal stability of the nanoparticles were improved, and the complexing properties of the cyclam core were retained and allowed the formation of copper-containing hydrogels [120].

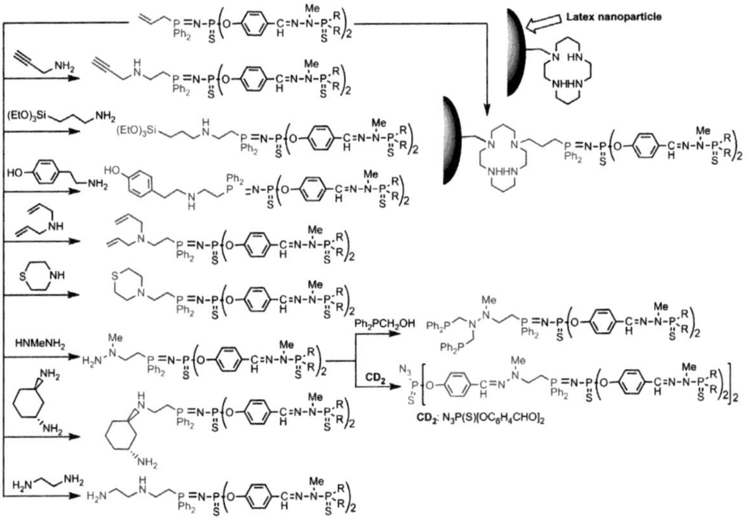

Figure 1.14 Examples of reactions of amines with the vinyl core of dendrons. These syntheses have been carried out in most cases up to generation 3 of dendrons. R corresponds to phosphorhydrazone branches bearing various types of terminal groups.

1.4 Hybrid Phosphorus–Viologen Dendrimers and Macromolecular Asterisks

There is continuous interest in extending the chemical skeleton feature of dendrimers in general and of phosphorus dendrimers in particular. This prompted us to design new dendritic phosphorus species offering diverse possibilities for their respective backbone chemical structures, including the core, branching points, internal branches, and outer shell. The previous paragraphs have already shown diverse possibilities; new and recent ones will be given in the next paragraphs.

Due to the numerous possible applications of viologen units (dialkylated 4,4-bipyridine units) in different fields, such as electron- and charge-storing devices, electron sponges, antimicrobial and antiviral agents, or sequential complexation agents as guest anions and for molecular recognition purposes [121–123], branches incorporating these active linkages were also added stepwise, for the preparation of a very few types of purely organic dendrimers. In light of these properties and the properties of phosphorus dendrimers, it appeared interesting to develop new methodologies for the preparation of dendrimers by mixing viologen and phosphorus linkages in the same framework, in order to propose fruitful nano-objects for new applications. For this purpose, new symmetric or asymmetric viologen monomers, dimers, or trimers were prepared, and mixed phosphorus viologens were obtained by using convergent and divergent strategies. The synthesis of viologen monomers is illustrated in Fig. 1.15 [124].

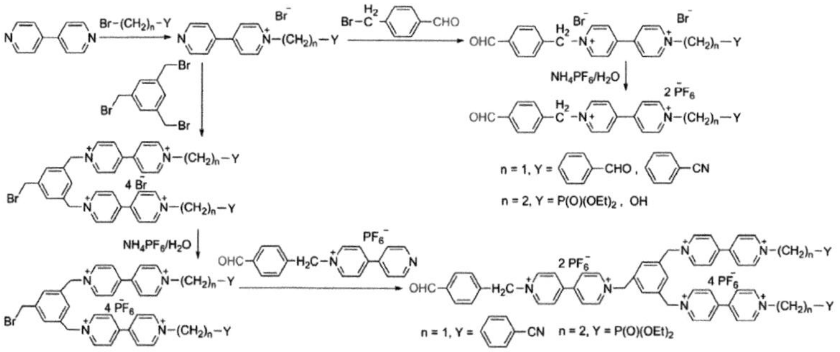

Figure 1.15 Synthesis of diverse viologen derivatives, in particular those functionalized by aldehydes, usable for the synthesis of dendrimers.

These functionalized viologen units, in particular those bearing and aldehyde, were used for the synthesis of the corresponding mix dendrimers, as shown in Fig. 1.16. Most of the reactions involved a condensation reaction with $(S)P(NMeNH_2)_3$ or $P_3N_3(NMeNH_2)_6$.

These strategies offer the possibility to incorporate positive charges not only at the surface of dendrimers but also within their cascade structures [124]. The biological properties of most of these dendrimers were tested. It was shown in particular that the poly(ethylene glycol) (PEG) derivative was not toxic toward normal cells, but toxic toward cancerous cells [125].

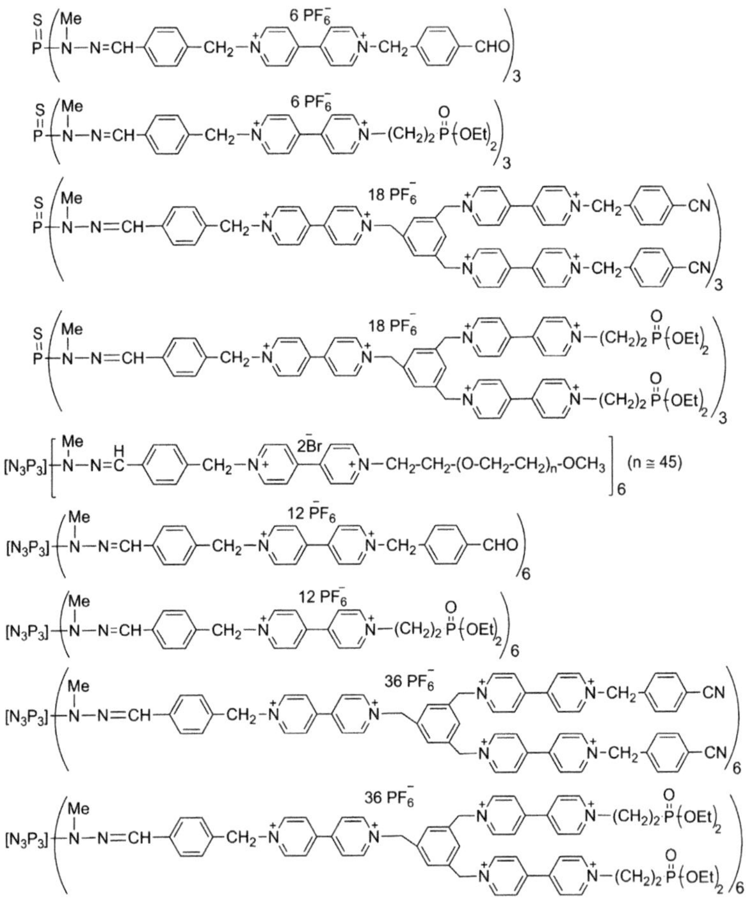

Figure 1.16 Small viologen dendrimers built from tri- or hexafunctional cores.

Such a strategy was recently developed for the design of new ambiphilic viologen-based dendritic-macromolecular asterisks incorporating three types of phosphorus units: a cyclotriphospha-zene core, phosphonate end groups, and hexafluorophosphate as counter anions [126]. Classical organic reactions and easy work-up procedures provide a library of mono-, bis-, tris-, and tetrakis-violo-gen-based molecular and macromolecular building blocks that can react with a functional cyclotriphosphazene core to generate photo-reactive phosphorus–viologen macromolecular asterisks. These soft scaffolds were used to efficiently stabilize nanosized gold particles up to 8 months. The structure of the mono-, bis-, and tris-viologen derivatives terminated in one side with aldehyde and on the other side with a phosphonate group is shown in Fig. 1.17, as well as the illustration of the methodology of synthesis of the macromolecular asterisk bearing up to 24 viologen linkages, the last step being a condensation reaction between $P_3N_3(NCH_3NH_2)_6$ and the tetrakis viologen monomer.

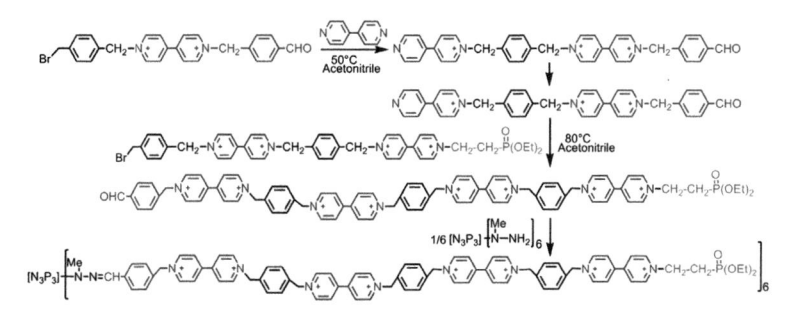

Figure 1.17 Synthesis of a macromolecular asterisk composed of four viologen units in each arm.

1.5 Onion Peel Dendritic Structures

An "onion peel" strategy for the divergent construction of glycodendrimers using different building blocks at each layer of the dendritic growth has been reported by Roy *et al.* [127, 128]. A combination of successive highly efficient and versatile chemical reactions, namely thiol–ene or thiol–yne, esterification, and azide–alkyne click chemistry, have been used to form heterogeneous layers. The dendrimers prepared using this strategy are fundamentally different from conventional dendrimers. Similarly, phosphorus dendrimers constituted with heterogeneous layers have been also reported, as can be seen in many of the previous figures. In fact, the very first example of layered dendrimer was presented a long time ago; it consisted in using in alternation the classical dichlorothiophosphorhydrazide $(S)PCl_2(NMeNH_2)$ and the corresponding oxo derivative $(O)PCl_2(NMeNH_2)$. The dendrimers have been built up to generation 4, exhibiting two layers of P(O) and three layers of P(S) functions, as shown in Fig. 1.18 [129].

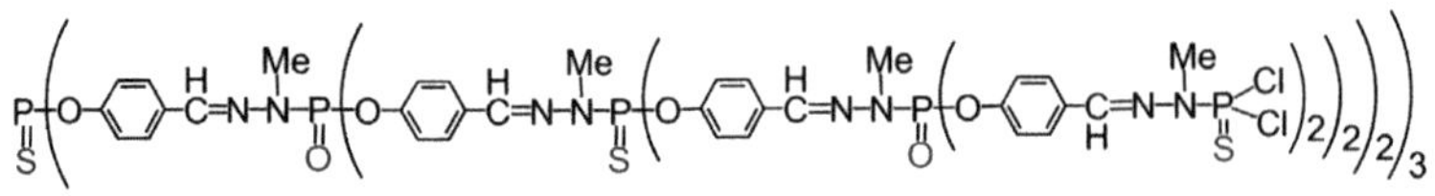

Figure 1.18 The first layered phosphorus dendrimer, built in alternation of PS and PO units.

Another example of this onion peel strategy was grounded on a convergent strategy by combination of double alkylation of viologen units with two different halogenated reagents, one of them based on a carbosilane dendron, and the subsequent ligation to a hexafunctionalized phosphorus core through an amine–aldehyde condensation reaction. This strategy allows combining the structural diversity of the three building blocks based on the lipophilicity of the carbosilane scaffold, the polarity imposed by the viologen branches, and the rigidity of the phosphorus-based core, along with their individually potential biological uses. Namely, hybrid systems containing carbosilane, viologen, and phosphorus dendritic scaffolds into one single molecule have been designed. Starting from the hexafunctionalized core $[(P_3N_3)(NMeNH_2)_6]$, dendrimers containing two kinds of cations were obtained. One is formed by viologen quaternized units located at inner branches while the other is ammonium groups at the surface of the carbosilane wedges (Fig. 1.19). This situation makes them unique and interesting, to be explored from the biological point of view [130].

Similarly, efforts were turned toward the design of unprecedented "onion peel" nanodendritic phosphorus structures, in which a large variety of different phosphorus units were regioselectively incorporated stepwise, each of them bringing the possibility to increase the functionalities of the final macromolecules or affording new perspectives for development. In addition, the repeating branches of each generation are generally not identical. A general strategy for the straightforward preparation of various onion peel nanodendritic structures, incorporating up to seven different types of phosphorus units, which, to our knowledge, is unprecedented for all classes of macromolecules and polymers, was recently proposed [131]. For such a purpose, a variety of cores and building blocks were prepared from which onion peel dendritic structures of generations 2 and 3 were obtained (Fig. 1.20).

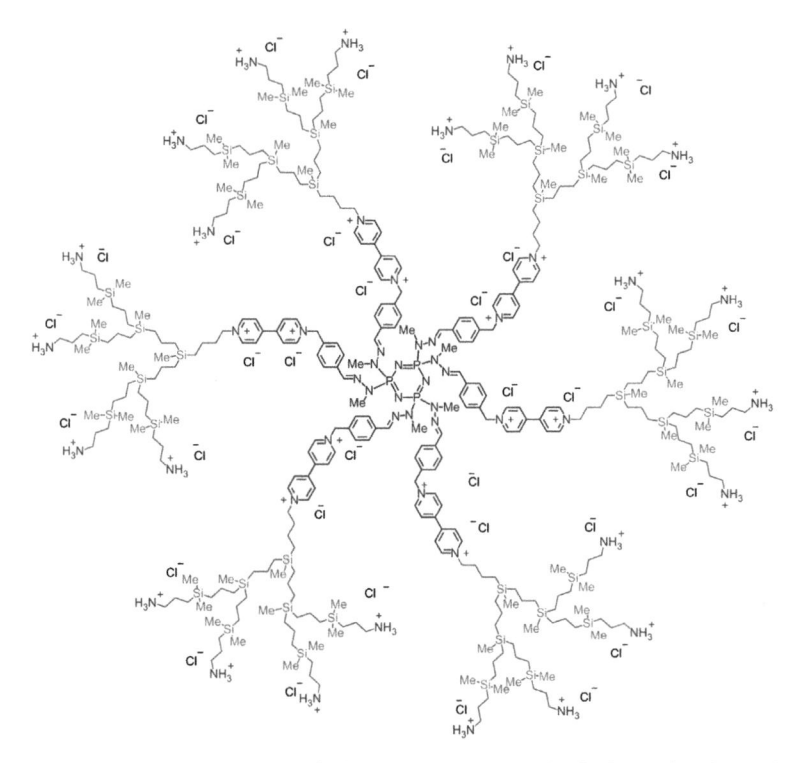

Figure 1.19 An onion peel dendrimer composed of three families of dendrimers: phosphorhydrazone, viologen, and carbosilane.

1.6 Janus Dendrimers

Janus dendrimers are formed with two dendrimeric wedges linked by their core, and having different terminal functions. Several reviews from our group already detailed the use of dendrons for the preparation of a great number of bisdendrons [132]. Only three examples will be mentioned in this chapter.

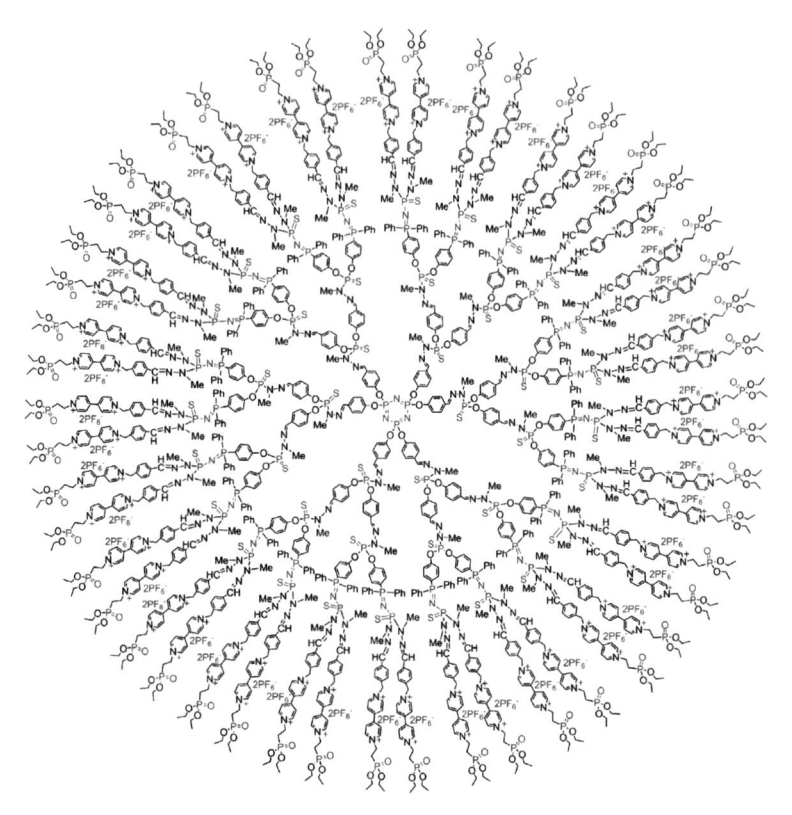

Figure 1.20 An onion peel dendrimer having seven types of phosphorus units in its structure.

The first example was elaborated with dendrons up to generation 3 bearing an activated vinyl group at the core, and different terminal functions. One of the dendrons was reacted with a diamine by Michael-like reaction, affording a dendron with a primary amine at the core (see Fig. 1.14), suitable for the reaction with another dendron having an activated vinyl group as core, and different terminal functions. Various combinations of terminal functions were obtained in this way, such as nitrile and tertiary amine [118], triphenyl phosphine (free or oxidized) and phenyl [105], or tertiary amine and carboxylate of different generations [133] (Fig. 1.21).

The Staudinger reaction between azide and phosphine was also used for coupling two dendritic wedges having a very different structure. On one side, a carbosilane dendron with a phosphine at the core, and on the other side, a phosphorhydrazone dendron with a thiophosphoryl azide at the core and P(S)Cl$_2$ terminal functions were readily associated. The Staudinger "click" reaction afforded a new type of Janus dendrimers, in which not only the terminal groups but also the full structure of the dendrons are entirely different. Furthermore, the P(S)Cl$_2$ terminal functions can be used for further functionalizations of the Janus dendrimer. Aldehydes, triphenyl phosphines, and azabisdiphosphines have been used to functionalize these Janus dendrimers (Fig. 1.22) [134].

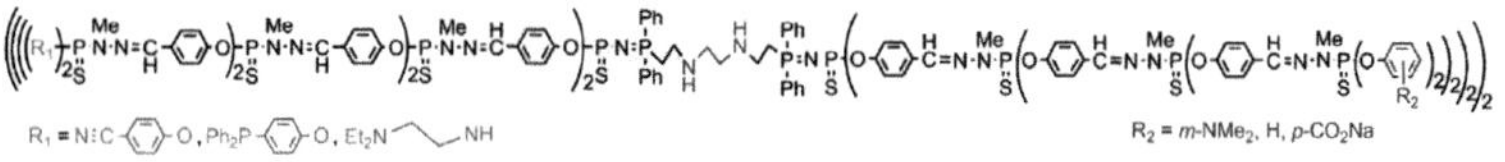

Figure 1.21 Janus dendrimers obtained after two consecutive Michael-type additions of ethylenediamine to the vinyl core of two dendrons.

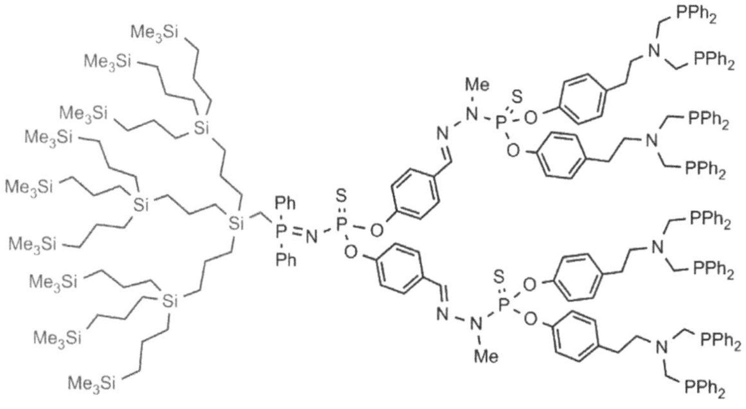

Figure 1.22 A Janus dendrimer obtained by Staudinger reactions between a carbosilane dendron and a phosphorus dendron, ended by P(S)Cl$_2$ groups, then functionalized by phosphines.

Several Janus dendrimers were also obtained by coupling two off-center dendrimers (see Fig. 1.5). Two examples of these Janus dendrimers are shown in Fig. 1.23. The one on the left was obtained by peptide coupling between a carboxylic acid and a primary amine; the one on the right was obtained by condensation reaction between a hydrazide and an aldehyde. In both cases, the coupling was carried out with the fluorescent dansyl on one side and Boc-protected tyramine on the other side, which were deprotected after the coupling to afford water-soluble Janus dendrimers [24].

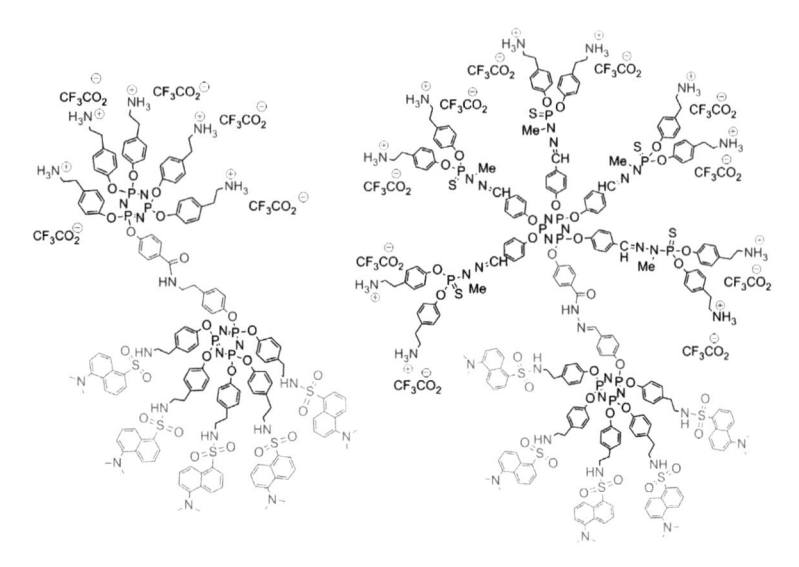

Figure 1.23 Fluorescent water-soluble Janus dendrimers synthesized by coupling two off-center dendrimers.

1.7 Miscellenous Methods

The very first example of phosphorus dendrimer was synthetized by the group of Engel in 1990. It was based on phosphonium salts at each branching point, which induce a multiplication by 3 of the number of terminal groups at each generation (Fig. 1.24) [135]. Insolubility of these polycationic dendrimers prevents from the extension of the methodology and the preparation of a variety of them.

Salamonczyk *et al.* developed the use of phosphoramidites as building blocks for the synthesis of phosphorus dendrimers constituted with phosphate repeating units. This is based on the reaction first of a phosphoramidite owing three acetate groups with a triol, followed by oxidation with elemental sulfur. Deprotection of the acetates leads to the corresponding polyols resulting in the formation of a new generation. Such a method allowed the authors to prepare dendrimers up to generation 5. Addition of selenium instead of elemental sulfur or direct oxidation permitted the synthesis of the corresponding dendrimers bearing P=Se or P=O groups (Fig. 1.24) [136].

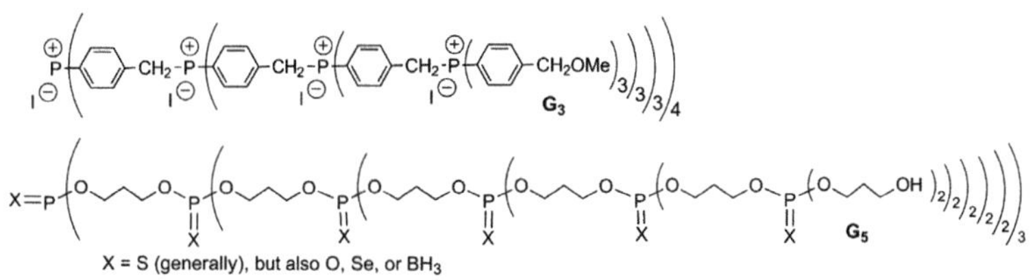

X = S (generally), but also O, Se, or BH$_3$

Figure 1.24 Phosphonium dendrimer proposed by Engel (G3) and phosphate dendrimer proposed by Salamonczyk (G5).

1.8 Conclusion

The versatility of the synthesis of phosphorus-containing dendrimers, due to the possibility to take profit of the rich organochemistry of phosphorus, is illustrated with a few limited examples reported above. This is just a partial view of the emerged iceberg concerning what is possible to synthetically develop with phosphorus for the creation of multi-dendritic macromolecules.

A number of these dendrimers present fascinating properties in different fields ranging from nanosciences to nanomedicine [137], and already some applications are in the way to be developed in two small companies.

We do believe that this is just a start considering that many other ways of synthesis of new phosphorus dendrimers are underway, which should lead to the design of nano-objects suitable for many applications. Indeed, the possibility to tailor at will not only the core but also the internal branches, the branching points and the surface, the possibility to graft regioselectively diverse functional groups within the cascade structure or to create a variety of multidendritic macromolecules, the easy way to modify their character (hydrophilic/ hydrophobic character) offer fascinating perspectives in the field of fundamental and applied research.

References

1. Launay, N., Caminade, A. M., Lahana, R., and Majoral, J. P. (1994). A general synthetic strategy for neutral phosphorus-containing dendrimers, *Angew. Chem. Int. Ed. Engl.*, **33**, pp. 1589–1592.

2. Lartigue, M. L., Donnadieu, B., Galliot, C., Caminade, A. M., Majoral, J. P., and Fayet, J. P. (1997). Large dipole moments of phosphorus-containing dendrimers, *Macromolecules*, **30**, pp. 7335–7337.

3. Launay, N., Caminade, A. M., and Majoral, J. P. (1997). Synthesis of bowl-shaped dendrimers from generation 1 to generation 8, *J. Organomet. Chem.*, **529**, pp. 51–58.

4. Le Berre, V., Trevisiol, E., Dagkessamanskaia, A., Sokol, S., Caminade, A. M., Majoral, J. P., Meunier, B., and Francois, J. (2003). Dendrimeric coating of glass slides for sensitive DNA microarrays analysis, *Nucleic Acids Res.*, **31**, pp. 8.

5. Trevisiol, E., Le Berre-Anton, V., Leclaire, J., Pratviel, G., Caminade, A. M., Majoral, J. P., Francois, J. M., and Meunier, B. (2003). Dendrislides, dendrichips: A simple chemical functionalization of glass slides with phosphorus dendrimers as an effective means for the preparation of biochips, *New J. Chem.*, **27**, pp. 1713–1719.

6. Turrin, C. O., Chiffre, J., de Montauzon, D., Daran, J. C., Caminade, A. M., Manoury, E., Balavoine, G., and Majoral, J. P. (2000). Phosphorus-containing dendrimers with ferrocenyl units at the core, within the branches, and on the periphery, *Macromolecules*, **33**, pp. 7328–7336.

7. Turrin, C. O., Chiffre, J., Daran, J. C., de Montauzon, D., Caminade, A. M., Manoury, E., Balavoine, G., and Majoral, J. P. (2001). New chiral phosphorus-containing dendrimers with ferrocenes on the periphery, *Tetrahedron*, **57**, pp. 2521–2536.

8. Routaboul, L., Vincendeau, S., Turrin, C. O., Caminade, A. M., Majoral, J. P., Daran, J. C., and Manoury, E. (2007). New phosphorus dendrimers with chiral ferrocenyl phosphine-thioether ligands on the periphery for asymmetric catalysis, *J. Organomet. Chem.*, **692**, pp. 1064–1073.

9. Neumann, P., Dib, H., Sournia-Saquet, A., Grell, T., Handke, M., Caminade, A. M., and Hey-Hawkins, E. (2015). Ruthenium complexes with dendritic ferrocenyl phosphanes: Synthesis, characterization, and application in the catalytic redox isomerization of allylic alcohols, *Chem. Eur. J.*, **21**, pp. 6590–6604.

10. Neumann, P., Dib, H., Caminade, A. M., and Hey-Hawkins, E. (2015). Redox control of a dendritic ferrocenyl-based homogeneous catalyst, *Angew. Chem. Int. Ed.*, **54**, pp. 311–314.

11. Sebastian, R. M., Caminade, A. M., Majoral, J. P., Levillain, E., Huchet, L., and Roncali, J. (2000). Electrogenerated poly(dendrimers) containing conjugated poly(thiophene) chains, *Chem. Commun.*, pp. 507–508.

12. Caminade, A. M., Ouali, A., Laurent, R., Turrin, C. O., and Majoral, J. P. (2016). Coordination chemistry with phosphorus dendrimers. Applications as catalysts, for materials, and in biology, *Coord. Chem. Rev.*, **308**, pp. 478–497.

13. Keller, M., Colliere, V., Reiser, O., Caminade, A. M., Majoral, J. P., and Ouali, A. (2013). Pyrene-tagged dendritic catalysts noncovalently grafted onto magnetic Co/C nanoparticles: An efficient and recyclable system for drug synthesis, *Angew. Chem. Int. Ed.*, **52**, pp. 3626–3629.

14. Lacour, M. A., Zablocka, M., Caminade, A. M., Taillefer, M., and Majoral, J. P. (2009). Design of phosphonium ended dendrimers bearing functionalized amines, *Tetrahedron Lett.*, **50**, pp. 4870–4873.

15. Keller, M., Hameau, A., Spataro, G., Ladeira, S., Caminade, A. M., Majoral, J. P., and Ouali, A. (2012). An efficient and recyclable dendritic catalyst able to dramatically reduce palladium leaching in Suzuki couplings, *Green Chem.*, **14**, pp. 2807–2815.

16. Koprowski, M., Sebastian, R. M., Maraval, V., Zablocka, M., Cadierno, V., Donnadieu, B., Igau, A., Caminade, A. M., and Majoral, J. P. (2002). Iminophosphine palladium complexes in catalytic Stille coupling reactions: From monomers to dendrimers, *Organometallics*, **21**, pp. 4680–4687.

17. Servin, P., Laurent, R., Romerosa, A., Peruzzini, M., Majoral, J. P., and Caminade, A. M. (2008). Synthesis of dendrimers terminated by bis(diphenylphosphinomethyl)amino ligands and use of their palladium complexes for catalyzing C-C cross-coupling reactions, *Organometallics*, **27**, pp. 2066–2073.

18. Gissibl, A., Padie, C., Hager, M., Jaroschik, F., Rasappan, R., Cuevas-Yanez, E., Turrin, C. O., Caminade, A. M., Majoral, J. P., and Reiser, O. (2007). Synthesis and application of phosphorus dendrimer immobilized azabis(oxazolines), *Org. Lett.*, **9**, pp. 2895–2898.

19. Keller, M., Ianchuk, M., Ladeira, S., Taillefer, M., Caminade, A. M., Majoral, J. P., and Ouali, A. (2012). Synthesis of dendritic beta-diketones and their application in copper-catalyzed diaryl ether formation, *Eur. J. Org. Chem.*, **5**, pp. 1056–1062.

20. Ouali, A., Laurent, R., Caminade, A. M., Majoral, J. P., and Taillefer, M. (2006). Enhanced catalytic properties of copper in O- and N-arylation and vinylation reactions, using phosphorus dendrimers as ligands, *J. Am. Chem. Soc.*, **128**, pp. 15990–15991.

21. Perrier, A., Keller, M., Caminade, A. M., Majoral, J. P., and Ouali, A. (2013). Efficient and recyclable rare earth-based catalysts for Friedel–Crafts acylations under microwave heating: Dendrimers show the way, *Green Chem.*, **15**, pp. 2075–2080.

22. Rull, J., Casals, M., Sebastian, R. M., Vallribera, A., Majoral, J. P., and Caminade, A. M. (2015). (+)-Cinchonine-decorated dendrimers as recoverable organocatalysts, *ChemCatChem*, **7**, pp. 2698–2704.

23. Franc, G., Mazeres, S., Turrin, C. O., Vendier, L., Duhayon, C., Caminade, A. M., and Majoral, J. P. (2007). Synthesis and properties of dendrimers possessing the same fluorophore(s) located either peripherally or off-center, *J. Org. Chem.*, **72**, pp. 8707–8715.

24. Fuchs, S., Pla-Quintana, A., Mazeres, S., Caminade, A. M., and Majoral, J. P. (2008). Cationic and fluorescent "Janus" dendrimers, *Org. Lett.*, **10**, pp. 4751–4754.

25. Hameau, A., Fuchs, S., Laurent, R., Majoral, J. P., and Caminade, A. M. (2011). Synthesis of dye/fluorescent functionalized dendrons based on cyclotriphosphazene, *Beilstein J. Org. Chem.*, **7**, pp. 1577–1583.

26. Mongin, O., Krishna, T. R., Werts, M. H. V., Caminade, A. M., Majoral, J. P., and Blanchard-Desce, M. (2006). A modular approach to two-photon absorbing organic nanodots: Brilliant dendrimers as an alternative to semiconductor quantum dots? *Chem. Commun.*, pp. 915–917.

27. Terenziani, F., Parthasarathy, V., Pla-Quintana, A., Maishal, T., Caminade, A. M., Majoral, J. P., and Blanchard-Desce, M. (2009). Cooperative two-photon absorption enhancement by through-space interactions in multichromophoric compounds, *Angew. Chem. Int. Ed.*, **48**, pp. 8691–8694.

28. Fuks-Janczarek, I., Nunzi, J. M., Sahraoui, B., Kityk, I. V., Berdowski, J., Caminade, A. M., Majoral, J. P., Martineau, A. C., Frere, P., and Roncali, J. (2002). Third-order nonlinear optical properties and two-photon absorption in branched oligothienylenevinylenes, *Opt. Commun.*, **209**, pp. 461–466.

29. Hadad, C., Majoral, J. P., Muzart, J., Caminade, A. M., and Bouquillon, S. (2009). First phosphorous D-xylose-derived glycodendrimers, *Tetrahedron Lett.*, **50**, pp. 1902–1905.

30. Perez-Anes, A., Spataro, G., Coppel, Y., Moog, C., Blanzat, M., Turrin, C. O., Caminade, A. M., Rico-Lattes, I., and Majoral, J. P. (2009). Phosphonate terminated PPH dendrimers: Influence of pendant alkyl chains on the *in vitro* anti-HIV-1 properties, *Org. Biomol. Chem.*, **7**, pp. 3491–3498.

31. Griffe, L., Poupot, M., Marchand, P., Maraval, A., Turrin, C. O., Rolland, O., Metivier, P., Bacquet, G., Fournie, J. J., Caminade, A. M., Poupot, R., and Majoral, J. P. (2007). Multiplication of human natural killer cells by nanosized phosphonate-capped dendrimers, *Angew. Chem. Int. Ed.*, **46**, pp. 2523–2526.

32. Rolland, O., Turrin, C. O., Bacquet, G., Poupot, R., Poupot, M., Caminade, A. M., and Majoral, J. P. (2009). Efficient synthesis of phosphorus-containing dendrimers capped with isosteric functions of amino-bismethylene phosphonic acids, *Tetrahedron Lett.*, **50**, pp. 2078–2082.

33. Poupot, M., Griffe, L., Marchand, P., Maraval, A., Rolland, O., Martinet, L., L'Faqihi-Olive, F. E., Turrin, C. O., Caminade, A. M., Fournié, J. J., Majoral, J. P., and Poupot, R. (2006). Design of phosphorylated dendritic architectures to promote human monocyte activation, *FASEB J.*, **20**, pp. 2339–2351.

34. Marchand, P., Griffe, L., Poupot, M., Turrin, C. O., Bacquet, G., Fournie, J. J., Majoral, J. P., Poupot, R., and Caminade, A. M. (2009). Dendrimers ended by non-symmetrical azadiphosphonate groups: Synthesis and immunological properties, *Bioorg. Med. Chem. Lett.*, **19**, pp. 3963–3966.

35. Hayder, M., Poupot, M., Baron, M., Nigon, D., Turrin, C. O., Caminade, A. M., Majoral, J. P., Eisenberg, R. A., Fournie, J. J., Cantagrel, A., Poupot, R., and Davignon, J. L. (2011). A phosphorus-based dendrimer targets inflammation and osteoclastogenesis in experimental arthritis, *Sci. Transl. Med.*, **3**, pp. 11.

36. Rolland, O., Griffe, L., Poupot, M., Maraval, A., Ouali, A., Coppel, Y., Fournie, J. J., Bacquet, G., Turrin, C. O., Caminade, A. M., Majoral, J. P., and Poupot, R. (2008). Tailored control and optimisation of the number of phosphonic acid termini on phosphorus-containing dendrimers for the ex-vivo activation of human monocytes, *Chem. Eur. J.*, **14**, pp. 4836–4850.

37. Caminade, A. M., Fruchon, S., Turrin, C. O., Poupot, M., Ouali, A., Maraval, A., Garzoni, M., Maly, M., Furer, V., Kovalenko, V., Majoral, J. P., Pavan, G. M., and Poupot, R. (2015). The key role of the scaffold on the efficiency of dendrimer nanodrugs, *Nature Comm.*, **6**, pp. 7722.

38. El Brahmi, N., El Kazzouli, S., Mignani, S. M., Essassi, E., Aubert, G., Laurent, R., Caminade, A. M., Bousmina, M. M., Cresteil, T., and Majoral, J. P. (2013). Original multivalent copper(II)-conjugated phosphorus dendrimers and corresponding mononuclear copper(II) complexes with antitumoral activities, *Mol. Pharm.*, **10**, pp. 1459–1464.

39. El Brahmi, N., Mignani, S. M., Caron, J., El Kazzouli, S., Bousmina, M. M., Caminade, A. M., Cresteil, T., and Majoral, J. P. (2015). Investigations on dendrimer space reveal solid and liquid tumor growth-inhibition by original phosphorus-based dendrimers and the corresponding monomers and dendrons with ethacrynic acid motifs, *Nanoscale*, **7**, pp. 3915–3922.

40. Mignani, S., El Brahmi, N., El Kazzouli, S., Eloy, L., Courilleau, D., Caron, J., Bousmina, M. M., Caminade, A. M., Cresteil, T., and Majoral, J. P. (2016). A novel class of ethacrynic acid derivatives as promising drug-like potent generation of anticancer agents with established mechanism of action, *Eur. J. Med. Chem.*, **122**, pp. 656–673.

41. Launay, N., Caminade, A. M., and Majoral, J. P. (1995). Synthesis and reactivity of unusual phosphorus dendrimers: A useful divergent growth approach up to the 7th generation, *J. Am. Chem. Soc.*, **117**, pp. 3282–3283.

42. Lartigue, M. L., Slany, M., Caminade, A. M., and Majoral, J. P. (1996). Phosphorus-containing dendrimers: Synthesis of macromolecules with multiple tri- and tetrafunctionalization, *Chem. Eur. J.*, **2**, pp. 1417–1426.

43. Prevote, D., Caminade, A. M., and Majoral, J. P. (1997). Phosphate-, phosphite-, ylide-, and phosphonate-terminated dendrimers, *J. Org. Chem.*, **62**, pp. 4834–4841.

44. Marmillon, C., Gauffre, F., Gulik-Krzywicki, T., Loup, C., Caminade, A. M., Majoral, J. P., Vors, J. P., and Rump, E. (2001). Organophosphorus dendrimers as new gelators for hydrogels, *Angew. Chem. Int. Ed.*, **40**, pp. 2626–2629.

45. Le Derf, F., Levillain, E., Trippe, G., Gorgues, A., Salle, M., Sebastian, R. M., Caminade, A. M., and Majoral, J. P. (2001). Immobilization of redox-active ligands on an electrode: The dendrimer route, *Angew. Chem. Int. Ed.*, **40**, pp. 224–227.

46. Prevote, D., LeRoy-Gourvennec, S., Caminade, A. M., Masson, S., and Majoral, J. P. (1997). Application of the Horner–Wadsworth–Emmons reaction to the functionalization of dendrimers: Synthesis of amino acid terminated dendrimers, *Synthesis-Stuttgart*, pp. 1199–1207.

47. Servin, P., Laurent, R., Gonsalvi, L., Tristany, M., Peruzzini, M., Majoral, J. P., and Caminade, A. M. (2009). Grafting of water-soluble phosphines to dendrimers and their use in catalysis: Positive dendritic effects in aqueous media, *Dalton Trans.*, **23**, pp. 4432–4434.

48. Rull, J., Jara, J. J., Sebastian, R. M., Vallribera, A., Najera, C., Majoral, J. P., and Caminade, A. M. (2016). Recoverable dendritic phase-transfer

catalysts that contain (+)-cinchonine-derived ammonium salts, *ChemCatChem*, **8**, pp. 2049–2056.

49. Marchand, P., Griffe, L., Caminade, A. M., Majoral, J. P., Destarac, M., and Leising, F. (2004). Thioacylation reactions for the surface functionalization of phosphorus-containing dendrimers, *Org. Lett.*, **6**, pp. 1309–1312.

50. Darcos, V., Dureault, A., Taton, D., Gnanou, Y., Marchand, P., Caminade, A. M., Majoral, J. P., Destarac, M., and Leising, F. (2004). Synthesis of hybrid dendrimer-star polymers by the RAFT process, *Chem. Commun.*, pp. 2110–2111.

51. Riegert, D., Bareille, L., Laurent, R., Majoral, J. P., Caminade, A. M., and Chaumonnot, A. (2016). Silica functionalized by bifunctional dendrimers: Hybrid nanomaterials for trapping CO_2, *Eur. J. Inorg. Chem.*, pp. 3103–3110.

52. Blattes, E., Vercellone, A., Eutamene, H., Turrin, C. O., Theodorou, V., Majoral, J. P., Caminade, A. M., Prandi, J., Nigou, J., and Puzo, G. (2013). Mannodendrimers prevent acute lung inflammation by inhibiting neutrophil recruitment, *Proc. Natl. Acad. Sci. USA*, **110**, pp. 8795–8800.

53. Franc, G., Turrin, C. O., Cavero, E., Costes, J. P., Duhayon, C., Caminade, A. M., and Majoral, J. P. (2009). Gem-bisphosphonate-ended group dendrimers: Design and gadolinium complexing properties, *Eur. J. Org. Chem.*, pp. 4290–4299.

54. Folgado, E., Guerre, M., Bijani, C., Ladmiral, V., Caminade, A. M., Ameduri, B., and Ouali, A. (2016). Well-defined poly(vinylidene fluoride) (PVDF) based-dendrimers synthesized by click chemistry: Enhanced crystallinity of PVDF and increased hydrophobicity of PVDF films, *Polymer Chem.*, **7**, pp. 5625–5629.

55. Launay, N., Slany, M., Caminade, A. M., and Majoral, J. P. (1996). Phosphorus-containing dendrimers. Easy access to new multi-difunctionalized macromolecules, *J. Org. Chem.*, **61**, pp. 3799–3805.

56. Loup, C., Zanta, M. A., Caminade, A. M., Majoral, J. P., and Meunier, B. (1999). Preparation of water-soluble cationic phosphorus-containing dendrimers as DNA transfecting agents, *Chem. Eur. J.*, **5**, pp. 3644–3650.

57. Kim, D. H., Karan, P., Goring, P., Leclaire, J., Caminade, A. M., Majoral, J. P., Gosele, U., Steinhart, M., and Knoll, W. (2005). Formation of dendrimer nanotubes by layer-by-layer deposition, *Small*, **1**, pp. 99–102.

58. Feng, C. L., Zhong, X. H., Steinhart, M., Caminade, A. M., Majoral, J. P., and Knoll, W. (2007). Graded-bandgap quantum-dot-modified nanotubes:

A sensitive biosensor for enhanced detection of DNA hybridization, *Adv. Mater.*, **19**, pp. 1933–1936.

59. Kim, B. S., Lebedeva, O. V., Kim, D. H., Caminade, A. M., Majoral, J. P., Knoll, W., and Vinogradova, O. I. (2005). Assembly and mechanical properties of phosphorus dendrimer/polyelectrolyte multilayer microcapsules, *Langmuir*, **21**, pp. 7200–7206.

60. Feng, C. L., Yin, M. Z., Zhang, D., Zhu, S. M., Caminade, A. M., Majoral, J. P., and Mullen, K. (2011). Fluorescent core-shell star polymers based bioassays for ultrasensitive DNA detection by surface plasmon fluorescence spectroscopy, *Macromol. Rapid Commun.*, **32**, pp. 679–683.

61. Solassol, J., Crozet, C., Perrier, V., Leclaire, J., Beranger, F., Caminade, A. M., Meunier, B., Dormont, D., Majoral, J. P., and Lehmann, S. (2004). Cationic phosphorus-containing dendrimers reduce prion replication both in cell culture and in mice infected with scrapie, *J. Gen. Virol.*, **85**, pp. 1791–1799.

62. Wasiak, T., Ionov, M., Nieznanski, K., Nieznanska, H., Klementieva, O., Granell, M., Cladera, J., Majoral, J. P., Caminade, A. M., and Klajnert, B. (2012). Phosphorus dendrimers affect Alzheimer's (A beta(1-28)) peptide and MAP-tau protein aggregation, *Mol. Pharm.*, **9**, pp. 458–469.

63. Lazniewska, J., Milowska, K., Zablocka, M., Mignani, S., Caminade, A. M., Majoral, J. P., Bryszewska, M., and Gabryelak, T. (2013). Mechanism of cationic phosphorus dendrimer toxicity against murine neural cell lines, *Mol. Pharm.*, **10**, pp. 3484–3496.

64. Padie, C., Maszewska, M., Majchrzak, K., Nawrot, B., Caminade, A. M., and Majoral, J. P. (2009). Polycationic phosphorus dendrimers: Synthesis, characterization, study of cytotoxicity, complexation of DNA, and transfection experiments, *New J. Chem.*, **33**, pp. 318–326.

65. Prevote, D., Donnadieu, B., Moreno-Manas, M., Caminade, A. M., and Majoral, J. P. (1999). Grafting of tetraazamacrocycles on the surface of phosphorus-containing dendrimers, *Eur. J. Org. Chem.*, pp. 1701–1708.

66. Badetti, E., Caminade, A. M., Majoral, J. P., Moreno-Manas, M., and Sebastian, R. M. (2008). Palladium(0) nanoparticles stabilized by phosphorus dendrimers containing coordinating 15-membered triolefinic macrocycles in periphery, *Langmuir*, **24**, pp. 2090–2101.

67. Franc, G., Badetti, E., Duhayon, C., Coppel, Y., Turrin, C. O., Majoral, J. P., Sebastian, R. M., and Caminade, A. M. (2010). An efficient synthesis combining phosphorus dendrimers and 15-membered triolefinic

azamacrocycles: Towards the stabilization of platinum nanoparticles, *New J. Chem.*, **34**, pp. 547–555.

68. Franc, G., Badetti, E., Colliere, V., Majoral, J. P., Sebastian, R. M., and Caminade, A. M. (2009). Dendritic structures within dendritic structures: Dendrimer-induced formation and self-assembly of nanoparticle networks, *Nanoscale*, **1**, pp. 233–237.

69. Hincapie, C. A., Sebastian, R. M., Barbera, J., Serrano, J. L., Sierra, T., Majoral, J. P., and Caminade, A. M. (2014). Supermolecular columnar liquid-crystalline phosphorus dendrimers decorated with sulfonamide, *Chem. Eur. J.*, **20**, pp. 17047–17058.

70. Severac, M., Leclaire, J., Sutra, P., Caminade, A. M., and Majoral, J. P. (2004). A new way for the internal functionalization of dendrimers, *Tetrahedron Lett.*, **45**, pp. 3019–3022.

71. Riegert, D., Pla-Quintana, A., Fuchs, S., Laurent, R., Turrin, C. O., Duhayon, C., Majoral, J. P., Chaumonnot, A., and Caminade, A. M. (2013). Diversified strategies for the synthesis of bifunctional dendrimeric structures, *Eur. J. Org. Chem.*, **24**, pp. 5414–5422.

72. Leclaire, J., Dagiral, R., Fery-Forgues, S., Coppel, Y., Donnadieu, B., Caminade, A. M., and Majoral, J. P. (2005). Octasubstituted metal-free phthalocyanine as core of phosphorus dendrimers: A probe for the properties of the internal structure, *J. Am. Chem. Soc.*, **127**, pp. 15762–15770.

73. Leclaire, J., Coppel, Y., Caminade, A. M., and Majoral, J. P. (2004). Nanometric sponges made of water-soluble hydrophobic dendrimers, *J. Am. Chem. Soc.*, **126**, pp. 2304–2305.

74. Maszewska, M., Leclaire, J., Cieslak, M., Nawrot, B., Okruszek, A., Caminade, A. M., and Majoral, J. P. (2003). Water-soluble polycationic dendrimers with a phosphoramidothioate backbone: Preliminary studies of cytotoxicity and oligonucleotide/plasmid delivery in human cell culture, *Oligonucleotides*, **13**, pp. 193–205.

75. Krishna, T. R., Parent, M., Werts, M. H. V., Moreaux, L., Gmouh, S., Charpak, S., Caminade, A. M., Majoral, J. P., and Blanchard-Desce, M. (2006). Water-soluble dendrimeric two-photon tracers for *in vivo* imaging, *Angew. Chem. Int. Ed.*, **45**, pp. 4645–4648.

76. Mongin, O., Rouxel, C., Robin, A. C., Pla-Quintana, A., Krishna, T. R., Recher, G., Tiaho, F., Caminade, A. M., Majoral, J. P., and Blanchard-Desce, M. (2008). Brilliant organic nanodots: Novel nano-objects for bionanophotonics, in: *Nanobiosystems: Processing, Characterization, and Applications*, E. M. Heckman, T. B. Singh, and J. Yoshida (Eds.), SPIE-Int Soc Optical Engineering, Bellingham, 7040.

77. Caminade, A. M., Hameau, A., and Majoral, J. P. (2016). The specific functionalization of cyclotriphosphazene for the synthesis of smart dendrimers, *Dalton Trans.*, **45**, pp. 1810–1822.

78. Cardona, C. M., Alvarez, J., Kaifer, A. E., McCarley, T. D., Pandey, S., Baker, G. A., Bonzagni, N. J., and Bright, F. V. (2000). Dendrimers functionalized with a single fluorescent dansyl group attached "off center": Synthesis and photophysical studies, *J. Am. Chem. Soc.*, **122**, pp. 6139–6144.

79. Tristany, M., Laurent, R., Dib, H., Gonsalvi, L., Peruzzini, M., Majoral, J. P., and Caminade, A. M. (2014). Bifunctional metallodendrimers based on AB(5) derivatives of cyclotriphosphazene as core and P,N ligands as terminal functions, *Inorg. Chim. Acta*, **409**, pp. 121–126.

80. Martinez-Ferrero, E., Franc, G., Mazeres, S., Turrin, C. O., Boissiere, U., Caminade, A. M., Majoral, J. P., and Sanchez, C. (2008). Optical properties of hybrid dendritic-mesoporous titania nanocomposite films, *Chem. Eur. J.*, **14**, pp. 7658–7669.

81. de Jong, E. R., Deloch, N., Knoll, W., Turrin, C. O., Majoral, J. P., Caminade, A. M., and Koper, I. (2015). Synthesis and characterization of bifunctional dendrimers: Preliminary use for the coating of gold surfaces and the proliferation of human osteoblasts (HOB), *New J. Chem.*, **39**, pp. 7194–7205.

82. Maraval, V., Caminade, A. M., Majoral, J. P., and Blais, J. C. (2003). Dendrimer design: How to circumvent the dilemma of a reduction of steps or an increase of function multiplicity? *Angew. Chem. Int. Ed.*, **42**, pp. 1822–1826.

83. Kazmierczak-Baranska, J., Pietkiewicz, A., Janicka, M., Wei, Y. Q., Turrin, C. O., Majoral, J. P., Nawrot, B., and Caminade, A. M. (2010). Synthesis of a fluorescent cationic phosphorus dendrimer and preliminary biological studies of its interaction with DNA, *Nucleosides Nucleotides Nucleic Acids*, **29**, pp. 155–167.

84. Magro, G., Marchand, P., Sebastian, R. M., Guyard-Duhayon, C., Caminade, A. M., and Majoral, J. P. (2005). Synthesis and characterization of phosphorus dendrimers containing long, conjugated branches, *Eur. J. Org. Chem.*, pp. 1340–1347.

85. Turrin, C. O., Chiffre, J., Daran, J. C., de Montauzon, D., Balavoine, G., Manoury, E., Caminade, A. M., and Majoral, J. P. (2002). New phosphorus-containing dendrimers with ferrocenyl units in each layer, *C. R. Chimie*, **5**, pp. 309–318.

86. Turrin, C. O., Chiffre, J., de Montauzon, D., Balavoine, G., Manoury, E., Caminade, A. M., and Majoral, J. P. (2002). Behavior of an optically

active ferrocene chiral shell located within phosphorus-containing dendrimers, *Organometallics*, **21**, pp. 1891–1897.

87. Sebastian, R. M., Blais, J. C., Caminade, A. M., and Majoral, J. P. (2002). Synthesis and photochemical behavior of phosphorus dendrimers containing azobenzene units within the branches and/or on the surface, *Chem. Eur. J.*, **8**, pp. 2172–2183.

88. Mongin, O., Rouxel, C., Vabre, J. M., Mir, Y., Pla-Quintana, A., Wei, Y. Q., Caminade, A. M., Majoral, J. P., and Blanchard-Desce, M. (2009). Customized multiphotonics nanotools for bioapplications: Soft organic nanodots as an eco-friendly alternative to quantum dots, in: *Nanobiosystems: Processing, Characterization, and Applications II Book series*, Proceedings of SPIE -Int. Soc. Optical Engineering, San Diego, CA, USA, N. Kobayashi, F. Ouchen, and I. Rau (Eds.), SPIE -Int. Soc. Optical Engineering; Bellingham, WA USA, **7403**, pp. 740303-1–740303-12.

89. Shakhbazau, A., Mishra, M., Chu, T. H., Brideau, C., Cummins, K., Tsutsui, S., Shcharbin, D., Majoral, J. P., Mignani, S., Blanchard-Desce, M., Bryszewska, M., Yong, V. W., Stys, P. K., and van Minnen, J. (2015). Fluorescent phosphorus dendrimer as a spectral nanosensor for macrophage polarization and fate tracking in spinal cord injury, *Macromol. Biosci.*, **15**, pp. 1523–1534.

90. Servin, P., Rebout, C., Laurent, R., Peruzzini, M., Caminade, A. M., and Majoral, J. P. (2007). Reduced number of steps for the synthesis of dense and highly functionalized dendrimers, *Tetrahedron Lett.*, **48**, pp. 579–583.

91. Chen, H. T., Neerman, M. F., Parrish, A. R., and Simanek, E. E. (2004). Cytotoxicity, hemolysis, and acute *in vivo* toxicity of dendrimers based on melamine, candidate vehicles for drug delivery, *J. Am. Chem. Soc.*, **126**, pp. 10044–10048.

92. Lai, L. L., Wang, L. Y., Lee, C. H., Lin, Y. C., and Cheng, K. L. (2006). Nanomaterials of triazine-based dendrons: Convergent synthesis and their physical studies, *Org. Lett.*, **8**, pp. 1541–1544.

93. Dib, H., Rebout, C., Laurent, R., Mallet-Ladeira, S., Sournia-Saquet, A., Sarosi, M. B., Hey-Hawkins, E., Majoral, J. P., Delavaux-Nicot, B., and Caminade, A. M. (2016). Ordered layered dendrimers constructed from two known dendrimer families: Inheritance and emergence of properties, *Chem. Eur. J.*, **22**, pp. 10736–10742.

94. Larre, C., Donnadieu, B., Caminade, A. M., and Majoral, J. P. (1999). N-thiophosphorylated and N-phosphorylated iminophosphoranes R3P=N-P(X)R′(2); X = O, S as models for dendrimers: Synthesis, reactivity and crystal structures, *Eur. J. Inorg. Chem.*, pp. 601–611.

95. Maraval, V., Laurent, R., Marchand, P., Caminade, A. M., and Majoral, J. P. (2005). Accelerated methods of synthesis of phosphorus-containing dendrimers, *J. Organomet. Chem.*, **690**, pp. 2458–2471.

96. Brauge, L., Magro, G., Caminade, A. M., and Majoral, J. P. (2001). First divergent strategy using two AB(2) unprotected monomers for the rapid synthesis of dendrimers, *J. Am. Chem. Soc.*, **123**, pp. 6698–6699.

97. Maraval, V., Pyzowski, J., Caminade, A. M., and Majoral, J. P. (2003). "Lego" chemistry for the straightforward synthesis of dendrimers, *J. Org. Chem.*, **68**, pp. 6043–6046.

98. Sebastian, R. M., Magro, G., Caminade, A. M., and Majoral, J. P. (2000). Dendrimers with N,N-disubstituted hydrazines as end groups, useful precursors for the synthesis of water-soluble dendrimers capped with carbohydrate, carboxylic or boronic acid derivatives, *Tetrahedron*, **56**, pp. 6269–6277.

99. Galliot, C., Prevote, D., Caminade, A. M., and Majoral, J. P. (1995). Polyaminophosphines containing dendrimers: Synthesis and characterizations, *J. Am. Chem. Soc.*, **117**, pp. 5470–5476.

100. Furer, V. L., Vandyukov, A. E., Majoral, J. P., Caminade, A. M., Gottis, S., Laurent, R., and Kovalenko, V. I. (2015). Comparative DFT study of structure, reactivity and IR spectra of phosphorus-containing dendrons with P=N–P=S linkages, vinyl and azide functional groups, *J. Mol. Struct.*, **1091**, pp. 6–15.

101. Larre, C., Caminade, A. M., and Majoral, J. P. (1997). Chemoselective polyalkylations of phosphorus-containing dendrimers, *Angew. Chem. Int. Ed. Engl.*, **36**, pp. 596–599.

102. Larre, C., Donnadieu, B., Caminade, A. M., and Majoral, J. P. (1998). Phosphorus-containing dendrimers: Chemoselective functionalization of internal layers, *J. Am. Chem. Soc.*, **120**, pp. 4029–4030.

103. Larre, C., Donnadieu, B., Caminade, A. M., and Majoral, J. P. (1998). Regioselective gold complexation within the cascade structure of phosphorus-containing dendrimers, *Chem. Eur. J.*, **4**, pp. 2031–2036.

104. Galliot, C., Larre, C., Caminade, A. M., and Majoral, J. P. (1997). Regioselective stepwise growth of dendrimer units in the internal voids of a main dendrimer, *Science*, **277**, pp. 1981–1984.

105. Maraval, V., Laurent, R., Merino, S., Caminade, A. M., and Majoral, J. P. (2000). Michael-type addition of amines to the vinyl core of dendrons: Application to the synthesis of multidendritic systems, *Eur. J. Org. Chem.*, **21**, pp. 3555–3568.

106. Larre, C., Bressolles, D., Turrin, C., Donnadieu, B., Caminade, A. M., and Majoral, J. P. (1998). Chemistry within megamolecules: Regiospecific functionalization after construction of phosphorus dendrimers, *J. Am. Chem. Soc.*, **120**, pp. 13070–13082.

107. Cadierno, V., Igau, A., Donnadieu, B., Caminade, A. M., and Majoral, J. P. (1999). Dendrimers containing zwitterionic phosphonium anionic zirconocene(IV) complexes, *Organometallics*, **18**, pp. 1580–1582.

108. Brauge, L., Caminade, A. M., Majoral, J. P., Slomkowski, S., and Wolszczak, M. (2001). Segmental mobility in phosphorus-containing dendrimers. Studies by fluorescent spectroscopy, *Macromolecules*, **34**, pp. 5599–5606.

109. Merino, S., Brauge, L., Caminade, A. M., Majoral, J. P., Taton, D., and Gnanou, Y. (2001). Synthesis and characterization of linear, hyperbranched, and dendrimer-like polymers constituted of the same repeating unit, *Chem. Eur. J.*, **7**, pp. 3095–3105.

110. Balueva, A., Merino, S., Caminade, A. M., and Majoral, J. P. (2002). Synthesis of dendrimers with phosphine end groups at each generation, *J. Organomet. Chem.*, **643**, pp. 112–124.

111. Magro, G., Donnadieu, B., Caminade, A. M., and Majoral, J. P. (2003). The first linear multiphosphazene having five different types of side groups and its use as the core of a dendrimeric species, *Chem. Eur. J.*, **9**, pp. 2151–2159.

112. Badetti, E., Franc, G., Majoral, J. P., Caminade, A. M., Sebastian, R. M., and Moreno-Manas, M. (2011). Macrocyclic core phosphorus dendrimers covered on the surface by N,P ligands, *Eur. J. Org. Chem.*, **7**, pp. 1256–1265.

113. Rodriguez, L. I., Zablocka, M., Caminade, A. M., Seco, M., Rossell, O., and Majoral, J. P. (2010). Phosphorus dendrimers and dendrons functionalized with the cage ligand tris(1,2-dimethylhydrazino) diphosphane, *Heteroat. Chem.*, **21**, pp. 290–297.

114. Maraval, V. R., Prevote-Pinet, D., Laurent, R., Caminade, A. M., and Majoral, J. P. (2000). Choice of strategies for the divergent synthesis of phosphorus-containing dendrons, depending on the function located at the core, *New J. Chem.*, **24**, pp. 561–566.

115. Sebastian, R. M., Griffe, L., Turrin, C. O., Donnadieu, B., Caminade, A. M., and Majoral, J. P. (2004). Synthesis and core and surface reactivity of phosphorus-based dendrons, *Eur. J. Inorg. Chem.*, **12**, pp. 2459–2466.

116. Caminade, A. M., Maraval, A., and Majoral, J. P. (2006). Phosphorus-containing dendrons: Synthesis, reactivity, properties, and use as

building blocks for various dendritic architectures, *Eur. J. Inorg. Chem.*, **5**, pp. 887–901.

117. Turrin, C. O., Maraval, V., Caminade, A. M., Majoral, J. P., Mehdi, A., and Reye, C. (2000). Organic-inorganic hybrid materials incorporating phosphorus-containing dendrimers, *Chem. Mater.*, **12**, pp. 3848–3856.

118. Maraval, V., Laurent, R., Donnadieu, B., Mauzac, M., Caminade, A. M., and Majoral, J. P. (2000). Rapid synthesis of phosphorus-containing dendrimers with controlled molecular architectures: First example of surface-block, layer-block, and segment-block dendrimers issued from the same dendron, *J. Am. Chem. Soc.*, **122**, pp. 2499–2511.

119. Maraval, V., Laurent, R., Caminade, A. M., and Majoral, J. P. (2000). Phosphorus-containing dendrimers and their transition metal complexes as efficient recoverable multicenter homogeneous catalysts in organic synthesis, *Organometallics*, **19**, pp. 4025–4029.

120. Larpent, C., Genies, C., Delgado, A. P. D., Caminade, A. M., Majoral, J. P., Sassi, J. F., and Leising, F. (2004). Giant dendrimer-like particles from nanolatexes, *Chem. Commun.*, pp. 1816–1817.

121. Alvaro, M., Ferrer, B., Fornes, V., and Garcia, H. (2001). A periodic mesoporous organosilica containing electron acceptor viologen units, *Chem. Commun.*, pp. 2546–2547.

122. Li, H., Chen, D. X., Sun, Y. L., Zheng, Y. B., Tan, L. L., Weiss, P. S., and Yang, Y. W. (2013). Viologen-mediated assembly of and sensing with carboxylatopillar[5]arene-modified gold nanoparticles, *J. Amer. Chem. Soc.*, **135**, pp. 1570–1576.

123. Asaftei, S., Huskens, D., and Schols, D. (2012). HIV-1 X4 activities of polycationic "viologen" based dendrimers by interaction with the chemokine receptor CXCR4: Study of structure–activity relationship, *J. Med. Chem.*, **55**, pp. 10405–10413.

124. Katir, N., Majoral, J. P., El Kadib, A., Caminade, A. M., and Bousmina, M. (2012). Molecular and macromolecular engineering with viologens as building blocks: Rational design of phosphorus-viologen dendritic structures, *Eur. J. Org. Chem.*, pp. 269–273.

125. Ciepluch, K., Katir, N., El Kadib, A., Felczak, A., Zawadzka, K., Weber, M., Klajnert, B., Lisowska, K., Caminade, A. M., Bousmina, M., Bryszewska, M., and Majoral, J. P. (2012). Biological properties of new viologen-phosphorus dendrimers, *Mol. Pharm.*, **9**, pp. 448–457.

126. Katir, N., El Kadib, A., Colliere, V., Majoral, J. P., and Bousmina, M. (2014). Viologen-based dendritic macromolecular asterisks: Synthesis and interplay with gold nanoparticles, *Chem. Commun.*, **50**, pp. 6981–6983.

127. Sharma, R., Kottari, N., Chabre, Y. M., Abbassi, L., Shiao, T. C., and Roy, R. (2014). A highly versatile convergent/divergent "onion peel" synthetic strategy toward potent multivalent glycodendrimers, *Chem. Commun.*, **50**, pp. 13300–13303.

128. Sharma, R., Zhang, I., Abbassi, L., Rej, R., Maysinger, D., and Roy, R. (2015). A fast track strategy toward highly functionalized dendrimers with different structural layers: An "onion peel approach," *Polymer Chem.*, **6**, pp. 1436–1444.

129. Lartigue, M. L., Launay, N., Donnadieu, B., Caminade, A. M., and Majoral, J. P. (1997). First 'layer-block' dendrimer built with a regular alternation of two types of repeat units up to the fourth generation, *Bull. Soc. Chim. Fr.*, **134**, pp. 981–988.

130. Moreno, S., Szwed, A., El Brahmi, N., Milowska, K., Kurowska, J., Fuentes-Paniagua, E., Pedziwiatr-Werbicka, E., Gabryelak, T., Katir, N., de la Mata, F. J., Munoz-Fernandez, M. A., Gomez-Ramirez, R., Caminade, A. M., Majoral, J. P., and Bryszewska, M. (2015). Synthesis, characterization and biological properties of new hybrid carbosilane-viologen-phosphorus dendrimers, *RSC Adv.*, **5**, pp. 25942–25958.

131. Katir, N., El Brahmi, N., El Kadib, A., Mignani, S., Caminade, A. M., Bousmina, M., and Majoral, J. P. (2015). Synthesis of onion-peel nanodendritic structures with sequential functional phosphorus diversity, *Chem. Eur. J.*, **21**, pp. 6400–6408.

132. Caminade, A. M., Laurent, R., Delavaux-Nicot, B., and Majoral, J. P. (2012). "Janus" dendrimers: Syntheses and properties, *New J. Chem.*, **36**, pp. 217–226.

133. Maraval, V., Maraval, A., Spataro, G., Caminade, A. M., Majoral, J. P., Kim, D. H., and Knoll, W. (2006). Design of tailored multi-charged phosphorus surface-block dendrimers, *New J. Chem.*, **30**, pp. 1731–1736.

134. Gottis, S., Rodriguez, L. I., Laurent, R., Angurell, I., Seco, M., Rossell, O., Majoral, J. P., and Caminade, A. M. (2013). Janus carbosilane/phosphorhydrazone dendrimers synthesized by the 'click' Staudinger reaction, *Tetrahedron Lett.*, **54**, pp. 6864–6867.

135. Rengan, K. and Engel, R. (1990). Phosphonium cascade molecules, *J. Chem. Soc. Chem. Commun.*, pp. 1084–1085.

136. Salamonczyk, G. M., Kuznikowski, M., and Poniatowska, E. (2001). Synthesis and oxygenation of selenophosphate dendrimers, *Chem. Commun.*, pp. 2202–2203.

137. Caminade, A. M. (2017). Phosphorus dendrimers for nanomedicine, *Chem. Commun.*, **53**, 9830–9838.

Chapter 2

Methods for Characterizing (Phosphorus) Dendrimers

Anne-Marie Caminade and Régis Laurent
Laboratoire de Chimie de Coordination, CNRS, 205 Route de Narbonne, BP 44099, 31077 Toulouse Cedex 4, France
anne-marie.caminade@lcc-toulouse.fr

2.1 Introduction

In view of the large number of applications of dendrimers in various fields, in particular for biology, there is a critical need for techniques to characterize them and ascertain their purity. This task is not trivial due to their very peculiar structure. Dendrimers pertain to molecular chemistry by virtue of their step-by-step controlled synthesis, and they pertain to polymers because of their repetitive structure constituted of monomers; thus, they should benefit from analytical techniques used for both types of compounds. Not only their chemical composition but also their morphology, shape, and homogeneity must be determined. Their theoretically perfect and monodisperse structure can be questionable and has to be proved,

Phosphorus Dendrimers in Biology and Nanomedicine: Synthesis, Characterization, and Properties
Edited by Anne-Marie Caminade, Cédric-Olivier Turrin, and Jean-Pierre Majoral
Copyright © 2018 Pan Stanford Publishing Pte. Ltd.
ISBN 978-981-4774-33-8 (Hardcover), 978-1-315-11085-1 (eBook)
www.panstanford.com

especially for dendrimers built by a divergent process. Indeed, the yield in perfect dendrimer at each step depends on the percentage of conversion per terminal group. High generations are only attainable if the percentage of conversion per terminal group is higher than 99.999%, a percentage rare in chemistry, which explains why the number of methods for synthesizing large dendrimers is still limited.

Several thousands of publications are related to the characterization of dendrimers, but among them, only very few general reviews have appeared, essentially one in 1999 from Meijer *et al.* [1] and two from our group in 2005 [2] and 2011 [3]. The techniques for characterizing dendrimers are highly diversified, but they can be gathered under a limited number of types of method. We will consider essentially in this chapter the characterization of phosphorus-containing dendrimers (see Chapter 1 for their synthesis). However, it must be emphasized that the methods used for characterizing them are generally very useful also for characterizing all the other types of dendrimers. This chapter will display first the use of spectrometry and spectroscopy (NMR, mass, X-ray, IR, Raman, UV, fluorescence, chirality measurements, electron paramagnetic resonance (EPR), magnetometry, electrochemistry, light scattering), then microscopy (TEM, AFM, POM), and physical characterizations (viscosity, DSC, TGA, dielectric spectroscopy, dipole moments).

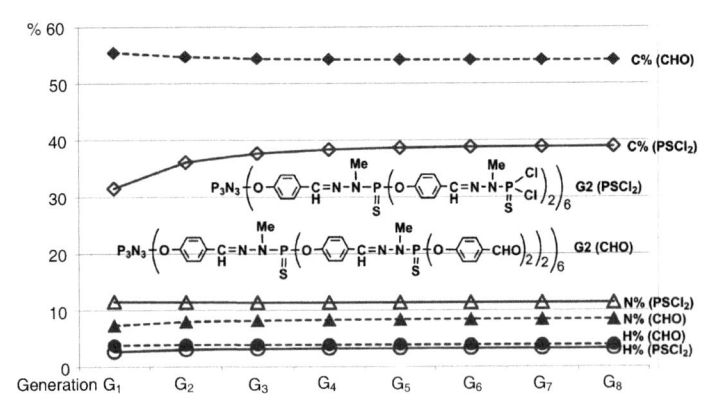

Figure 2.1 Theoretical percentage of C, N, and H in phosphorhydrazone (PPH) dendrimers depending on the generation and the type of terminal groups. Structure of the second generation ended by either P(S)Cl$_2$ or aldehyde functions.

Of course, elemental analyses are usually performed with dendrimers, but due to their repetitive structure, this technique is uninformative, especially for high generations, as illustrated in Fig. 2.1 for phosphorhydrazone (PPH) dendrimers. All generations have the same percentage of carbon, hydrogen, and nitrogen; thus, even if a branch is missing, the defect will be undetectable by elemental analyses. Besides, dendrimers very often trap solvents and this can result in incorrect elemental analyses even for a chemically pure dendrimers.

2.2   Spectroscopy and Spectrometry Techniques

Spectroscopy and spectrometry techniques are mostly used to ascertain the chemical composition of dendrimers, and to detect the presence of defects in the structure. In some cases, they are used also for determining their three-dimensional structure.

2.2.1   Nuclear Magnetic Resonance

Nuclear magnetic resonance is certainly the most widely used technique in routine analysis for characterizing dendrimers, but special NMR techniques have also been used to probe their size and morphology. All types of dendrimers are characterized by ^{1}H NMR, frequently also by ^{13}C NMR and, depending on their chemical structure, by ^{31}P or ^{29}Si NMR; ^{2}H, ^{11}B, ^{15}N, ^{19}F, ^{119}Sn, ^{195}Pt NMR are also used as the need arises. Routine NMR analyses are especially useful for characterizing the step-by-step growth of dendrimers, even up to higher generations. Indeed, they afford information about the transformation undergone by the terminal groups. ^{1}H and ^{13}C NMR are generally the most used for such purpose. The completion of the condensation step in the synthesis of poly(phosphorhydrazone) (PPH) dendrimers is easily demonstrated by ^{1}H NMR, with the disappearance of the aldehyde signal. Obviously, ^{31}P NMR is the most useful technique for characterizing phosphorus-containing dendrimers [4]. Indeed, ^{31}P NMR is so sensitive to small changes in the environment that it allows one to differentiate each layer up to the fourth generation [5] and at least the three most external layers for higher generations, up to G7 [6], and even G12 [7]. It is particularly useful to ascertain the completion of reactions, as signals corresponding to intermediates are very different from those of the starting and final products. As illustrated in Fig. 2.2, the ^{31}P NMR spectrum taken during the course of the reaction for the synthesis of a first-generation dendrimer ended by aldehydes, starting from P(S)Cl$_2$ terminal functions, displays a large difference between mono- and di-substituted terminal functions. Even highly sophisticated structures can be fully characterized by ^{31}P NMR [8].

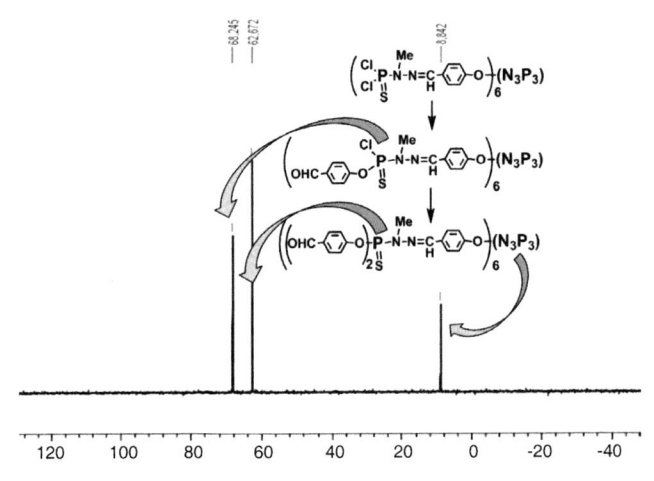

Figure 2.2 ^{31}P NMR spectrum taken during the course of the substitution reaction undergone by P(S)Cl$_2$ terminal groups. The monosubstitution reaction gives a signal very different from that of the disubstitution.

Depending on the type of terminal or internal functions of phosphorus dendrimers, other nucleus have been studied. This includes ^{15}N NMR [9], ^{19}F NMR [10, 11], and ^{195}Pt NMR [12].

Besides the chemical characterization, NMR gives access to the morphology of dendrimers, and eventually to the dynamics of their aggregation processes, by measuring relaxation times. In particular, pulse field-gradient spin echo (PGSE or PFGSE) ^{1}H NMR gives the size of dendrimers in solution, through the molecular diffusion coefficient. This technique was applied in water to a generation 5 of poly(phosphorhydrazone) dendrimer (G5 PPH) ended by ammonium groups [13], and in THF to a G4 PPH dendrimer ended by aldehydes [14]. It was shown that addition of water to THF induced a shrinkage of the dendrimeric structure, whereas addition of THF to water induced an expansion of the size, emphasizing the rather hydrophobic nature of the internal structure of PPH dendrimers. DOSY (diffusion ordered spectroscopy) experiments were carried out to determine the size of dendrimers ended by polymers such as PEG (glycol 550) [15], or poly(vinylidene fluoride) [16], often in association with dynamic laser light scattering techniques (see Section 2.2.11).

Most NMR experiments are carried out in solution, but magic angle spinning (MAS) NMR in the solid phase may also afford useful information. ^{31}P NMR MAS was used for detecting the presence of phosphorus dendrons inside silica [17], but also on the surface of silica nanoparticles [18]. The incorporation of PPH dendrimers inside hierarchically porous titanium dioxide materials [19], with eventual formation of discrete anatase nanocrystals [20], and of PPH dendrimers ended by ammonium groups, inside clays [21] was also assessed by MAS NMR of different nucleus (essentially ^{31}P and ^{13}C).

2.2.2 Mass Spectrometry

Mass spectrometry techniques developed for the characterization of high molecular weight compounds such as polymers and proteins are also potentially usable for the characterization of dendrimers. It is expected not only to obtain the molecular mass, but also to detect the presence of defects. Two major techniques are mainly used: electro-spray ionization (ESI) for dendrimers able to form stable multicharged species, and matrix-assisted laser desorption ionization time of flight (MALDI-TOF), which is theoretically able to analyze unlimited masses. However, great care should be taken to avoid false interpretation of the results, as some dendrimers can be broken by these techniques. In particular, the purity of poly(phosphorhydrazone) dendrimers is impossible to assess using these techniques, as both induce dramatic cleavages of their structure. Using MALDI-TOF, it was shown that the UV laser light used for desorption was not only absorbed by the matrix but also by the dendrimer, inducing fragmentation and rearrangements [22], and even precluding the observation of the molecular peak [23]. Only the use of a laser in the IR for the MALDI-TOF afforded clean spectra with only the molecular peak observed for a G2 PPH dendrimer with aldehyde terminations [3]. The specific design of dendrimers, including azobenzenes in their branches, that should absorb the UV light of the laser to preserve the structure, induced in fact more fragmentations [24].

2.2.3 X-Ray Diffraction

The molecular structure of dendrimers is generally impossible to determine by X-ray diffraction, except for lower generations (first, eventually second in case of very short branches). Indeed, many dendrimers are solids, but they are amorphous and lack long-range order in the condensed phase. In the case of phosphorus dendrimers, several first-generation dendrimers were characterized by X-ray diffraction. Their size is already large, and variable, depending on the nature of the core: (i) with three branches ended by $P(S)Cl_2$ [7] or $P(O)Cl_2$ [25] functions emanating from a P=S core, having size of about 1.7 nm; (ii) with six branches emanating from a cyclotriphosphazene core (N_3P_3), having size of about 2.3 nm [26]; and (iii) with four branches emanating from 1,8-diphosphino cores, having size of about 3.2 nm [27–29].

2.2.4 X-Ray Methods for Chemical (Surface) Analyses

Two methods based on X-rays are used for determining the chemical composition of materials or of compounds deposited on solid surfaces. X-ray photoelectron spectroscopy (XPS) is a quantitative spectroscopic technique that measures photoelectrons emitted from the sample, affording the elemental composition at the parts per thousand range, empirical formula, chemical state and electronic state of the elements that exist within a material. It was used for determining the chemical composition of poly(phosphorhydrazone) dendrimers with aldehyde terminal functions, deposited on quartz plates [30–32]. It was used also for characterizing a small dendrimer with maleimide terminal functions, grafted to a TiO_2 thin film [33].

Energy-dispersive X-ray spectroscopy (EDX) is also an analytical technique used for the elemental analysis or chemical characterization of a sample; it measures X-rays emitted from the sample and is based on the uniqueness of characteristic X-rays of each element. It was applied in particular for detecting the typical signals of the PPH dendrimers grafted onto silica nanoparticles [18], in nanoporous titanium dioxide materials [19], around anatase nanocrystals [20], and on graphene covering cobalt nanoparticles [34], but also in nanotubes elaborated by the alternate deposit of positively and negatively charged dendrimers [35]. The presence of PPH dendrimers was also detected in dendritic ribbons of Pt nanoparticles, which were wrapped by the dendrimers to ensure their cohesion. It was shown that large dendrimers wrap Pt nanoparticles more efficiently, inducing the creation of longer ribbons [36].

2.2.5 Infrared and Raman Spectroscopy

The role of infrared (IR) spectroscopy for the characterization of dendrimers is mainly limited to the routine analyses of the transformations occurring on the surface of dendrimers. For instance, the disappearance of the aldehyde terminal functions in the condensation step for the synthesis of phosphorus dendrimers is easily monitored by IR spectroscopy [37]. Detailed IR analyses combined with DFT (density functional theory) calculations were also carried out for poly(phosphorhydrazone) dendrimers of various generations [38], and built from various cores [39]. An additive behavior was observed for the intensity of the signals when the number of generations increased [40].

Raman spectroscopy yields similar information, but complementary to IR, about the vibrational modes in the system considered. In the case of PPH dendrimers, the FT-Raman spectra of generations 0 to 10 were recorded. It could be deduced from the different spectra that for generations higher than six, steric congestion disturbed the conformations of terminal groups, information that could not be obtained before with any other technique [41]. The different IR and Raman spectra of molecules built from the thiophosphoryl and phthalocyanine cores with the same repeating units and terminal groups were also studied in order to underline the role of core functionality on the dendrimer architecture [42].

2.2.6 Ultraviolet–Visible (UV-vis) and Fluorescence Spectroscopy

When chromophoric units constitute the terminal groups of dendrimers, their increasing number when the generation of the dendrimer increases generally induces an increase in the absorption intensity, which obeys the Beer–Lambert law. The UV-vis spectroscopy can be used to monitor the synthesis of dendrimers, as observed for instance for phosphorus dendrimers having azobenzenes within the branches [24]. UV-vis spectroscopy has also been used to get morphological information. An octa-substituted metal-free phthalocyanine located at the core of PPH dendrimers was used as a sensor and a probe for analyzing the properties of the internal structure. UV-visible spectra show both a hyperchromic and bathochromic effect on the Q-bands of the phthalocyanine with increasing generations. This finding indicates that the chromophore is more isolated when the generation increases and that the dendrimeric shell mimics a highly polar solvent, such as DMF, toward the core [14].

The role of fluorescence for biological imaging will be emphasized in Chapter 4; here we will consider only fluorescence as a technique of characterization of dendrimers. For instance, the large free space available inside dendrimers was shown by the possibility of formation of excimers between pyrene groups linked to the internal branches of PPH dendrimers [43]. The fluorescence intensity of a maleimide group linked "off-center" to the core of a series of phosphorhydrazone dendrimers was progressively quenched as the generation increased. This was an indication of the detrimental influence of the branches toward this particular fluorophore [44].

2.2.7 Characterizations Related to Chirality

Chiral entities located in different places of dendrimers may afford structural information, obtained by the measurement of optical rotation. Chiral benzylamine [45] or chiral ferrocenes [46] linked to the surface of phosphorhydrazone dendrimers simply gave additive optical rotation values, demonstrating the absence of interaction between the terminal groups. The chiral entities can also constitute the internal structure, at one or several layers. It was shown that the chiroptical properties of PPH dendrimers having one layer of chiral ferrocenes located inside the structure are not sensitive to the location of the chiral units, even for very high generations (up to G11) [47].

2.2.8 Electron Paramagnetic Resonance

EPR is used for studying compounds having one (or more) unpaired electron. Besides metallic radicals, which are mainly characterized by electrochemistry (see Section 2.2.10), the most widely used radicals are various nitroxides. The generation zero of PPH dendrimer functionalized by 6 TEMPO radicals as terminal groups was characterized by X-ray crystallography, which displayed the organization of three branches up and three branches down, relative to the cyclotriphosphazene core in the solid state. Characterization of the same compound by EPR in solution displayed the same geometry, as shown by seven lines centered at g = 2.0066 and separated by ca. 5.0 G in the EPR spectrum. This corresponds to a spectrum generated by the interaction of three TEMPO radicals [48].

Larger PPH dendrimers (up to generation 5) bearing the same nitroxide radical have been synthesized. It was shown that the radicals exhibit a strong exchange interaction, which depends on both the dendrimer generation and the temperature. The intramolecular origin of the interactions between radicals has been demonstrated, as well as a direct proportionality between the EPR intensity and the number of radicals by generation [49].

Cu(II)-conjugated phosphorus dendrimers bearing different ligand moieties have been studied also by EPR. It was shown that the coordination mode, the chemical structure, the flexibility, and the stability of these complexes strongly depend on different parameters such as the nature of the ligands, the size (generation) of the PPH dendrimer, and the molar ratio between Cu(II) and the ligands. To clarify the interaction mode of the dendrimeric Cu(II) complexes in a biological medium at different equilibration times, studies were performed in the presence of HCT-116 cancer cells and MRC-5 normal cells [50]. The dendrimer complex displaying the higher stability in these conditions was also the one having the highest antitumor properties [51]. The usefulness of this method is emphasized in Chapter 3.

2.2.9 Magnetometry (SQUID)

One of the most sensitive types of magnetometry is the SQUID (single/ superconducting quantum interface device), which can be used for characterizing dendrimers in which "magnetic entities" are included in the structure. It was used for characterizing the dendrimeric nitroxyl radicals studied by EPR in the previous paragraph (Section 2.2.8). The magnetic properties of the zero, first, and fourth generation of these dendrimers studied by SQUID magnetometry show antiferromagnetic interaction between radicals [49].

Generations 1 to 3 of PPH dendrimers capped with gadolinium(III) complexes of gem-bisphosphonates were also studied by SQUID. The magnetic measurements demonstrated clearly that the Gd ions were not coordinated to the gem-bisphosphonate pairs as isolated ions but that at least some of these ions are bridged through oxygen atoms [52].

2.2.10 Electrochemistry

Electrochemistry may afford three types of information when redox entities are linked somewhere in the structure of a dendrimer: the number of electroactive groups involved, the degree of burying of the electroactive groups, and the possibility to detect molecular recognition. Exhaustive coulometry is used to measure the number of electroactive groups. It was mainly applied in the case of ferrocenes linked to the surface of PPH dendrimers [53]. Most dendrimers having redox entities in their structure were analyzed by cyclic voltammetry [53], but this technique is particularly interesting for studying the degree of burying of electroactive groups inside dendrimers, which induces a progressive decrease in the electron-transfer rate constant, and thus of the intensity of the corresponding wave [47]. Water-soluble dendrimers having positive or negative charges on their terminal functions and ferrocenes inside their structure were tentatively characterized by electrochemistry, but a massive adsorption of the multicharged dendrimers onto the electrode was observed. Only small compounds could be characterized in this way [54]. Diverse types of ferrocenyl phosphines (different linkers between the ferrocene and the phosphines) were grafted on the surface of PPH dendrimers and were used for the complexation of ruthenium, and their electrochemical properties were studied (Fig. 2.3) [55]. These compounds were designed for studying their catalytic properties, in particular for catalyzing the isomerization of 1-octen-3-ol to 3-octanone. The catalysis can be switched ON or OFF, depending on the electronic state of the ferrocene (active) of ferrocenium (inactive). This is the first example of a molecular switch for catalysis, based on dendrimers [56].

All the above examples concerned electrochemistry of metallic entities, but organic entities can also afford interesting electrochemical information. Crown ether-TTF derivatives linked to the surface of PPH dendrimers were used for the detection of barium cations by electrochemistry. Indeed, the complexation in the macrocycle by Ba^{2+} induced a modification of the redox wave of TTF [57]. Recently, a new family of dendrimers, constituted of building blocks pertaining to poly(phosphorhydrazone) dendrimers and to poly(triazine) dendrimers was synthesized. These dendrimers display properties already known for their "parents," but also very new properties, in particular electrochemical properties, which allowed, for the first time, the monitoring of the growth of an organic dendrimer by electrochemistry while highlighting an even–odd generation behavior [58].

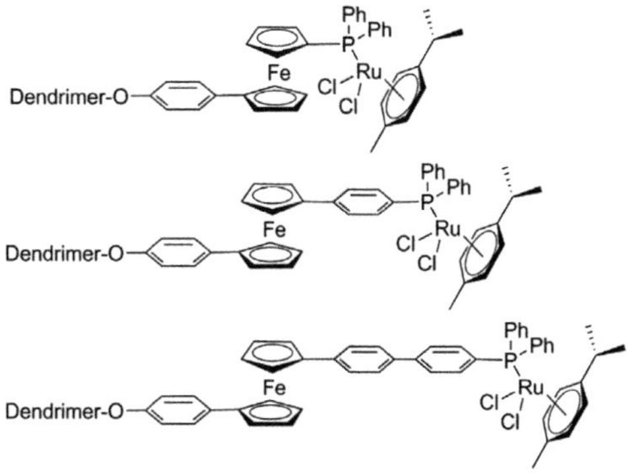

	E1/2/[V] Fe2+/Fe3+	E1/2/[V] Ru2+/Ru3+
M	0.46	irreversible
G1	0.54	irreversible
G2	0.55	1.23
G3	0.55	1.23
M	0.46	1.15
G1	0.52	1.16
G2	0.50	1.14
G3	0.51	1.16
M	0.42	1.14
G1	0.48	1.16
G2	0.47	1.14
G3	0.46	1.12

Figure 2.3 Two electroactive entities (Fe and Ru) separated by different linkers on monomers (M, with Me instead of dendrimer) and on the surface of generations 1 to 3 of PPH dendrimers, and their cyclic voltammetry data (GC working electrode/SCE reference electrode).

2.2.11 Laser Light Scattering (LLS) and Dynamic Light Scattering (DLS) and Coupling with Size Exclusion Chromatography (SEC)

Scattering techniques are based on the deflection of a beam of an electromagnetic wave away from the straight trajectory after its interaction with the structure to be analyzed. They give information about the size and shape of structures. Hydrodynamic radius is obtained via DLS, and it is more often an SLS (static light scattering) detector that is coupled to a SEC apparatus; SLS gives gyration radius. A series of phosphorus-containing dendrimeric structures has been synthesized using a dendron as starting point. All these compounds have been characterized by SEC, which displayed polydispersity better than that of narrow distribution polystyrene standards. A plot of log molecular weight *versus* retention time for these dendrimeric structures gave a relatively straight line, but different from that of polystyrene standards, with an increasing deviation as the molecular weight increased [59]. Another family of phosphorus-containing dendrimers and related hyperbranched polymers was also characterized by SEC with an LLS detector. Large differences in the polydispersity index (PDI = Mw/Mn) were observed as expected (PDI = 1.008 for the third-generation dendrimer, 1.32 for the hyperbranched polymer of comparable molecular weight) [60]. PPH dendrimers bearing poly(vinylidene fluoride) as terminal functions were also characterized by SEC and DLS [16].

However, LLS/DLS has also been used for the direct analysis of samples of dendrimers in solution. It was used for determining the hydrodynamic radius of PPH dendrimers capped with either phosphonic acids or poly(ethylene glycol) (PEG) derivatives. Comparison with DOSY NMR experiments displayed a good correlation in water for the size of the third generation in both cases (Rh = 2.5 nm by DOSY, 2.2 nm by DLS with phosphonic acid terminal groups; Rh = 5.3 nm by DOSY, 5.1 nm by DLS with PEG terminal groups) [15]. Self-assemblies of dendrimers have been also detected by DLS. Electrostatic self-assembly between acidic terminal groups of PPH dendrimers and an aminolactitol in water-induced spontaneous aggregates, with two distinct populations of supramolecular objects centered on 40 and 200 nm, as detected by DLS [61]. The same process carried out with PPH dendrimer ended by phosphonic acid derivatives also led to various types of aggregates detected by DLS [62].

2.3 Microscopy Methods

Three main types of microscopy methods, very different in principle, have been used for imaging dendrimers: transmission electron microscopy, scanning microscopy such as AFM, and polarized optical microscopy.

2.3.1 Transmission Electron Microscopy

Transmission electron microscopy (TEM) afforded images of individual dendrimer molecules from generation 3 to generation 10 of poly(phosphorhydrazone) dendrimers having gold covalently attached to each terminal group. A strict linear correlation was observed between the size and the logarithm of the molecular weight [63]. TEM has also been frequently used for observing nanoparticles wrapped by dendrimers. Only the metallic nanoparticles could be detected by TEM, but the presence of the dendrimers could be detected by EDX (see Section 2.2.4).

2.3.2 Atomic Force Microscopy

In scanning microscopy such as atomic force microscopy (AFM), the images are produced by "touch contact" at a few angstroms of a sensitive cantilever arm with the sample. AFM was often used for the characterization of dendrimeric macromolecular thin films [64], but also thick films [65]. In the case of a wavy surface, even individual G4 dendrimers could be detected [31, 32]. Microcapsules elaborated with PPH dendrimers were also characterized by AFM [66, 67], as well as their behavior in the presence of THF [68]. A G4 PPH dendrimer has been grafted to the TIP of AFM, to be used as a sensor for detecting and quantifying single-molecule interactions by AFM. Using the functionalized-dendritip, single-molecule force interactions between glutathione-S-transferase (GST) and its cognate antibody were measured (67±11 pN for single interaction) [69].

2.3.3 Polarizing Optical Microscopy

Contrarily to TEM and AFM, the resolution of polarizing optical microscopy (POM) is not high enough to be used for characterizing single dendrimers. It is used for characterizing the self-assembly of liquid crystalline dendrimers. Introducing mesogen groups as constituents of the structure of dendrimers should lead both to self-organizing processes inside the dendrimers and to self-assemblies between dendrimers, which may afford new types of mesophases with uncommon morphologies. Many works in this field were carried out by Percec *et al.* [70].

In the case of poly(phosphorhydrazone) dendrimers, a series of compounds (generations 0, 1, and 4) having sulfonamide derivatives bearing four mesogenic units (long alkyl chains) as terminal functions were synthesized. A cylindrical symmetry of the molecules has been proposed to promote the supramolecular columnar arrangement observed in all cases in the mesophases [71].

2.4 "Physical" Characterizations

We will gather, in this part, the following methods applied to PPH dendrimers: intrinsic viscosity, differential scanning calorimetry (DSC), thermogravimetric analyses (TGA), dielectric spectroscopy (DS), and the measurement of dipole moments, in connection with the dielectric properties.

2.4.1 Intrinsic Viscosity

Dilute solution viscosimetry studies can be used as an analytical probe of the morphological structure of dendrimers. Dendrimers should exhibit a maximum in the dependence of the intrinsic viscosity [η] on generation because the volume grows faster with generation than the molecular weight for the low generations, whereas the opposite occurs after a certain generation. This behavior was experimentally observed for several series of dendrimers, including for phosphorus dendrimers with two types of end groups (free phosphines or phosphines complexing BH_3). For this series, the maximum of intrinsic viscosity was observed for the third-generation dendrimers [60].

2.4.2   Differential Scanning Calorimetry (DSC) and Thermogravimetric Analyses (TGA)

The DSC technique is generally used to detect the glass transition temperature (T_g), which depends on the molecular weight, entanglement, and chain-end composition of polymers. In the case of dendrimers, T_g is affected by the terminal group substitutions and by the molecular mass (the generation). For PPH dendrimers ended by aldehydes, T_g varies from 74.75°C for the first generation to 140.15°C for the fifth generation [72], and from 153°C for G3 to 243°C for G4 PPH dendrimers ended by pyrene derivatives [73]. For other types of phosphorus dendrimers (phosphine–borane complexes as terminal groups), T_g varies from 119.7°C for G1 to 148.2°C for G5 [60]. In both cases, T_g correlates with n_e/M (n_e is the number of chain ends). DSC experiments were also carried out with the PPH dendrimers having liquid crystal properties [71].

DSC can be also correlated with thermogravimetric analyses (TGA), which afford the decomposition curve upon heating. Twenty four different dendrimers and dendrons based on PPH structures were analyzed by TGA. It was shown that the internal structure of these PPH dendrimers is stable up to at least 376°C, and that there is practically no influence of the generation on the thermal stability. On the contrary, the nature of the terminal functions has a dramatic influence on the stability. The least stable compounds (225°C) are the cationic dendrimers soluble in water, particularly with pyridinium terminal functions, whereas most of the studied PPH dendrimers soluble in organic solvents are stable over 300°C [10, 73], as shown in Fig. 2.4.

The thermal stability of latex nanoparticles has been greatly improved when covered by PPH dendrons ended by ammonium groups: the nude latex nanoparticles are completely decomposed at 450°C, whereas those covered by the second-generation PPH dendrons retain 40–45% weight at 550°C [74]. The preservation of the structure of crystalline anatase, even after thermal treatment at 800°C, when protected by PPH dendrimers is another illustration of the thermal stability they can induce [19]. This improved stability might be due to ring-opening polymerization upon heat treatment of the cyclotriphosphazene core [20].

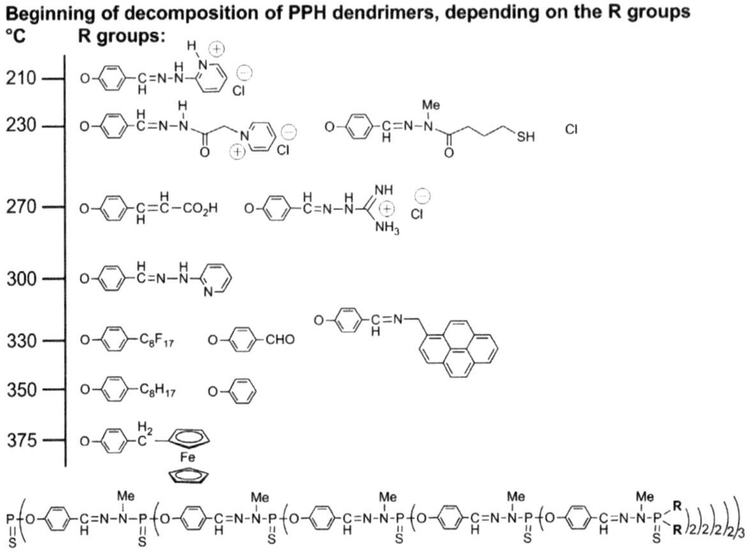

Figure 2.4 Examples of terminal functions of PPH dendrimers, and temperature at which the decomposition of the G5 dendrimers (shown in the lower part) begins, depending on the type of terminal functions.

TGA has also been used several times to detect and possibly quantify the presence of PPH dendrimers in materials. The presence of PPH dendrons in silica xerogels [17], of PPH dendrimers with ammonium terminal groups inside periodic mesoporous silica of type MCM-41 [75], and of PPH dendrimers with aldehyde or PEG terminal functions on silica nanoparticles [18] was ascertained in this way.

2.4.3 Dielectric Spectroscopy

Dielectric spectroscopy gives information about molecular dynamic processes in polymers (α-, β-, γ-, and δ-relaxation). This technique was applied to various types of dendrimers, and it was generally found that the α-relaxation values obtained by DS agree well with those obtained in differential scanning calorimetry measurements. Poly(phosphorhydrazone) dendrimers with aldehyde terminal functions were studied by dynamic dielectric spectroscopy (DDS) and thermostimulated currents (TSC), to analyze the evolution of molecular mobility upon increasing of generation (β-relaxation mode), first for generations 0 to 2 [76, 77], then up to generation 5 [78].

2.4.4 Dipole Moments

In connection with the dielectric properties, dipole moment values of some dendrimers were calculated, in particular from measurements of capacitance and refractive index. It might be anticipated that fully symmetrical entities such as dendrimers should have 0 as the dipole moment value. However, application of an electric field results in significant distortion of the molecules because the polar units of the structure may align in the direction of the field. In the case of poly(phosphorhydrazone) dendrimers (PPH) built from a trifunctional core, and having $P(S)Cl_2$ or CHO terminal functions, it was shown that the dipole moment values increased exponentially from 8.43 D for G1 up to 328 D for G11. Moreover, plotting the dipole moment ratio Dr = $\mu^2/N(\mu_0)^2$ (where μ is the dipole moment of the dendrimer, N is the number of polar monomeric units, and μ_0 is the dipole moment of the monomeric units) *versus* the molecular weight gives a constant of value 2.3 [7].

2.5 Conclusion

Most of the methods shown in this chapter for the characterization of phosphorus dendrimers have been applied also for the characterization of other types of dendrimers. A few particular methods of analyses have not been used for PPH dendrimers but for other types of dendrimers. This include in particular electrophoresis for assessing the purity and homogeneity of water-soluble dendrimers [79–83], circular dichroism (CD), which may afford information about the structure of chiral dendrimers [84, 85], and Mössbauer spectroscopy used for characterizing the local environment in some iron-containing dendrimers [86–88]. Various scattering techniques have also been applied to dendrimers. Small-angle neutron scattering (SANS) may give access to the radius of gyration, the molecular weight, and the location of the terminal groups of dendrimers [89–95]. Small-angle X-ray scattering (SAXS) affords information about the radius of gyration, and the segment density distribution inside the dendrimers [96–98], and wide-angle X-ray scattering (WAXS) was applied to characterize the mesophase of liquid crystal dendrimers [99].

All these methods are issued from methods well known for the characterization of small molecules, in particular most of the spectroscopic and spectrometric techniques. On the other hand, most scattering techniques, microscopy methods, and physical methods are issued from the work on macromolecules such as polymers or proteins. It must also be emphasized that most of these techniques are not only used for characterizing dendrimers but also for characterizing their interactions with their environment, for example for creation of networks, for the encapsulation of guests (including nanoparticles), or for the interaction with biological entities (in particular DNA). Several examples of such dendrimers will be given in the forthcoming chapters.

Acknowledgments

Thanks are due to the CNRS and to the COST action CM1302 (SIPs) for financial support.

References

1. Bosman, A. W., Janssen, H. M., and Meijer, E. W. (1999). About dendrimers: Structure, physical properties, and applications, *Chem. Rev.*, **99**, pp. 1665–1688.

2. Caminade, A. M., Laurent, R., and Majoral, J. P. (2005). Characterization of dendrimers, *Adv. Drug Deliv. Rev.*, **57**, pp. 2130–2146.

3. Caminade, A. M., Turrin, C. O., Laurent, R., Ouali, A., and Delavaux-Nicot, B. (2011). Methods of characterization of dendrimers, in: *Dendrimers: Towards Catalytic, Material and Biomedical Uses*, Caminade, A. M. (Ed.) (John Wiley & Sons Ltd, Chichester, UK), pp. 35–66.

4. Caminade, A. M., Laurent, R., Turrin, C. O., Rebout, C., Delavaux-Nicot, B., Ouali, A., and Majoral, J. P. (2010). Phosphorus dendrimers as viewed by 31P NMR spectroscopy: Synthesis and characterization, *C. R. Chimie*, **13**, pp. 1006–1027.

5. Launay, N., Caminade, A. M., Lahana, R., and Majoral, J. P. (1994). A general synthetic strategy for neutral phosphorus-containing dendrimers, *Angew. Chem. Int. Ed. Engl.*, **33**, pp. 1589–1592.

6. Launay, N., Caminade, A. M., and Majoral, J. P. (1995). Synthesis and reactivity of unusual phosphorus dendrimers: A useful divergent growth approach up to the 7th generation, *J. Amer. Chem. Soc.,* **117**, pp. 3282–3283.

7. Lartigue, M. L., Donnadieu, B., Galliot, C., Caminade, A. M., Majoral, J. P., and Fayet, J. P. (1997). Large dipole moments of phosphorus-containing dendrimers, *Macromolecules,* **30**, pp. 7335–7337.

8. Galliot, C., Larre, C., Caminade, A. M., and Majoral, J. P. (1997). Regioselective stepwise growth of dendrimer units in the internal voids of a main dendrimer, *Science,* **277**, pp. 1981–1984.

9. Deloncle, R., Coppel, Y., Rebout, C., Majoral, J. P., and Caminade, A. M. (2008). Characterization of two series of nitrogen-containing dendrimers by natural abundance 15N NMR, *Magn. Reson. Chem.,* **46**, pp. 493–496.

10. Turrin, C. O., Maraval, V., Leclaire, J., Dantras, E., Lacabanne, C., Caminade, A. M., and Majoral, J. P. (2003). Surface, core, and structure modifications of phosphorus-containing dendrimers. Influence on the thermal stability, *Tetrahedron,* **59**, pp. 3965–3973.

11. Caminade, A. M., Turrin, C. O., Sutra, P., and Majoral, J. P. (2003). Fluorinated dendrimers, *Curr. Opin. Colloid Interface Sci.,* **8**, pp. 282–295.

12. Bardaji, M., Kustos, M., Caminade, A. M., Majoral, J. P., and Chaudret, B. (1997). Phosphorus-containing dendrimers as multidentate ligands: Palladium, platinum, and rhodium complexes, *Organometallics,* **16**, pp. 403–410.

13. Leclaire, J., Coppel, Y., Caminade, A. M., and Majoral, J. P. (2004). Nanometric sponges made of water-soluble hydrophobic dendrimers, *J. Am. Chem. Soc.,* **126**, pp. 2304–2305.

14. Leclaire, J., Dagiral, R., Fery-Forgues, S., Coppel, Y., Donnadieu, B., Caminade, A. M., and Majoral, J. P. (2005). Octasubstituted metal-free phthalocyanine as core of phosphorus dendrimers: A probe for the properties of the internal structure, *J. Am. Chem. Soc.,* **127**, pp. 15762–15770.

15. Hameau, A., Fruchon, S., Bijani, C., Barducci, A., Blanzat, M., Poupot, R., Pavan, G. M., Caminade, A. M., and Turrin, C. O. (2015). Theoretical and experimental characterization of amino-PEG-phosphonate-terminated poly(phosphorhydrazone) dendrimers: Influence of size and PEG capping on cytotoxicity profiles, *J. Polym. Sci. A,* **53**, pp. 761–774.

16. Folgado, E., Guerre, M., Bijani, C., Ladmiral, V., Caminade, A. M., Ameduri, B., and Ouali, A. (2016). Well-defined poly(vinylidene fluoride) (PVDF) based-dendrimers synthesized by click chemistry: Enhanced crystallinity of PVDF and increased hydrophobicity of PVDF films, *Polymer Chem.* **7**, pp. 5625–5629.

17. Turrin, C. O., Maraval, V., Caminade, A. M, Majoral, J. P., Mehdi, A., and Reye, C. (2000). Organic–inorganic hybrid materials incorporating phosphorus-containing dendrimers, *Chem. Mater.*, **12**, pp. 3848–3856.

18. Hameau, A., Colliere, V., Grimoud, J., Fau, P., Roques, C., Caminade, A. M., and Turrin, C. O. (2013). PPH dendrimers grafted on silica nanoparticles: Surface chemistry, characterization, silver colloids hosting and antibacterial activity, *RSC Adv.* **3**, pp. 19015–19026.

19. Brahmi, Y., Katir, N., Hameau, A., Essoumhi, A., Essassi, E., Caminade, A. M., Bousmina, M., Majoral, J. P., and El Kadib, A. (2011). Hierarchically porous nanostructures through phosphonate-metal alkoxide condensation and growth using functionalized dendrimeric building blocks, *Chem. Comm.*, **47**, pp. 8626–8628.

20. Brahmi, Y., Katir, N., Ianchuk, M., Colliere, V., Essassi, E., Ouali, A., Caminade, A. M., Bousmina, M., Majoral, J. P., and El Kadib, A. (2013). Low temperature synthesis of ordered mesoporous stable anatase nanocrystals: The phosphorus dendrimer approach, *Nanoscale*, **5**, pp. 2850–2856.

21. Beraa, A., Hajjaji, M., Laurent, R., Delavaux-Nicot, B., and Caminade, A. M. (2016). Removal of chromate from aqueous solutions by dendrimers-clay nanocomposites, *Desalination Water Treatment*, **57**, pp. 14290–14303.

22. Blais, J. C., Turrin, C. O., Caminade, A. M., and Majoral, J. P. (2000). MALDI-TOF mass spectrometry for the characterization of phosphorus-containing dendrimers. Scope and limitations, *Anal. Chem.*, **72**, pp. 5097–5105.

23. Maraval, V., Caminade, A. M., Majoral, J. P., and Blais, J. C. (2003). Dendrimer design: How to circumvent the dilemma of a reduction of steps or an increase of function multiplicity? *Angew. Chem. Int. Ed.*, **42**, pp. 1822–1826.

24. Sebastian, R. M., Blais, J. C., Caminade, A. M., and Majoral, J. P. (2002). Synthesis and photochemical behavior of phosphorus dendrimers containing azobenzene units within the branches and/or on the surface, *Chem. Eur. J.*, **8**, pp. 2172–2183.

25. Lartigue, M. L., Launay, N., Donnadieu, B., Caminade, A. M., and Majoral, J. P. (1997). First 'layer-block' dendrimer built with a regular

alternation of two types of repeat units up to the fourth generation, *Bull. Soc. Chim. Fr.,* **134**, pp. 981–988.

26. Riegert, D., Pla-Quintana, A., Fuchs, S., Laurent, R., Turrin, C. O., Duhayon, C., Majoral, J. P., Chaumonnot, A., and Caminade, A. M. (2013). Diversified strategies for the synthesis of bifunctional dendrimeric structures, *Eur. J. Org. Chem.,* pp. 5414–5422.

27. Larre, C., Donnadieu, B., Caminade, A. M., and Majoral, J. P. (1998). Phosphorus-containing dendrimers: Chemoselective functionalization of internal layers, *J. Am. Chem. Soc.,* **120**, pp. 4029–4030.

28. Larre, C., Bressolles, D., Turrin, C., Donnadieu, B., Caminade, A. M., and Majoral, J. P. (1998). Chemistry within megamolecules: Regiospecific functionalization after construction of phosphorus dendrimers, *J. Am. Chem. Soc.,* **120**, pp. 13070–13082.

29. Larre, C., Donnadieu, B., Caminade, A. M., and Majoral, J. P. (1998). Regioselective gold complexation within the cascade structure of phosphorus-containing dendrimers, *Chem. Eur. J.,* **4**, pp. 2031–2036.

30. Demathieu, C., Chehimi, M. M., Lipskier, J. F., Caminade, A. M., and Majoral, J. P. (1999). Characterization of dendrimers by X-ray photoelectron spectroscopy, *Appl. Spectrosc.,* **53**, pp. 1277–1281.

31. Slomkowski, S., Miksa, B., Chehimi, M. M., Delamar, M., Cabet-Deliry, E., Majoral, J. P., and Caminade, A. M. (1999). Inorganic-organic systems with tailored properties controlled on molecular, macromolecular and microscopic level, *React. Funct. Polym.,* **41**, pp. 45–57.

32. Miksa, B., Slomkowski, S., Chehimi, M. M., Delamar, M., Majoral, J. P., and Caminade, A. M. (1999). Tailored modification of quartz surfaces by covalent immobilization of small molecules (gamma-aminopropyl-triethoxysilane), monodisperse macromolecules (dendrimers), and poly(styrene/acrolein/divinylbenzene) microspheres with narrow diameter distribution, *Colloid Polym. Sci.,* **277**, pp. 58–65.

33. Martinez-Ferrero, E., Franc, G., Mazeres, S., Turrin, C. O., Boissiere, U., Caminade, A. M., Majoral, J. P., and Sanchez, C. (2008). Optical properties of hybrid dendritic-mesoporous titania nanocomposite films, *Chem. Eur. J.,* **14**, pp. 7658–7669.

34. Keller, M., Colliere, V., Reiser, O., Caminade, A. M., Majoral, J. P., and Ouali, A. (2013). Pyrene-tagged dendritic catalysts non-covalently grafted onto magnetic Co/C nanoparticles: An efficient and recyclable system for drug synthesis, *Angew. Chem. Int. Ed.,* **52**, pp. 3626–3629.

35. Kim, D. H., Karan, P., Goring, P., Leclaire, J., Caminade, A. M., Majoral, J. P., Gosele, U., Steinhart, M., and Knoll, W. (2005). Formation of dendrimer nanotubes by layer-by-layer deposition, *Small*, **1**, pp. 99–102.

36. Franc, G., Badetti, E., Colliere, V., Majoral, J. P., Sebastian, R. M., and Caminade, A. M. (2009). Dendritic structures within dendritic structures: Dendrimer-induced formation and self-assembly of nanoparticle networks, *Nanoscale*, **1**, pp. 233–237.

37. Galliot, C., Prevote, D., Caminade, A. M., and Majoral, J. P. (1995). Polyaminophosphines containing dendrimers: Syntheses and characterizations, *J. Am. Chem. Soc.*, **117**, pp. 5470–5476.

38. Furer, V. L., Vandukova, I. I., Padie, C., Majoral, J. P., Caminade, A. M., and Kovalenko, V. I. (2007). FTIR spectroscopy studies of dendrimers built from cyclophosphazene core, *Vib. Spectrosc.*, **44**, pp. 89–93.

39. Furer, V. L., Vandyukov, A. E., Vandyukova, I. I., Majoral, J. P., Caminade, A. M., and Kovalenko, V. I. (2009). Comparative IR spectroscopic study of phosphorus-containing dendrimers built of thiophosphoryl, cyclophosphazene and phthalocyanine cores, *Vib. Spectrosc.*, **51**, pp. 326–332.

40. Furer, V. L., Vandukova, I. I., Majoral, J. P., Caminade, A. M., and Kovalenko, V. I. (2007). Spectral additive properties of phosphorus-containing dendrimers, *Vib. Spectrosc.*, **43**, pp. 351–357.

41. Furer, V. L., Majoral, J. P., Caminade, A. M., and Kovalenko, V. I. (2004). Elementoorganic dendrimer characterization by Raman spectroscopy, *Polymer*, **45**, pp. 5889–5895.

42. Furer, V. L., Vandyukova, I. I., Vandyukov, A. E., Majoral, J. P., Caminade, A. M., and Kovalenko, V. I. (2009). DFT study of structure, IR and Raman spectra of P'(0) and P'(4) dendrimers built from octasubstituted metal-free phthalocyanine core, *Chem. Phys.*, **358**, pp. 177–183.

43. Brauge, L., Caminade, A. M., Majoral, J. P., Slomkowski, S., and Wolszczak, M. (2001). Segmental mobility in phosphorus-containing dendrimers. Studies by fluorescent spectroscopy, *Macromolecules*, **34**, pp. 5599–5606.

44. Franc, G., Mazères, S., Turrin, C. O., Vendier, L., Duhayon, C., Caminade, A. M., and Majoral, J. P. (2007). Synthesis and properties of dendrimers possessing the same fluorophore(s) located either peripherally or off-center, *J. Org. Chem.*, **72**, pp. 8707–8715.

45. Lartigue, M. L., Caminade, A. M., and Majoral, J. P. (1997). Chiroptical properties of dendrimers with stereogenic end groups, *Tetrahedron – Asym.*, **8**, pp. 2697–2708.

46. Turrin, C. O., Chiffre, J., Daran, J. C., de Montauzon, D., Caminade, A. M., Manoury, E., Balavoine, G., and Majoral, J. P. (2001). New chiral phosphorus-containing dendrimers with ferrocenes on the periphery, *Tetrahedron*, **57**, pp. 2521–2536.

47. Turrin, C. O., Chiffre, J., de Montauzon, D., Balavoine, G., Manoury, E., Caminade, A. M., and Majoral, J. P. (2002). Behavior of an optically active ferrocene chiral shell located within phosphorus-containing dendrimers, *Organometallics*, **21**, pp. 1891–1897.

48. Badetti, E., Lloveras, V., Wurst, K., Sebastian, R. M., Caminade, A. M., Majoral, J. P., Veciana, J., and Vidal-Gancedo, J. (2013). Synthesis and structural characterization of a dendrimer model compound based on a cyclotriphosphazene core with TEMPO radicals as substituents, *Org. Lett.*, **15**, pp. 3490–3493.

49. Badetti, E., Lloveras, V., Munoz-Gomez, J. L., Sebastian, R. M., Caminade, A. M., Majoral, J. P., Veciana, J., and Vidal-Gancedo, J. (2014). Radical dendrimers: A family of five generations of phosphorus dendrimers functionalized with TEMPO radicals, *Macromolecules,* **47**, pp. 7717–7724.

50. Ottaviani, M. F., El Brahmi, N., Cangiotti, M., Coppola, C., Buccella, F., Cresteil, T., Mignani, S., Caminade, A. M., Costes, J. P., and Majoral, J. P. (2014). Comparative EPR studies of Cu(II)-conjugated phosphorous-dendrimers in the absence and presence of normal and cancer cells, *RSC Adv.*, **4**, pp. 36573–36583.

51. El Brahmi, N., El Kazzouli, S., Mignani, S. M., Essassi, E., Aubert, G., Laurent, R., Caminade, A. M., Bousmina, M. M., Cresteil, T., and Majoral, J. P. (2013). Original multivalent copper(II)-conjugated phosphorus dendrimers and corresponding mononuclear copper(II) complexes with antitumoral activities, *Mol. Pharm.,* **10**, pp. 1459–1464.

52. Franc, G., Turrin, C. O., Cavero, E., Costes, J. P., Duhayon, C., Caminade, A. M., and Majoral, J. P. (2009). Gem-bisphosphonate-ended group dendrimers: Design and gadolinium complexing properties, *Eur. J. Org. Chem.*, pp. 4290–4299.

53. Turrin, C. O., Chiffre, J., de Montauzon, D., Daran, J. C., Caminade, A. M., Manoury, E., Balavoine, G., and Majoral, J. P. (2000). Phosphorus-containing dendrimers with ferrocenyl units at the core, within the branches, and on the periphery, *Macromolecules,* **33**, pp. 7328–7336.

54. de Jong, E. R., Manoury, E., Daran, J. C., Turrin, C. O., Chiffre, J., Sournia-Saquet, A., Knoll, W., Majoral, J. P., and Caminade, A. M. (2012). Synthesis and characterization of water-soluble ferrocene-dendrimers, *J. Organomet. Chem.*, **718**, pp. 22–30.

55. Neumann, P., Dib, H., Sournia-Saquet, A., Grell, T., Handke, M., Caminade, A. M., and Hey-Hawkins, E. (2015). Ruthenium complexes with dendritic ferrocenyl phosphanes: Synthesis, characterization, and application in the catalytic redox isomerization of allylic alcohols, *Chem. Eur. J.*, **21**, pp. 6590–6604.

56. Neumann, P., Dib, H., Caminade, A. M., and Hey-Hawkins, E. (2015). Redox control of a dendritic ferrocenyl-based homogeneous catalyst, *Angew. Chem. Int. Ed.*, **54**, pp. 311–314.

57. Le Derf, F., Levillain, E., Trippe, G., Gorgues, A., Salle, M., Sebastian, R. M., Caminade, A. M., and Majoral, J. P. (2001). Immobilization of redox-active ligands on an electrode: The dendrimer route, *Angew. Chem. Int. Ed.*, **40**, pp. 224–227.

58. Dib, H., Rebout, C., Laurent, R., Mallet-Ladeira, S., Sournia-Saquet, A., Sarosi, M., Hey-Hawkins, E., Majoral, J. P., Delavaux-Nicot, B., and Caminade, A. M. (2016). Ordered layered dendrimers constructed from two known dendrimer families. Inheritance and emergence of properties, *Chem. Eur. J.*, **22**, pp. 10736–10742.

59. Maraval, V., Laurent, R., Donnadieu, B., Mauzac, M., Caminade, A. M., and Majoral, J. P. (2000). Rapid synthesis of phosphorus-containing dendrimers with controlled molecular architectures: First example of surface-block, layer-block, and segment-block dendrimers issued from the same dendron, *J. Am. Chem. Soc.*, **122**, pp. 2499–2511.

60. Merino, S., Brauge, L., Caminade, A. M., Majoral, J. P., Taton, D., and Gnanou, Y. (2001). Synthesis and characterization of linear, hyperbranched, and dendrimer-like polymers constituted of the same repeating unit, *Chem. Eur. J.*, **7**, pp. 3095–3105.

61. Blanzat, M., Turrin, C. O., Perez, E., Rico-Lattes, I., Caminade, A. M., and Majoral, J. P. (2002). Phosphorus-containing dendrimers bearing galactosylceramide analogs: self-assembly properties, *Chem. Commun.*, pp. 1864–1865.

62. Perez-Anes, A., Rodrigues, F., Caminade, A. M., Stefaniu, C., Tiersch, B., Turrin, C. O., and Blanzat, M. (2015). Influence of structural parameters on the self-association properties of anti-HIV catanionic dendrimers, *ChemPhysChem.*, **16**, pp. 3433–3437.

63. Slany, M., Bardaji, M., Casanove, M. J., Caminade, A. M., Majoral, J. P., and Chaudret, B. (1995). Dendrimer surface chemistry: Facile route to polyphosphines and their gold complexes, *J. Am. Chem. Soc.*, **117**, pp. 9764–9765.

64. Lazzara, T. D., Lau, K. H. A., Abou-Kandil, A. I., Caminade, A. M., Majoral, J. P., and Knoll, W. (2010). Polyelectrolyte layer-by-layer deposition in cylindrical nanopores, *ACS Nano*, **4**, pp. 3909–3920.

65. Gerasimov, A. V., Ziganshin, M. A., Vandyukov, A. E., Kovalenko, V. I., Gorbatchuk, V. V., Caminade, A. M., and Majoral, J. P. (2011). Specific vapor sorption properties of phosphorus-containing dendrimers, *J. Colloid Interface Sci.*, **360**, pp. 204–210.

66. Kim, B. S., Lebedeva, O. V., Kim, D. H., Caminade, A. M., Majoral, J. P., Knoll, W., and Vinogradova, O. I. (2005). Assembly and mechanical properties of phosphorus dendrimer/polyelectrolyte multilayer microcapsules, *Langmuir*, **21**, pp. 7200–7206.

67. Kim, B. S., Lebedeva, O. V., Koynov, K., Gong, H. F., Caminade, A. M., Majoral, J. P., and Vinogradova, O. I. (2006). Effect of dendrimer generation on the assembly and mechanical properties of DNA/phosphorus dendrimer multilayer microcapsules, *Macromolecules*, **39**, pp. 5479–5483.

68. Kim, B. S., Lebedeva, O. V., Park, M. K., Knoll, W., Caminade, A. M., Majoral, J. P., and Vinogradova, O. I. (2010). THF-induced stiffening of polyelectrolyte/phosphorus dendrimer multilayer microcapsules, *Polymer*, **51**, pp. 4525–4529.

69. Jauvert, E., Dague, E., Severac, M., Ressier, L., Caminade, A. M., Majoral, J. P., and Trevisiol, E. (2012). Probing single molecule interactions by AFM using bio-functionalized dendritips, *Sensors Actuators B Chem.*, **168**, pp. 436–441.

70. Rosen, B. M., Wilson, C. J., Wilson, D. A., Peterca, M., Imam, M. R., and Percec, V. (2009). Dendron-mediated self-assembly, disassembly, and self-organization of complex systems, *Chem. Rev.*, **109**, pp. 6275–6540.

71. Hincapie, C. A., Sebastian, R. M., Barbera, J., Serrano, J. L., Sierra, T., Majoral, J. P., and Caminade, A. M. (2014). Supermolecular columnar liquid-crystalline phosphorus dendrimers decorated with sulfonamide, *Chem. Eur. J.*, **20**, pp. 17047–17058.

72. Dantras, E., Dandurand, J., Lacabanne, C., Caminade, A. M., and Majoral, J. P. (2002). Enthalpy relaxation in phosphorus-containing dendrimers, *Macromolecules*, **35**, pp. 2090–2094.

73. Brauge, L., Veriot, G., Franc, G., Deloncle, R., Caminade, A. M., and Majoral, J. P. (2006). Synthesis of phosphorus dendrimers bearing chromophoric end groups: Toward organic blue light-emitting diodes, *Tetrahedron*, **62**, pp. 11891–11899.

74. Larpent, C., Genies, C., Delgado, A. P. D., Caminade, A. M., Majoral, J. P., Sassi, J. F., and Leising, F. (2004). Giant dendrimer-like particles from nanolatexes, *Chem. Commun.*, pp. 1816–1817.

75. Reinert, P., Chane-Ching, J. Y., Bull, L., Dagiral, R., Batail, P., Laurent, R., Caminade, A. M., and Majoral, J. P. (2007). Influence of cationic phosphorus dendrimers on the surfactant-induced synthesis of mesostructured nanoporous silica, *New J. Chem.*, **31**, pp. 1259–1263.

76. Dantras, E., Lacabanne, C., Caminade, A. M., and Majoral, J. P. (2001). TSC and broadband dielectric spectroscopy studies of beta relaxation in phosphorus-containing dendrimers, *Macromolecules*, **34**, pp. 3808–3811.

77. Dantras, E., Caminade, A. M., Majoral, J. P., and Lacabanne, C. (2002). Dielectric study of local relaxations in dendritic macromolecules, *J. Phys. D-Appl. Phys.*, **35**, pp. 5–8.

78. Dantras, E., Dandurand, J., Lacabanne, C., Caminade, A. M., and Majoral, J. P. (2004). TSC and broadband dielectric spectroscopy studies of the α-relaxation in phosphorus-containing dendrimers, *Macromolecules*, **37**, pp. 2812–2816.

79. Hudson, R. H. E. and Damha, M. J. (1993). Nucleic-acid dendrimers: Novel biopolymer structures, *J. Am. Chem. Soc.*, **115**, pp. 2119–2124.

80. Pesak, D. J., Moore, J. S., and Wheat, T. E. (1997). Synthesis and characterization of water-soluble dendritic macromolecules with a stiff, hydrocarbon interior, *Macromolecules*, **30**, pp. 6467–6482.

81. Welch, C. F. and Hoagland, D. A. (2003). The electrophoretic mobility of PPI dendrimers: Do charged dendrimers behave as linear polyelectro-lytes or charged spheres? *Langmuir*, **19**, pp. 1082–1088.

82. Shi, X. Y., Majoros, I. J., Patri, A. K., Bi, X. D., Islam, M. T., Desai, A., Ganser, T. R., and Baker, J. R. (2006). Molecular heterogeneity analysis of poly(amidoamine) dendrimer-based mono- and multifunctional nanodevices by capillary electrophoresis, *Analyst*, **131**, pp. 374–381.

83. Lalwani, S., Venditto, V. J., Chouai, A., Rivera, G. E., Shaunak, S., and Simanek, E. E. (2009). Electrophoretic behavior of anionic triazine and PAMAM dendrimers: Methods for improving resolution and assessing purity using capillary electrophoresis, *Macromolecules*, **42**, pp. 3152–3161.

84. Murer, P. and Seebach, D. (1995). Synthesis and properties of first-generation to 3rd-generation dendrimers with doubly and triply branched chiral building-blocks, *Angew. Chem. Int. Ed. Engl.*, **34**, pp. 2116–2119.

85. Rosini, C., Superchi, S., Peerlings, H. W. I., and Meijer, E. W. (2000). Enantiopure dendrimers derived from the 1,1'-binaphthyl moiety: A correlation between chiroptical properties and conformation of the 1,1'-binaphthyl template, *Eur. J. Org. Chem.*, **1**, pp. 61–71.

86. Daniel, M. C., Ruiz, J., Blais, J. C., Daro, N., and Astruc, D. (2003). Synthesis of five generations of redox-stable pentamethylamidoferrocenyl dendrimers and comparison of amidoferrocenyl- and pentamethylamidoferrocenyl dendrimers as electrochemical exoreceptors for the selective recognition of $H_2PO_4^-$, HSO_4^-, and adenosine 5'-triphosphate (ATP) anions: Stereoelectronic and hydrophobic roles of cyclopentadienyl permethylation, *Chem. Eur. J.*, **9**, pp. 4371–4379.

87. Zhao, M., Helms, B., Slonkina, E., Friedle, S., Lee, D., DuBois, J., Hedman, B., Hodgson, K. O., Frechet, J. M. J., and Lippard, S. J. (2008). Iron complexes of dendrimer-appended carboxylates for activating dioxygen and oxidizing hydrocarbons, *J. Am. Chem. Soc.*, **130**, pp. 4352–4363.

88. Ochi, Y., Suzuki, M., Imaoka, T., Murata, M., Nishihara, H., Einaga, Y., and Yamamoto, K. (2010). Controlled storage of ferrocene derivatives as redox-active molecules in dendrimers, *J. Am. Chem. Soc.*, **132**, pp. 5061–5069.

89. Potschke, D., Ballauff, M., Lindner, P., Fischer, M., and Vogtle F. (1999). Analysis of the structure of dendrimers in solution by small-angle neutron scattering including contrast variation, *Macromolecules*, **32**, pp. 4079–4087.

90. Topp, A., Bauer, B. J., Tomalia, D. A., and Amis, E. J. (1999). Effect of solvent quality on the molecular dimensions of PAMAM dendrimers, *Macromolecules*, **32**, pp. 7232–7237.

91. Topp, A., Bauer, B. J., Klimash, J. W., Spindler, R., Tomalia, D. A., and Amis, E. J. (1999). Probing the location of the terminal groups of dendrimers in dilute solution, *Macromolecules*, **32**, pp. 7226–7231.

92. Rosenfeldt, S., Dingenouts, N., Ballauff, M., Werner, N., Vogtle, F., and Lindner, P. (2002). Distribution of end groups within a dendritic structure: A SANS study including contrast variation, *Macromolecules*, **35**, pp. 8098–8105.

93. Chen, W. R., Porcar, L., Liu, Y., Butler, P. D., and Magid, L. J. (2007). Small angle neutron scattering studies of the counterion effects on the molecular conformation and structure of charged G4 PAMAM dendrimers in aqueous solutions, *Macromolecules*, **40**, pp. 5887–5898.

94. Li, T. F., Hong, K., Porcar, L., Verduzco, R., Butler, P. D., Smith, G. S., Liu, Y., and Chen, W. R. (2008). Assess the intramolecular cavity of a PAMAM dendrimer in aqueous solution by Small-Angle Neutron Scattering, *Macromolecules*, **41**, pp. 8916–8920.

95. Liu, Y., Bryantsev, V. S., Diallo, M. S., and Goddard, W. A. (2009). PAMAM dendrimers undergo pH responsive conformational changes without swelling, *J. Am. Chem. Soc.*, **131**, pp. 2798–2799.

96. Omotowa, B. A., Keefer, K. D., Kirchmeier, R. L., and Shreeve, J. M. (1999). Preparation and characterization of nonpolar fluorinated carbosilane dendrimers by APcI mass spectrometry and small-angle X-ray scattering, *J. Am. Chem. Soc.*, **121**, pp. 11130–11138.

97. Prosa, T. J., Bauer, B. J., and Amis, E. J. (2001). From stars to spheres: A SAXS analysis of dilute dendrimer solutions, *Macromolecules*, **34**, pp. 4897–4906.

98. Lombardo D. (2009). Liquid-like ordering of negatively charged poly(amidoamine) (PAMAM) dendrimers in solution, *Langmuir*, **25**, pp. 3271–3275.

99. Lorenz, K., Frey, H., Stuhn, B., and Mulhaupt, R. (1997). Carbosilane dendrimers with perfluoroalkyl end groups. Core-shell macromolecules with generation-dependent order, *Macromolecules*, **30**, pp. 6860–6868.

Chapter 3

EPR Characterization of Phosphorus Dendrimers as Drugs for Cancer and Neurodegenerative Diseases

Maria Francesca Ottaviani,[a] Michela Cangiotti,[a] Barbara Klajnert-Maculewicz,[b] Anne-Marie Caminade,[c] and Jean-Pierre Majoral[c]

[a]*Department of Pure and Applied Sciences, University of Urbino, Via Ca' le Suore, 61029 Urbino, Italy*
[b]*Department of General Biophysics, Faculty of Biology and Environmental Protection, University of Lodz, 12/16 Banacha St., 90-237 Lodz, Poland*
[c]*Laboratoire de Chimie de Coordination du CNRS, 205 route de Narbonne, 31077 Toulouse Cedex 4, France*
maria.ottaviani@uniurb.it

The electron paramagnetic resonance (EPR) technique is a precious tool to investigate biological systems at a molecular level with the purpose to obtain *in situ* information about the interactions between the different molecules and the chemical transformations occurring in the system under study. We used spin probes to analyze the interactions between phosphorus dendrimers and the amyloid and the prion peptides involved in Alzheimer and prion

Phosphorus Dendrimers in Biology and Nanomedicine: Synthesis, Characterization, and Properties
Edited by Anne-Marie Caminade, Cédric-Olivier Turrin, and Jean-Pierre Majoral
Copyright © 2018 Pan Stanford Publishing Pte. Ltd.
ISBN 978-981-4774-33-8 (Hardcover), 978-1-315-11085-1 (eBook)
www.panstanford.com

neurodegenerative diseases. It was found that selected spin probes are able to monitor the peptide–dendrimer interactions indicating the involvement of charged sites. We also followed the kinetics of amyloid and prion peptides aggregation to form the fibrils that are responsible for the senile plaques. It was found that amyloid fibrils form after 220 min, while less packed prion aggregates were formed after about 90 min. P-dendrimers with different functions at the external surface of dendrimers at different generation were characterized in the absence and presence of cancer cells by adding Cu(II) ions, which enhance anti-cancer activity. The dendrimer termed G3B showed a particular stability of the Cu(II) complex, which may be related to its peculiar anti-cancer action. The different Cu(II) complex formed in the presence of the cells also showed a particular stabilization in the presence of cancer cells.

3.1 Introduction

Dendrimers are examples of polymers that consist of a core molecule and layers of branched monomers. Each layer is called generation (G). Therefore, the dendrimers are characterized by a globular structure that contains empty cavities and bear an increasingly large number of functional groups on the surface with the increase in the G number.

In recent years, based on the huge therapeutic applications of biocompatible dendrimers, both active *per se* or as drug carriers, the use of dendrimers in nanomedicine has rapidly grown [1–5].

The increase in interest on dendrimers as drugs and drug-carrier candidates can be explained by their unique and tunable properties: (i) well-defined globular structures, predictable molecular weights, and monodispersity, which favor reproducible pharmacokinetics; (ii) the generation-dependent size, which fits various biomedical purposes; (iii) the lack of immunogenicity, which renders the dendrimers preferable *versus* synthesized peptide or natural protein carriers; (iv) the high penetration ability through the cell membranes, which allows high cellular uptake, preferential by cancer cells and inflamed tissues; (v) the variety of routes of administration, including non-classical routes as trans-dermal diffusion, trans-nasal diffusion, and ocular delivery; (vi) the size, shape, and surface properties, which influence pharmacokinetic/pharmacodynamics (PK/PD) behaviors, etc.

The possibility to use dendrimers as active *per se* drugs for curing both cancer and neurodegenerative diseases is well documented in recent literature [6–8], but, mostly, recent studies separately deal on cancer therapy [9, 10] or on curing neurodegenerative diseases, mainly Alzheimer [11–14]. The ability of dendrimers as drug-delivery agents for anti-cancer and Alzheimer therapies has also been deeply debated in recent literature [15–19].

Alzheimer's disease is characterized by the presence of amyloid plaques and neurofibrillar tangles in the brain tissue [20]. It has been found that aggregates of β-amyloid peptides ($A\beta$) are neurotoxic both *in vitro* and *in vivo* [21–26]. This holds more for the oligomer form than for mature fibrils. The mechanism responsible of $A\beta$-aggregates neurotoxicity is still unclear, but some evidences indicate the involvement of decreased acetylcholinesterase activity, generation of reactive oxygen species, neuroinflammation, mitochondria damage, and destabilization of intercellular Ca(II) homeostasis in Alzheimer pathogenesis [27–31]. The process of aggregation can be followed by observation of changes in the secondary structure from α-helical structure to β-sheet-rich organization [32, 33].

The presence of amyloids is a common feature for prion and Alzheimer's diseases. Prion diseases are fatal neurodegenerative disorders that result from conformational changes from a normal cellular form of prion proteins (PrP^C) to an infectious scrapie isoform (PrP^{Sc}) [34]. The infectious form has a changed secondary structure from α-helical into β-sheets, and it results in the formation of fibrils—amyloid-like structures, similar to Alzheimer's disease.

Several studies have demonstrated the ability of different types of dendrimers to prevent the aggregation of amyloid peptide ($A\beta$ 1-28) and prion peptide (PrP 185-208), both responsible for neurodegenerative disorders [35–42]. These two sequences not only contain the fibrilization sites but also present a structural homology, which could play an important role in the amyloidogenic process [43].

The role of dendrimers to disturb fibril formation has been mainly studied by fluorescence, using the thioflavine T (ThT) assay, and by monitoring changes in the secondary structure of peptides by FTIR. To obtain further and unique *in situ* information at a molecular level about the interactions occurring between the dendrimers and the amyloid and prion peptides, we made use of the EPR technique.

It has been already demonstrated that the computer-aided analysis of the EPR spectra of properly selected spin probes and spin labels provides unique information on the interactions occurring between dendrimers and biomolecules or biostructures [44–49].

This report first resumes the EPR studies performed to characterize the interactions occurring between monomers of Alzheimer's Aβ 1-28 and prion PrP 106-126 peptides and the phosphorus dendrimers (P-dendrimers, Fig. 3.1a) [50], showing the selectivity of interaction of the peptides with these dendrimers. These interactions allow preventing peptide aggregation and conversion into fibrils.

In most experiments where dendrimers were proved to be effective inhibitors of fibril aggregation, heparin was added to the system. Heparin has been found to induce amyloid aggregation and β-sheet formation [51]. However, there are contradictory hypotheses about the role of heparin in the infection, since both enhancing and inhibiting effects have been identified [52]. We studied—by means of EPR, supported by fluorescence and zeta potential measurements [53]—the interactions between heparin and dendrimers that have shown to possess anti-prion activity [38–40]. It was found that heparin–dendrimer interactions were indirectly responsible for the inhibition or enhancement of peptide-fibril formation by dendrimers. In this case too, in the present report we will underline the peculiar behavior of P-dendrimers (Fig. 3.1a), which have shown, by means of spin-probe EPR analysis, the strongest interactions with heparin among the different studied dendrimers [53].

Based on the fluorescence and FTIR results about the kinetics of formation of the amyloid and prion fibrils in the absence and presence of the dendrimers [35, 37–41], further EPR studies were carried out to analyze the aggregation behavior of the peptides involved in Alzheimer's and prion diseases [54–56]. The use of a selected spin probe allowed us to follow the aggregation process of the peptides over time, at heparin concentration and pH characteristic of the physiological conditions, thus providing precious information on the kinetics of aggregation and the type of interactions occurring in the system. The time evolution of the spectra was followed also in the presence of P-dendrimers to demonstrate their ability to prevent fibril formation [54]. In the present report, these results are described and discussed on the basis of the peculiar role of the dendrimer.

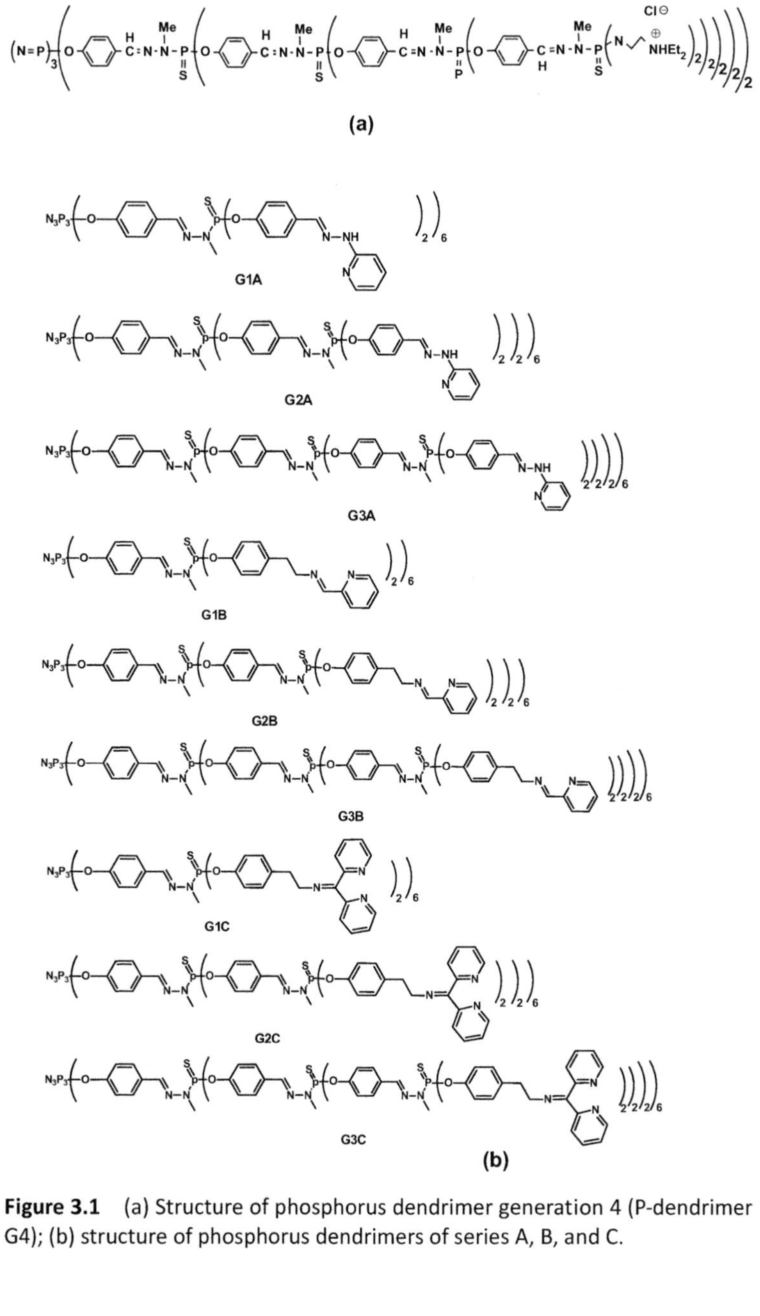

(a)

(b)

Figure 3.1 (a) Structure of phosphorus dendrimer generation 4 (P-dendrimer G4); (b) structure of phosphorus dendrimers of series A, B, and C.

Finally, the present report also describes and discuss EPR analyses, which help to clarify the role of phosphorus dendrimers in cancer therapy. Recent studies have shown that phosphorus dendrimers may be successfully functionalized to be used as anti-cancer drugs [57–66].

Based on the widespread success of cisplatin and derivatives in the clinical treatment of various types of cancers, metal-drugs are in pole position to tackle cancer progression. However, the antitumoral properties of dendrimer-conjugated metallodrugs for nanotherapy in oncology are not so intensively reported. Today, Pt and Ru metallodendrimers are the most representative examples of potential anti-cancer therapeutic agents [67, 68]. In addition to these two metals, copper (I/II) complexes represent very interesting alternative anti-cancer strategies [68]. Many copper complexes have been proposed as promising cytotoxic agents based on *in vitro* assays, but most of them use small ligands [68]. Surprisingly, in our knowledge, very few examples deal on the formation and the antitumoral properties of Cu(II)-conjugated dendrimers. Indeed, a PAMAM-based heptanuclear Cu(II) metallodendrimer shows a strong *in vitro* cytotoxicity against leukemia (MOLT-4) and breast cancer MCF-7 cell lines [69].

Recently, Cu(II)-conjugated phosphorus biocompatible dendrimers with a cyclotriphosphazene ring as core (Fig. 3.1b) were synthesized and their excellent antitumor activities were studied and verified against both solid and liquid tumor cell lines and the first structure activity relationships of cell growth inhibition against several cancer cell lines [65] (see also Chapter 9). The data suggested that cytotoxicity increased with generation and was enhanced by complexed Cu(II) ions. The most potent antiproliferative effects have been obtained by functionalizing the external surface of G3 dendrimers with the *N*-(di(pyridine-2-yl)methylene)ethanamine moiety (termed B)—as host–guest complexation chelator (Fig. 3.1). Two other chelators have been studied: 2-(2-methylenehydrazinyl)-pyridine (termed A: Fig. 3.1) and *N*-(di(pyridine-2-yl)methylene) ethanamine (termed C: Fig. 3.1). To clarify the complexation process of these dendrimers together with the structural and dynamical properties of the obtained metallodendrimers and their interactions with cancer cells, we performed a computer-aided EPR analysis of the Cu(II) dendritic complexes for G1–G3 dendrimers in the following steps and conditions [66]: (a) changing the Cu(II)/chelator molar ratio; (b) comparing the dendrimer–Cu(II) complexation behavior to that of the corresponding "monomeric" Cu(II) complexes; (c) changing temperature (mainly, the structural and dynamical parameters were obtained by computing the spectra at 298 K and 150 K); (d) due to the peculiar anti-cancer properties of Cu(II)–G3B complex, HCT-116 cancer cells and MRC-5 normal cells (as reference) were added to this complex at selected concentrations; (e) finally, computations were performed and structural and dynamical information were obtained by comparing the obtained parameters with those from previous EPR studies on other Cu(II)–dendrimer complexes [70–86].

The results obtained from the different EPR studies will be described and discussed separately in the following and final comments will be provided.

3.2 Interactions between P-Dendrimers and Peptides Involved in Alzheimer's and Prion Diseases

The spin-probe 4-trimethylammonium, 2,2,6,6-tetramethyl-piperidine-1oxyl Bromide (CAT1) was used for studying the interactions between P-dendrimers and the synthetic peptides $A\beta$ 1-28 [DAEFRHDSGYEVHHQKLVFFAEDVGSNK], simply termed $A\beta$, and PrP 106-126 [KTNMKHMAGAAAAGAVVGGLG], simply termed PrP; this spin probe was found to be informative on the interactions occurring between the dendrimers and their environmental molecules.

Figure 3.2a shows, as examples, the experimental spectra obtained at 255 K for the CAT1 probe in the presence of the P-dendrimer, the $A\beta$ peptide, and both P-dendrimer and $A\beta$ peptide. CAT1 concentration was 0.5 mM; the peptide concentration was 0.5 mM, and the P-dendrimer concentration was 0.01 mM. Therefore, the molar ratio peptide:dendrimer equaled to 50 and corresponded to the conditions that were applied previously in spectrofluorimetric experiments [37–39].

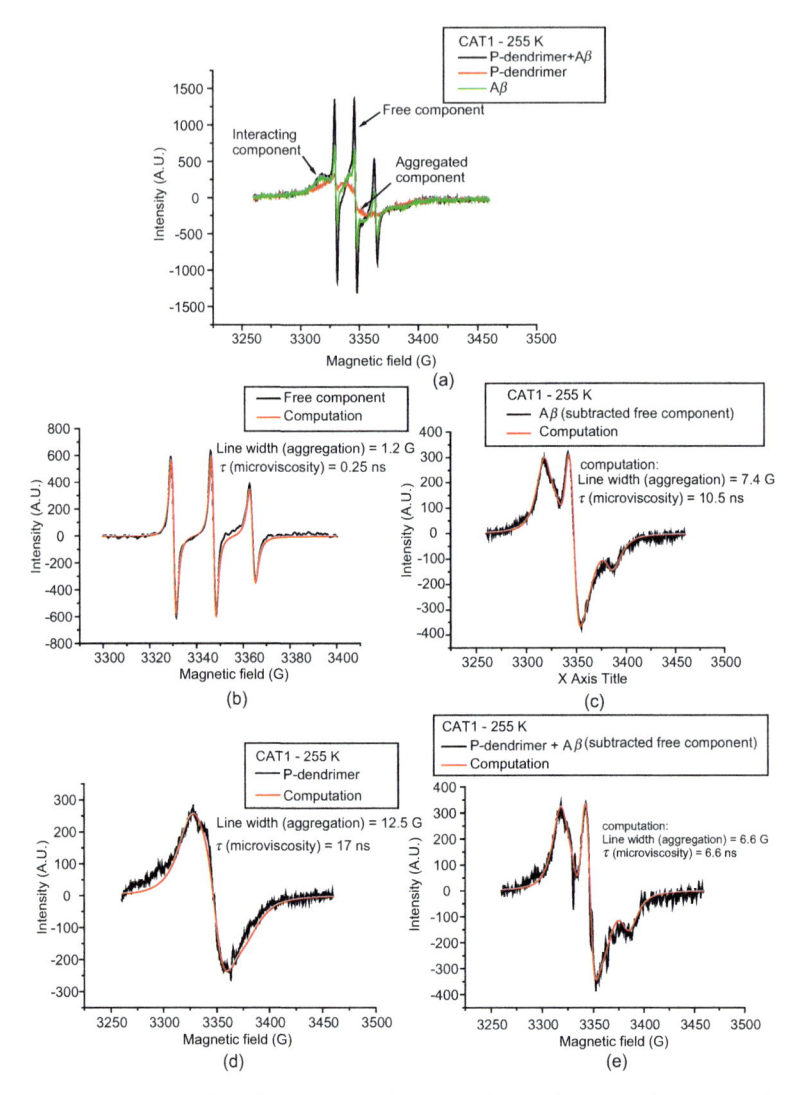

Figure 3.2 Examples of experimental spectra obtained at 255 K for CAT1 with P-dendrimer, with $A\beta$, and with both P-dendrimer and $A\beta$ (a); experimental and computed free component (b); experimental and computed components obtained after subtraction of the free component from the spectra of CAT1 with $A\beta$ (c); P-dendrimer (d); and $A\beta$ + P-dendrimer (e).

We selected a temperature of 255 K since it is just below the freezing temperature of CAT1-alone solutions in the EPR tube. At this temperature, CAT1-alone "disappears" from the spectrum since it separates as a salt, while the various differently interacting components in the solution separate into different fractions, each showing, on the basis of the EPR analysis, a different probe environment (corresponding to a different spectral component). This is the reason we identified three components in the spectra, which are indicated with arrows in Fig. 3.2a.

The three spectral components were extracted by a subtraction procedure between experimental spectra. Then, each component was computed, as shown in Figs. 3.2b–e. The computations, performed using the program by Budil&Freed [87] provided two main parameters selected to describe these systems, that is, the line width, which is a measure of dipolar spin–spin interactions between probes in vicinity to each other, and the correlation time for the rotational motion, τ, which is a measure of the microviscosity of the probe environment, in turn measuring the interactions occurring at the spin-probe level (accuracy 2% for both parameters). These three components were, therefore, characterized by different line width and τ values, as shown in Figs. 3.2b–e, but also their relative amounts (percentages) were different from one to another system:

- The **free component**, constituted by three hyperfine lines, shows low line width and τ values, which are characteristic of fast moving probes in solution. We have to note that this free component cannot come from CAT1 free in solution, since at 155 K the free-CAT1 alone is frozen and does not contribute any more to the EPR spectrum. Therefore, this component comes from CAT1 in interfacial solution where the rheological properties of water are modified. The relative amount of this free component significantly changes under the different experimental conditions, as shown in Table 3.1 where the relative percentage of the free component is listed.

- In the **interacting component**, the anisotropic components of the magnetic parameters are resolved due to the interactions of the probes with the molecules in solution. The correlation time for motion, τ, increases due to the increased strength of interactions. This value is reported in Table 3.1 for the different samples.

- The **aggregated component** is constituted by a single unresolved line, due to probes close to each other. Interactions of the probes with close sites of the peptides originated an aggregated component, but the probe density and freedom changes from one to the other situation. As described above, when aggregation occurs, the line width increases due to spin–spin interactions among close probes that are cooperatively interacting with another molecule or a surface.

Table 3.1 Line width measuring the aggregation, correlation time for motion of the interacting component and percentage of the free component, obtained from the analysis and computations of the spectral components

Sample	Line Width (G)	τ (ns)	%
P-dendrimer	12.5	17	5
$A\beta$	7.4	10.5	61
PrP	9	10.5	72
P-dendrimer + $A\beta$	6.6	6.6	55
P-dendrimer + PrP	10	11	32

From the data reported in Table 3.1, we extract the following information:

- A cooperative interaction of a large fraction of probes at the P-dendrimer surface occurs as evidenced by the high τ and line width values and the low amount (relative %) of free probes.
- When the CAT1 probes interact with the peptides, the line width and τ values decrease if compared to the CAT1-dendrimer system, but the interaction remains quite strong ($\tau = 10.5$ ns). However, for $A\beta$, the percentage, line width, and τ values are lower than obtained for PrP. This means that the interacting sites for $A\beta$ are more in number, but better distributed and less interacting than for PrP.
- When both the dendrimer and the peptides are present, the situation is further changing, monitoring the peptide–dendrimer interactions.
  - Mainly, we found that, for the $A\beta$ case, the co-presence of the dendrimer slightly increases the percentage of

interacting probes with respect to the absence of the dendrimer, but these probes are less interacting and better distributed at the surface because the dendrimer–peptide interaction expels the probes from the interacting sites that are available when only one of the two other ingredients is present. Other interacting sites, less interacting and quite far from each other, get occupied by the probes when both dendrimers and peptides are present. These sites are mainly polar instead of charged.

o For the PrP case, the mobility and line width parameters are quite similar as those for PrP alone, but the percentage is almost as high as for the dendrimer alone. So, in this case, the CAT probes are captured and partially concentrated at the dendrimer–PrP interface, where the freedom degree is quite low.

So we found a quite different behavior for the two peptides, indicating a stronger and more perturbative (regarding the probe) interaction between the P-dendrimer and $A\beta$ with respect to the P-dendrimer and PrP.

3.3 Interactions between P-Dendrimers and Heparin Affecting Prion Diseases

The effect of heparin in the P-dendrimer (G4, Fig. 3.1) solutions was also investigated by means of EPR using the CAT1 probe and decreasing the temperature down to 255 K to eliminate the contribution of freezable probes and distinguish among different interacting situations [53]. EPR spectra were recorded changing the dendrimer concentration (10, 20, and 30 µM), and the heparin concentration (0.2, 0.4, 0.6 mg/mL). We also tried different spin probes and different generations, but we found CAT1 and G4 providing the most interesting information about the dendrimer–heparin interactions.

Figure 3.3a shows as an example the EPR experimental spectrum recorded at 255 K for CAT1 probe (0.5 mM) in the system P-dendrimer and heparin at the concentrations of 20 µM and

0.4 mg/mL, respectively. In this case too, as for the P-dendrimer and peptide solutions, we may recognize in the spectrum (main features indicated with arrows) the three components termed free, interacting, and aggregated, which were first extracted by subtracting different experimental spectra and then computed as shown in Figs. 3.3b–d, respectively. The correlation time for motion, τ, obtained from the computations is also shown in the figures. The line width is only shown for the aggregated component, since in the other cases it is quite small (about 1 G) and almost invariant in the different experimental conditions.

Table 3.2 Different percentages of the three components indicated as "inter" (interacting), "free," and "agg" (aggregated), and the τ values obtained for the free component

P-dend µM	Heparin mg/mL	% Inter	% Free	% Agg	τ Free 10^{-10} s
0	0.2	13	7	80	2.0
0	0.4	0	90	10	1.0
0	0.6	15	5	80	(1)
10	0	16	4	80	(1)
20	0	25	7	68	3.5
30	0	37	11	52	3.55
10	0.2	22	7	71	4.15
10	0.4	20	12	68	3.65
10	0.6	19	5	76	4.3
20	0.4	24	11	65	4.2
30	0.4	25	15	60	4.5

Note: The values in parenthesis account for the low accuracy in the calculation due to a very small percentage of this component.

Table 3.2 resumes the different percentages of the three components, for simplicity indicated as "inter" (interacting), "free," and "agg" (aggregated), and the τ values obtained for the free component. Few values are in parenthesis to account for the low accuracy in the calculation due to a very small percentage of this component.

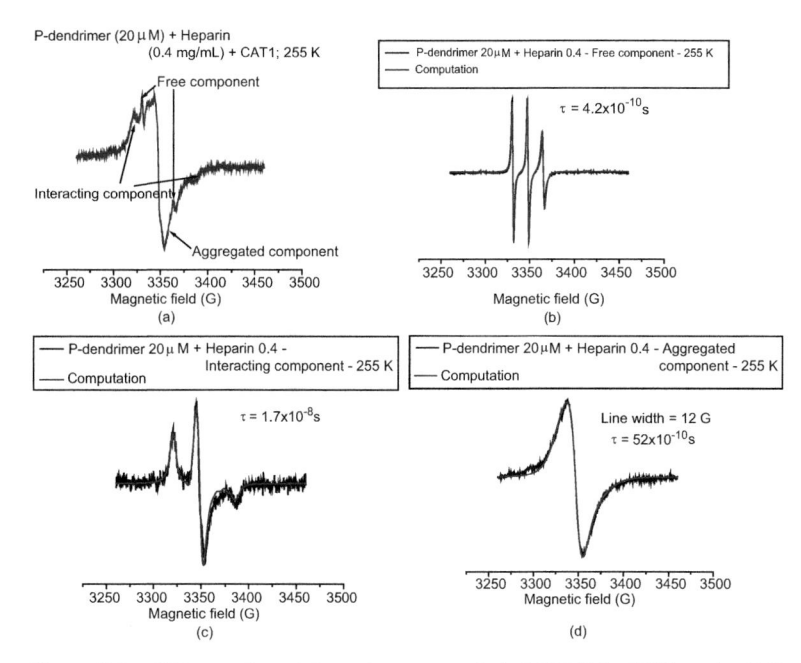

Figure 3.3 EPR experimental spectrum recorded at 255 K for CAT1 probe (0.5 mM) in the system P-dendrimer and heparin at the concentrations of 20 μM and 0.4 mg/mL, respectively (a); experimental and computed free component (b); interacting component (c); and aggregated component (d) constituting the overall EPR spectrum. The correlation time for motion, τ, obtained from the computations is also shown in the figures. The line width is only shown for the aggregated component.

The analysis of the EPR data suggests the following:

- In the presence of P-dendrimers as in their absence, the relative percentage of the free component is higher at 0.4 mg/mL heparin than at 0.2 and 0.6 mg/mL and is lowest at 0.6 mg/mL. This is in line with two effects: (i) disaggregation of the probes in the hydration layer of heparin when the heparin concentration increases from 0.2 to 0.4 mg/mL; (ii) aggregation of the probes when heparin concentration is 0.6 mg/mL, due to a competition between CAT1 and heparin counter ions to interact with the highly charged heparin.

- For the free component, the higher the relative percentage, the higher the mobility, because a higher amount of probes locates into the hydration layer of heparin. However, the mobility is lower in all solutions containing the dendrimer than in pure heparin solutions, indicating that the hydration layer becomes a dendrimer/heparin interphase. We have to take into account that CAT1 positive charge is neutralized by the heparin negatively charged sites; therefore, it is not repulsed by positively charged amino groups at the dendrimer surface.

- However, P-dendrimers interact quite strongly with heparin and show a poor variation in the EPR parameters with experimental conditions. Only a small fraction of the probes remains free in the dendrimer/heparin interphase, with relatively slow mobility and showing little change in response to differences in heparin and dendrimer concentrations. Therefore, by interacting with the dendrimer, the heparin amount available to interact with the prion or the amyloid peptides decreases, thus preventing the formation of fibrils responsible of neurodegenerative diseases.

3.4 Kinetics of the Aggregation Process of Prion and Amyloid Peptides in the Absence and Presence of P-Dendrimers

Finally, we wanted to follow the aggregation process of the prion and amyloid peptides by means of EPR; therefore, we performed a computer-aided EPR analysis of a selected nitroxide spin probe in water solutions of the β-amyloid peptide Aβ 1-28 (simply termed Aβ) and the prion peptide PrP 185-208 (simply termed PrP), which contain the fibril nucleation sites, in the absence and in the presence of the P-dendrimers (Fig. 3.1) [54].

A careful analysis of the process in different experimental conditions was performed to find the optimal conditions that allow aggregation to occur and to be monitored by EPR analysis over time. 4-octyl-dimethylammonium,2,2,6,6-tetramethyl-piperidine-1oxyl bromide (CAT8) spin probe was selected. In this case, CAT1 probe was poorly informative and we found CAT8 as the best probe for this kind of analysis. CAT8 (0.05 mM) was added to the peptide at a concentration of 0.5 mM, while 0.04 mg/mL of heparin and pH = 5 were used to trigger the aggregation. The experiments were performed both in the absence and presence of the dendrimer, which was added at a peptide/dendrimer molar ratio of 50.

In this case too, we recorded EPR spectra at 255 K to well differentiate in the spectra the interacting and non-interacting probes and eliminate the freezable ones. The goal to follow the aggregation process over time was accomplished by taking portions of each peptide solution at subsequent times from the mixture that was left equilibrating at 310 K [54]. The starting time (t = 0) corresponds to the time of heparin addition at pH = 5. The experiment was repeated in the absence and in the presence of the dendrimers.

Figure 3.4 shows as examples the experimental EPR spectra obtained at t = 150 min, and 255 K in the EPR cavity (equilibrated outside the cavity at 310 K) for CAT8 in the P-dendrimer solution (bottom), in the $A\beta$ peptide solution (middle), and in the $A\beta$ + P-dendrimer solution (top). The peptide aggregation process was generated adding 0.04 mg/mL of heparin at pH = 5.

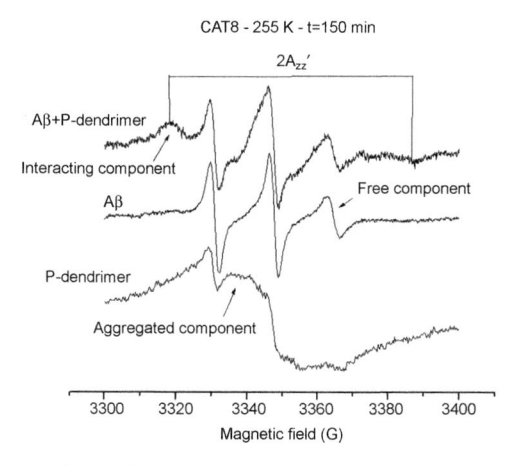

Figure 3.4 Experimental EPR spectra at t = 150 min, and 255 K in the EPR cavity (equilibrated at 310 K) for CAT8 (0.05 mM) in the $A\beta$ peptide solution (0.5 mM), in the P-dendrimer solution (0.01 mM), and in the $A\beta$ + P-dendrimer solution. The peptide aggregation process was generated adding 0.04 mg/mL of heparin at pH = 5.

As in the previous studies described in the present report, in this case too, the spectra are constituted by three components, termed free, interacting, and aggregated (indicated with arrows in Fig. 3.4). In the absence of the peptides, probe aggregation was evidenced by a single broad line (the aggregate component). But, since no single broad line was recorded for CAT8-peptide solutions both in the absence and in the presence of the dendrimer, the interacting and the free components may only arise from the probes localized at the surface of the peptides or at the peptide/dendrimer interphase. Precisely, the slow motion signal, termed interacting, is ascribed to the probes (the charged CAT group) interacting (ion–dipole) with the peptides (mainly at the polar –NH-CO– groups or the termini groups) and with the peptide–dendrimer adducts. On the contrary, the fast motion signal at 255 K may be ascribed to the probes at the water/peptide or dendrimer/water/peptide interphases, where the rheological properties of water are modified and, consequently, the water itself cannot freeze.

The analysis of the spectra was performed by computing (using the Budil&Freed program [87]) each spectral component extracted after a subtraction procedure among different experimental spectra. For the free component obtained for the $A\beta$ solution in the absence and presence of the P-dendrimer, the following parameters were plotted as a function of time in Fig. 3.5: (a) the relative percentage, which increases if the probes are expelled by their interacting sites due to other interactions like those forming the fibrils; and (b) the correlation time for motion, τ, which measures the weak interactions occurring at the probe environments; this parameter is poorly affected by the peptide–peptide interactions.

For the interacting component, we calculated the A'_{zz} distance (indicated in Fig. 3.4), which is a measure of the strength of interaction of the probe with peptides and/or dendrimers: A'_{zz} is reported for $A\beta$ solutions as a function of the aggregation time in Fig. 3.5c.

Also the absolute intensity of the spectra is a good parameter to obtain information about the system: The intensity may decrease mainly because of condensation–aggregation of probes at the surface of peptides and/or dendrimers. The condensation–aggregation may be promoted by the tendency of the probes to self-aggregate at a surface, and by the presence of close interacting sites at the surface of the peptides and/or the dendrimers (cooperative interaction).

As we see in the graphs in Fig. 3.5, all the parameters show different trends over time in the absence and presence of the dendrimers, which are summarized and discussed as follows.

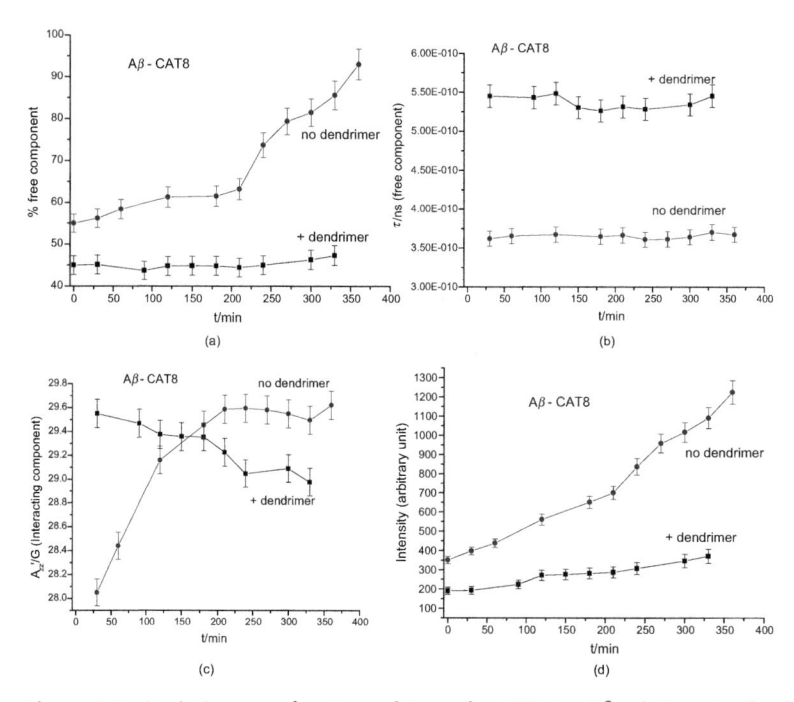

Figure 3.5 Variation as a function of time, for CAT8 in $A\beta$ solutions in the absence and presence of P-dendrimers, of (a) the relative percentage of free component; (b) the correlation time for the rotational motion of the free probes; (c) the A'_{zz} distance (Fig. 3.4) measuring the interaction strength of the interacting probes; and (d) the total intensity of the EPR spectra.

Initially, for the $A\beta$ peptide solution, the intensity is quite low since the probes self-aggregate in solution and at the peptide interacting sites. In the presence of the dendrimers, the intensity is even lower due to further self-aggregation at the dendrimer surface or at the dendrimer–peptide interphase. About half of the remaining probes distribute at the interphase with weak interactions (free component). The mobility (measured by τ) of the free component for $A\beta$ poorly changed over time, being lower in the presence then in the absence of the dendrimer (τ slightly increased upon addition of P-dendrimers). This is in agreement with the peptide/dendrimer interactions and the consequent decreased freedom of motion of the free probe in the water layer at the $A\beta$/dendrimer interphase. However, over time, both the intensity and the free component percentage increased, mainly after 220 min. We interpret this effect as a consequence of $A\beta$ fibril formation. The peptide aggregation provoked the extrusion of the probe from the peptide surface and consequently broke down the peptide-CAT8 bond. The probe migrated in the rheologically modified water/peptide interphase, where it gained freedom. When the fibrils are formed (after 220 min), the interacting sites available for a cooperative interaction with CAT8 are largely engaged in the peptide–peptide interactions and the probe is extracted in the fluid interphase. Conversely, in the presence of the dendrimer, which interacted with $A\beta$, the probe remained trapped at the dendrimer/peptide interphase and both the overall spectral intensity and the relative amount of the free component remained small over time.

The A'_{zz} value increased over time for $A\beta$ in the absence of the dendrimer. This change may be ascribed to the progressive formation–stabilization of peptide–probe strong interactions. When the fibrils are forming (after 220 min), the probe mobility did not change anymore since the peptide interacting sites become engaged in the peptide–peptide interactions. On the contrary, in the presence of the dendrimer, the stabilization of the $A\beta$/dendrimer binding led to a small increase in mobility (decrease in A'_{zz}) for the interacting probe, because the dendrimer interferes in the probe–peptide binding.

For the PrP peptide, the EPR analysis (results not shown) indicated the formation of low packed aggregates after about 90 min. However, the binding organization of the prion peptide poorly changed upon aggregation in comparison to $A\beta$ and the effect of the dendrimer was less evident than for $A\beta$. It is proposed that dendrimers mainly interfere in the lag (nucleation) phase of the prion peptide.

3.5 EPR Studies of Cu(II)-Conjugated Phosphorus Dendrimers in the Absence and Presence of Normal and Cancer Cells

We studied and compared the EPR results obtained for Cu(II)-conjugated phosphorus dendrimers from G1 to G3, decorated with 2-(2-methylenehydrazinyl)-pyridine (termed A, Fig. 3.1b), *N*-(pyridin-2-ylmethylene)ethanamine (termed B, Fig. 3.1b), and *N*-(di(pyridin-2-yl)methylene)ethanamine (termed C, Fig. 3.1b).

Figure 3.6 shows, as examples, the experimental and computed EPR spectra obtained for the B-dendrimer series for a 1:1 molar ratio between dendrimer surface sites and Cu(II) ions at 298 K and 150 K.

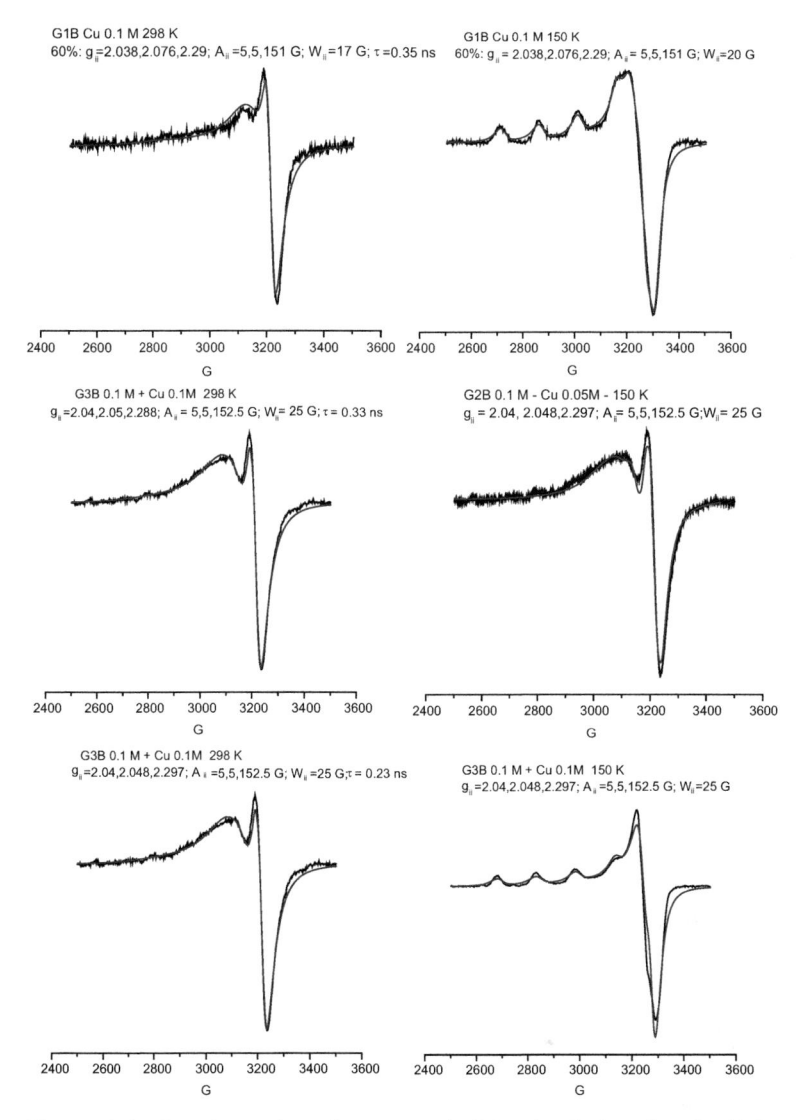

Figure 3.6 Experimental and computed EPR signal for the Cu–N_2O_2 coordination obtained for the B-dendrimer series for a 1:1 molar ratio between dendrimer surface sites and Cu(II) ions at 298 K and 150 K.

The figure legends also report the main parameters used for the computation of the spectra at both low and room temperatures (using Budil&Freed program [87]): (a) the g_{ii} components (accuracy in the third decimal, on the basis of the computation itself) for the coupling between the electron spin and the magnetic field; (b) the A_{ii} components (accuracy of about ±0.5 G) for the coupling between the electron spin and the copper nuclear spin ($I_{Cu} = 3/2$); (c) the correlation time for the diffusion rotational motion of the complexed Cu(II) ions, τ, (accuracy 2%); and (d) the line widths W_{ii} of the x, y, and z lines (accuracy 2%). The magnetic parameters extracted from the computation were then compared with equivalent parameters from previous studies on Cu(II)–dendrimer complexes [70–86]. This allowed us to assign the signals in Fig. 3.6 to the Cu–N$_2$O$_2$ coordination and also get information about a quite high dendrimer-complex flexibility from the τ values. It was found that this Cu–N$_2$O$_2$ coordination is very stable for G3B.

For the A-dendrimer series (G1A, G2A, G3A) at the 1:1 dendrimer surface sites:Cu(II) molar ratio, the Cu–O4 coordination using the solvent molecules predominated. The same holds for G1C and G2C, while for G3C the Cu–N$_2$O$_2$ coordination again prevails but in a short range of stability as a function of the molar ratio.

When the Cu(II) ions are added to the dendrimer + cells (MRC-5 and HCT-116) systems, the spectra completely changed with respect to the binary systems (Fig. 3.7), being constituted by a single component characteristic of a Cu–N$_4$ coordination in fast motion conditions (Fig. 3.8).

Therefore, the binding between the dendrimer and the cells modifies the structure of the Cu(II)–dendrimer complex favoring the coordination of Cu(II) with four nitrogen sites in a fluid condition (fast mobility). Furthermore, the spectra become much less intense. This means that a fraction of ions remains trapped at the dendrimer/cell interphase and strong spin–spin interactions let the EPR signal disappearing.

Some interesting differences were found between the Cu(II) + MRC-5 + G3B and the Cu(II) + HCT-116 + G3B spectra (Fig. 3.7). Mainly, we noted that the spectrum of Cu(II) + MRC-5 + G3B is at lower intensity with respect to the spectrum of Cu(II) + HCT-116 + G3B.

This indicates a higher stability of the latter system. Furthermore, the Cu(II) binding is a little bit stronger and the complex mobility a little bit slower in the MRC-5 case with respect to the HCT-116 one, since the ions are squeezed at the less stable G3B/MRC-5 adduct interphase.

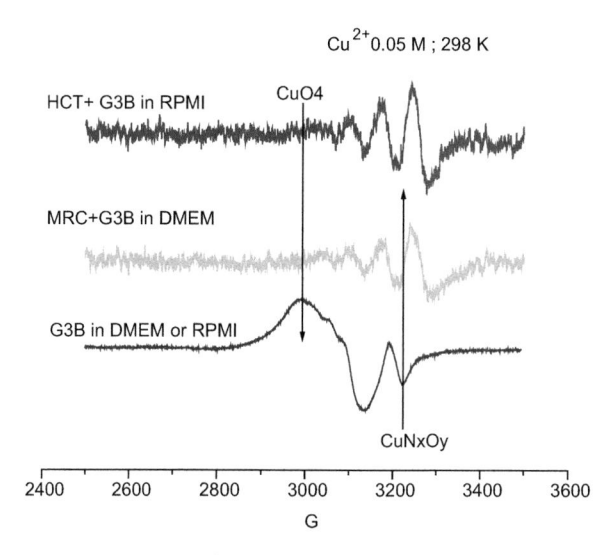

Figure 3.7 EPR experimental spectra obtained for Cu(II)–G3B complexes in the absence and presence of HCT-116 cells (simply termed HCT) and MRC-5 cells (simply termed MRC).

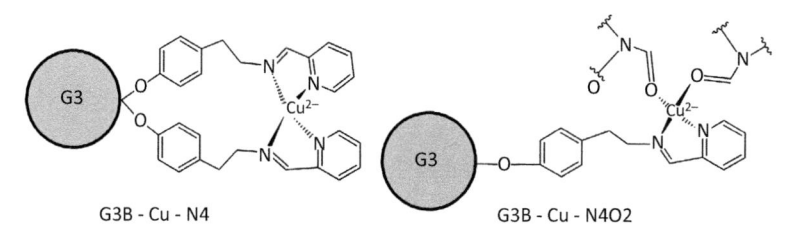

Figure 3.8 Main structures proposed for the Cu(II)–G3B complexes.

Definitely, the EPR analysis demonstrated to be useful to clarify the interaction modes of Cu(II) ions in biologically relevant systems like those containing healthy and cancer cells and dendrimers able to interact with the cells in a specific binding behavior.

3.6 Concluding Remarks

The present chapter describes some examples of the EPR characterization of P-dendrimers in the absence and presence of (a) peptides involved in neurodegenerative diseases, and (b) cancer cells.

In all cases, the results helped to clarify the interacting behavior of the dendrimers, which is of importance for a better understanding of the biochemical processes occurring *in situ* at a molecular level for a biomedical–pharmacological use of the dendrimers.

Acknowledgments

COST Actions MP1202 and TD0802 are acknowledged for supporting networking.

References

1. Khandare, J., Calderon, M., Dagia, N. M., and Haag, R. (2012). Multifunctional dendritic polymers in nanomedicine: Opportunities and challenges, *Chem. Soc. Rev.*, **41**, pp. 2824–2848.

2. Medina, S. H. and El-Sayed, M. E. H. (2009). Dendrimers as carriers for delivery of chemotherapeutic agents, *Chem. Rev.*, **109**, pp. 3141–3157.

3. Tekade, R. K., Kumar, P. V., and Jain, N. K. (2009). Dendrimers in oncology: An expanding horizon, *Chem. Rev.*, **109**, pp. 49–87.

4. Duncan, R. and Izzo, L. (2005). Dendrimer biocompatibility and toxicity, *Adv. Drug Delivery Rev.*, **57**, pp. 2215–2237.

5. Boas, U. and Heegaard, P. M. H. (2004). Dendrimers in drug research, *Chem. Soc. Rev.*, **33**, pp. 43–63.

6. Caminade, A. M. and Majoral, J. P. (2013). Positively charged phosphorus dendrimers. An overview of their properties, *New J. Chem.*, **37**, pp. 3358–3373.

7. Ghosh, S., Chatterjee, S., Roy, A., Ray, K., Swarnakar, S., Fujita, D., and Bandyopadhyay, A. (2015). Resonant oscillation language of a futuristic nano-machine-module: Eliminating cancer cells and Alzheimer Aβ plaques, *Curr. Top. Med. Chem.*, **15**, pp. 534–541.

8. Shcharbin, D., Shcharbina, N., and Bryszewska, M. (2014). Recent patents in dendrimers for nanomedicine: Evolution 2014, *Recent Pat. Nanomed.*, **4**, pp. 25–31.

9. Svenningsen, S. W., Janaszewska, A., Ficker, M., Petersen, J. F., Klajnert-Maculewicz, B., and Christensen, J. B. (2016). Two for the price of one: PAMAM-dendrimers with mixed phosphoryl choline and oligomeric poly(caprolactone) surfaces, *Bioconjug. Chem.*, **27**, pp. 1547–1557.

10. (a) Ionov, M., Lazniewska, J., Dzmitruk, V., Halets, I., Loznikova, S., Novopashina, D., Apartsin, E., Krasheninina, O., Venyaminova, A., Milowska, K., Nowacka, O., Gomez-Ramirez, R., de la Mata, F. J., Majoral, J. P., Shcharbin, D., and Bryszewska, M. (2015). Anticancer siRNA cocktails as a novel tool to treat cancer cells. Part (A). Mechanisms of interaction, *Int. J. Pharm.*, **485**, pp. 261–269. (b) Dzmitruk, V., Szulc, A., Shcharbin, D., Janaszewska, A., Shcharbina, N., Lazniewska, J., Novopashina, D., Buyanova, M., Ionov, M., Klajnert-Maculewicz, B., Gomez-Ramirez, R., Mignani, S., Majoral, J. P., Munoz-Fernandez, M. A., and Bryszewska, M. (2015). Anticancer siRNA cocktails as a novel tool to treat cancer cells. Part (B). Efficiency of pharmacological action, *Int. J. Pharm.*, **485**, pp. 288–294.

11. Stanczyk, M., Dziki, A., and Morawiec, Z. (2012). Dendrimers in therapy for breast and colorectal cancer, *Curr. Med. Chem.*, **19**, pp. 4896–4902.

12. (a)Appelhans, D., Benseny, N., Klementiveva, O., Bryszewska, M., Klajnert, B., and Cladera, J. (2013). Dendrimer-amyloid aggregates morphology and cell toxicity. In: *Dendrimers in Biomedical Applications*, Klajnert, B., Peng, L., and Cena, V. (Eds.), RSC Publishing, pp. 1–13. (b) Klementieva, O., Aso, E., Filippini, D., Benseny-Cases, N., Carmona, M., Juves, S., Appelhans, D., Cladera, J., and Ferrer, I. (2013). Effect of poly(propylene imine) glycodendrimers on β-amyloid aggregation *in vitro* and in APP/PS1 transgenic mice, as a model of brain amyloid deposition and Alzheimer's disease, *Biomacromolecules*, **14**, pp. 3570–3580. (c) Klementieva, O., Benseny-Cases, N., Gella, A., Appelhans, D., Voit, B., and Cladera, J. (2011). Dense shell glycodendrimers as potential nontoxic anti-amyloidogenic agents in Alzheimer's disease. Amyloid-dendrimer aggregates morphology and cell toxicity, *Biomacromolecules*, **12**, pp. 3903–3909.

13. Neelov, I. M., Janaszewska, A., Klajnert, B., Bryszewska, M., Makova, N. Z., Hicks, D., Pearson, H. A., Vlasov, G. P., Ilyash, M. Yu., Vasilev, D. S., Dubrovskaya, N. M., Tumanova, N. L., Zhuravin, I. A., Turner, A. J., and Nalivaeva, N. N. (2013). Molecular properties of lysine dendrimers and their interactions with Aβ-peptides and neuronal cells, *Curr. Med. Chem.*, **20**, pp. 134–143.

14. Klajnert, B., Wasiak, T., Ionov, M., Fernandez-Villamarin, M., Sousa-Herves, A., Correa, J., Riguera, R., and Fernandez-Megia, E. (2012).

Dendrimers reduce toxicity of Aβ 1-28 peptide during aggregation and accelerate fibril formation, *Nanomedicine,* **8**, pp. 1372–1378.

15. Liu, Y., Ng, Y., Toh, M. R., and Chiu, G. N. C. (2015). Lipid-dendrimer hybrid nanosystem as a novel delivery system for paclitaxel to treat ovarian cancer, *J. Control. Release,* **220**(Part A), pp. 438–446.

16. Subramanian, A. P., Jaganathan, S. K., Manikandan, A., Pandiaraj, K. N., Gomathi, N., and Supriyanto, E. (2016). Recent trends in nano-based drug delivery systems for efficient delivery of phytochemicals in chemotherapy, *RSC Adv.,* **6**, pp. 48294–48314.

17. Singh, K., Ahmad, Z., Shakya, P., Ansari, V. A., Kumar, A., Zishan, M., and Arif, M. (2016). Nano formulation: A novel approach for nose to brain drug delivery, *J. Chem: Pharm: Res.*, **8**, pp. 208–215.

18. Wong, H. L., Wu, X, Y., and Bendayan, R. (2012). Nanotechnological advances for the delivery of CNS therapeutics, *Adv. Drug Deliv. Rev.*, **64**, pp. 686–670.

19. Beg, S., Samad, A., Alam, M. I., and Nazish, I. (2011). Dendrimers as novel systems for delivery of neuropharmaceuticals to the brain, *CNS Neurol. Disord. Drug Targets,* **10**, pp. 576588.

20. Lahiri, D. K., Farlow, M. R., Sambamurti, K., Greig, N. H., Giacobin, E., and Schneider, L. S. (2003). A critical analysis of new molecular targets and strategies for drug developments in Alzheimer's disease, *Curr. Drug Targets,* **4**, pp. 97–112.

21. Lorenzo, A. and Yankner, B. A. *(*1994). Beta-amyloid neurotoxicity requires fibril formation and is inhibited by congo red, *Proc. Natl. Acad. Sci. U.S.A.*, **91**, pp. 12243–12247.

22. Bucciantini, M., Giannoni, E., Chiti, F., Baroni, F., Formigli, L., and Zurdo, J. S. (2002). Inherent toxicity of aggregates implies a common mechanism for protein misfolding diseases, *Nature*, **416**, pp. 507–511.

23. Caughey, B. and Lansbury, P. T. (2003). Protofibrils, pores, fibrils, and neurodegeneration: Separating the responsible protein aggregates from the innocent bystanders, *Annu. Rev. Neurosci.*, **26**, pp. 267–298.

24. Klein, W. L., Stine, W. B. Jr, and Teplow, D. B. (2004). Small assemblies of unmodified amyloid beta-protein are the proximate neurotoxin in Alzheimer's disease, *Neurobiol. Aging*, **25**, pp. 569–580.

25. Stefani, M. and Dobson, C. M. (2003). Protein aggregation and aggregate toxicity: New insights into protein folding, misfolding diseases and biological evolution, *J. Mol. Med.*, **81**, pp. 678–699.

26. Walsh, D. M. and Selkoe, D. J. (2004). Oligomers on the brain: The emerging role of soluble protein aggregates in neurodegeneration, *Protein Pept. Lett.*, **11**, pp. 213–228.

27. Bartolini, M., Bertucci, C., Cavrini, V., and Andrisano, V. (2003). Beta-amyloid aggregation induced by human acetylcholinesterase: Inhibition studies, *Biochem. Pharmacol.*, **65**, pp. 407–416.

28. Dyrks, T., Dyrks, E., Hartmann, T., Masters, C., and Beyreuther, K. (1992). Amyloidogenicity of beta A4 and beta A4-bearing amyloid protein precursor fragments by metal-catalyzed oxidation, *J. Biol. Chem.*, **267**, pp. 18210–18217.

29. Colell, A., Fernandez, A., and Fernandez-Checa, J. C. (2009). Mitochondria, cholesterol and amyloid beta peptide: A dangerous trio in Alzheimer disease, *J. Bioenerg. Biomembr.*, **41**, pp. 417–423.

30. Abramov, A. Y., Fraley, C., Diao, C. T., Winkfein, R., Colicos, M. A., Duchen, M. R., French, R. J., and Pavlo, E. (2007). Targeted polyphosphatase expression alters mitochondrial metabolism and inhibits calcium-dependent cell death, *Proc. Natl. Acad. Sci. U.S.A.*, **104**, pp. 18091–18096.

31. Bezprozvanny, I. and Mattso, M. P. (2008). Neuronal calcium mishandling and the pathogenesis of Alzheimer's disease, *Trends Neurosci.*, **31**, pp. 454–463.

32. Shibata, M., Yamada, S., Kumar, S. R., Calero, M., Bading, J., Frangione, B., Holtzman, D. M., Miller, C. A., Strickland, D. K., Ghiso, J., and Zlokovic, B. V. (2000). Clearance of Alzheimer's amyloid $\beta(1–40)$-peptide from brain by LDL receptor-related protein-1 at the blood-brain barrier, *J. Clin. Invest.*, **106**, pp. 1489–1499.

33. Casserly, I. and Topol, E. (2004). Convergence of atherosclerosis and Alzheimer's disease: Inflammation, cholesterol, and misfolded proteins, *Lancet*, **363**, pp. 1139–1146.

34. Prusiner, S. B. (1989). Scrapie prions, *Annu. Rev. Microbiol.*, **43**, pp. 345–374.

35. (a) Supattapone, S., Nguyen, H.O. B., Cohen, F. E., Prusiner, S. B., and Scott, M. R. (1999). Elimination of prions by branched polyamines and implications for therapeutics, *Proc. Natl. Acad. Sci. U.S.A.*, **96**, pp. 14529–14534. (b) Supattapone, S., Wille, H., Uyechi, L., Safar, J., Tremblay, P., Szoka, F. C., Cohen, F. E., Prusiner, S. B., and Scott, M. (2001). Branched polyamines cure prion-infected neuroblastoma cells, *J. Virol.*, **75**, pp. 3453–3461.

36. Solassol, J., Crozet, C., Perrier, V., Leclaire, J., Beranger, F., Caminade, A. M., Meunier, B., Dormont, D., Majoral, J. P., and Lehmann, S. (2004).

Cationic phosphorus-containing dendrimers reduced prion replication both in cell culture and in mice infected scrapie, *J. Gen. Virol.*, **85**, pp. 1791–1799.

37. Klajnert, B., Cortijo, M., Bryszewska, M., and Cladera, J. (2006). Influence of heparin and dendrimers on the aggregation of two amyloid peptides related to Alzheimer's and prion diseases, *Biochem. Biophys. Res. Commun.*, **339**, pp. 577–582.

38. Klajnert, B., Cortijo-Arellano, M., Cladera, J., and Bryszewska, M. (2006). Influence of dendrimer's structure on its activity against amyloid fibril formation, *Biochem. Biophys. Res. Commun.*, **345**, pp. 21–28.

39. Klajnert, B., Cladera, J., and Bryszewska, M. (2006). Molecular interactions of dendrimers with amyloid peptides: pH dependence, *Biomacromolecules*, **7**, pp. 2186–2191.

40. Klajnert, B., Cortijo-Arellano, M., Cladera, J., Majoral, J.-P., Caminade, A.-M., and Bryszewska, M. (2007). Influence of phosphorus dendrimers on the aggregation of the prion peptide PrP 185-208, *Biochem. Biophys. Res. Commun.*, **364**, pp. 20–25.

41. Klajnert, B., Appelhans, D., Komber, H., Morgner, N., Schwarz, S., Richter, S., Brutschy, B., Ionov, M., Tonkikh, A. K., Bryszewska, M., and Voit, B. (2008). The influence of densely organized maltose shells on the biological properties of poly(propylene imine) dendrimers: New effects dependent on hydrogen bonding, *Chem. Eur. J.*, **14**, pp. 7030–7041.

42. Wasiak, O., Ionov, M., Nieznanski, K., Nieznanska, H., Klementieva, O., Granell, M., Cladera, J., Majoral, J. P., Caminade, A. M., and Klajnert, B. (2012). Phosphorus dendrimers affect Alzheimer's (Aβ1-28) peptide and MAP-tau protein aggregation, *Mol. Pharmaceutics*, **9**, pp. 458–469.

43. Mahfoud, R., Garmy, N., Maresca, M., Yahi, N., Puigserver, A., and Fantini, J. (2002). Identification of a common sphingolipid-binding domain in Alzheimer, prion, and HIV-1 proteins, *J. Biol. Chem.*, **277**, pp. 11292–11296.

44. Ottaviani, M. F., Matteini, P., Brustolon, M., Turro, N. J., Jockusch, S., and Tomalia, D. A. (1998). Characterization of starburst dendrimers and vesicle solutions and their interactions by cw- and pulsed-EPR, TEM and dynamic light scattering, *J. Phys. Chem.*, **102**, pp. 6029–6039.

45. Ottaviani, M. F., Daddi, R., Brustolon, M., Turro, N. J., and Tomalia, D. A. (1999). Structural modifications of DMPC vesicles upon interaction with poly(amidoamine) dendrimers studied by cw-electron paramagnetic resonance and electron spin echo techniques, *Langmuir*, **15**, pp. 1973–1980.

46. Ottaviani, M. F., Sacchi, B., Turro, N. J., Chen, W., Jockusch, S., and Tomalia, D. A. (1999). An EPR study of the interactions between starburst dendrimers and polynucleotides, *Macromolecules*, **32**, pp. 2275–2282.

47. Ottaviani, M. F., Furini, F., Casini, A., Turro, N. J., Jockusch, S., Tomalia, D. A., and Messori, L. (2000). Formation of supramolecular structures between DNA and starburst dendrimers studied by EPR, CD, UV and melting profiles, *Macromolecules*, **33**, pp. 7842–7851.

48. Ottaviani, M. F., Jockusch, S., Turro, N. J., Tomalia, D. A., and Barbon, A. (2004). Interactions of dendrimers with selected amino acids and proteins studied by continuous wave EPR and Fourier transform EPR, *Langmuir*, **20**, pp. 10238–10245.

49. Ottaviani, M. F., Favuzza, P., Sacchi, B., Turro, N. J., Jockusch, S., and Tomalia, D. A. (2002). Interactions between starburst dendrimers and mixed DMPC/DMPA-Na vesicles studied by the spin label and the spin probe techniques, supported by TEM, *Langmuir*, **18**, p. 2347.

50. Klajnert, B., Cangiotti, M., Calici, S., Majoral, J. P., Caminade, A. M., Cladera, J., Bryszewska, M., and Ottaviani, M. F. (2007). EPR study of the interactions between dendrimers and peptides involved in Alzheimer's and prion diseases, *Macromol. Biosci.* **7**, pp. 1065–1074.

51. Gellermann, G. P., Ullrich, K., Unger, C., Fändrich, M., Sauter, S., and Diekmann, S. (2007). Identification of molecular compounds critical to Alzheimer's-like plaque formation, *J. Neuroscience Res.*, **85**, pp. 2037–2044.

52. Andrievskaia, O., Potetinova, Z., Balachandran, A., and Nielsen, K. (2007). Binding of bovine prion protein to heparin: A fluorescence polarization study, *Arch. Biochem. Biophys.*, **460**, pp. 10–16.

53. Klajnert, B., Cangiotti, M., Calici, S., Ionov, M., Majoral, J. P., Caminade, A. M., Cladera, J., Bryszewska, M., and Ottaviani, M. F. (2009). Interactions between dendrimers and heparin and their implications for the anti-prion activity of dendrimers, *New J. Chem.*, **33**, pp. 1087–1093.

54. Ottaviani, M. F., Mazzeo, R., Cangiotti, M., Fiorani, L., Majoral, J. P., Caminade, A. M., Pedziwiatr, E., Bryszewska, M., and Klajnert, B. (2010). Time evolution of the aggregation process of peptides involved in neurodegenerative diseases and preventing aggregation effect of phosphorus dendrimers studied by EPR, *Biomacromolecules*, **11**, pp. 3014–3021.

55. Ottaviani, M. F., Cangiotti, M., Fiorani, L., Fattori, A., Wasiak, T., Appelhans, D., and Klajnert, B. (2012). Kinetics of amyloid and prion

fibril formation in the absence and presence of dense shell sugar-decorated dendrimers, *Curr. Med. Chem.,* **19**, pp. 5907–5921.

56. Ottaviani, M. F., Appelhans, D., de la Mata, F. J., Garcia-Gallego, S., Fattori, A., Coppola, C., Cangiotti, M., Fiorani, L., Majoral, J. P., Caminade, A. M., Bryszewska, M., Smith, D. K., Garti, N., and Klajnert, B. (2013). Characterization of dendrimers and their interactions with biomolecules for medical use by means of electron magnetic resonance. In: *Dendrimers in Biomedical Applications,* Klajnert, B., Peng, L., and Cena, V. (Eds.), RSC Publishing, pp. 115–133.

57. Shcharbin, D., Shcharbina, N., Shakhbazau, A., Mignani, S., Majoral, J. P., and Bryszewska, M. (2015). Phosphorus-containing nanoparticles: Biomedical patents review, *Expert Opin. Ther. Pat.,* **25**, pp. 539–548.

58. Caminade, A. M., Turrin, C. O., and Majoral, J. P. (2010). Biological properties of phosphorus dendrimers, *New J. Chem.,* **34**, pp. 1512–1524.

59. Gomulak, P., Klajnert, B., Bryszewska, M., Majoral, J. P., Caminade, A. M., and Blasiak, J. (2012). Cytotoxicity and genotoxicity of cationic phosphorus-containing dendrimers, *Curr. Med. Chem.,* **19**, pp. 6233–6240.

60. Shcharbin, D., Dzmitruk, V., Shakhbazau, A., Goncharova, N., Seviaryn, I., Kosmacheva, S., Potapnev, M., Pedziwiatr-Werbicka, E., Bryszewska, M., Talabaev, M., Chernov, A., Kulchitsky, V., Caminade, A. M., and Majoral, J. P. (2011). Fourth generation phosphorus-containing dendrimers: Prospective drug and gene delivery carrier, *Pharmaceutics,* **3**, pp. 458–473.

61. Dabrzalska, M., Benseny-Cases, N., Barnadas-Rodriguez, R., Mignani, S., Zablocka, M., Majoral, J. P., Bryszewska, M., Klajnert-Maculewicz, B., and Cladera, J. (2016). Fourier transform infrared spectroscopy (FTIR) characterization of the interaction of anti-cancer photosensitizers with dendrimers, *Anal. Bioanal. Chem.,* **408**, pp. 535–544.

62. El Brahmi, N., Mignani, S. M., Caron, J., El Kazzouli, S., Bousmina, M. M., Caminade, A. M., Cresteil, T., and Majoral, J. P. (2015). Investigations on dendrimer space reveal solid and liquid tumor growth-inhibition by original phosphorus-based dendrimers and the corresponding monomers and dendrons with ethacrynic acid motifs, *Nanoscale,* **7**, pp. 3915–3922.

63. Szulc, A., Zablocka, M., Coppel, Y., Bijani, C., Dabkowski, W., Bryszewska, M., Klajnert-Maculewicz, B., and Majoral, J. P. (2014). A viologen phosphorus dendritic molecule as a carrier of ATP and Mant-ATP:

Spectrofluorimetric and NMR studies, *New J. Chem.*, **38**, pp. 6212–6222.

64. Caminade, A. M., Ouali, A., Laurent, R., Turrin, C. O., and Majoral, J. P. (2016). Coordination chemistry with phosphorus dendrimers. Applications as catalysts, for materials, and in biology, *Coord. Chem. Rev.*, **308(Part 2)**, pp. 478–497.

65. El Brahmi, N., El Kazzouli, S., Mignani, S. M., Essassi, E. M., Aubert, G., Laurent, R., Caminade, A. M., Bousmina, M. M., Cresteil, T., and Majoral, J. P. (2013). Original multivalent copper(II)-conjugated phosphorus dendrimers and corresponding mononuclear copper(II) complexes with antitumoral activities, *Mol. Pharm.*, **10**, pp. 1459–1464.

66. Ottaviani, M. F., El Brahmi, N., Cangiotti, M., Coppola, C., Buccella, F., Cresteil, T., Mignani, S., Caminade, A. M., Costes, J. P., and Majoral, J. P. (2014). Comparative EPR studies of Cu(II)-conjugated phosphorous-dendrimers in the absence and presence of normal and cancer cells, *RSC Adv.*, **4**, pp. 36573–36583.

67. El Kazzouli, S., El Brahmi, N., Mignani, S., Bousmina, M., and Majoral, J. P. (2012). From metallodrugs to metallodendrimers for nanotherapy in oncology: A concise overview, *Curr. Med. Chem.*, **19**, pp. 4995–5010.

68. Santini, C., Pellei, M., Gandin, V., Porchia, M., Tisato, F., and Marzano, C. (2014). Advances in copper complexes as anticancer agents, *Chem. Rev.*, **114**, pp. 815–862.

69. Zhao, X., Loo, S. C. J., Lee, P. P., Tan, T. T. Y., and Chu, C. K. (2010). Synthesis and cytotoxic activities of chloropyridylimineplatinum(II) and chloropyridyliminecopper(II) surface-functionalized poly(amidoamine) dendrimers, *J. Inorg. Biochem.*, **104**, pp. 105–110.

70. Ottaviani, M. F., Bossmann, S., Turro, N. J., and Tomalia, D. A. (1997). Characterization of starburst dendrimers by the EPR technique: 1. Copper complexes in water solution, *J. Am. Chem. Soc.*, **116**, pp. 661–671.

71. Ottaviani, M. F., Montalti, F., Turro, N. J., and Tomalia, D. A. (1997). Characterization of starburst dendrimers by the EPR technique. Copper(II) ions full generation dendrimers, *J. Phys. Chem. B*, **101**, pp. 158–166.

72. Ottaviani, M. F., Valluzzi, R., and Balogh, L., (2002). Internal structure of silver-poly(amidoamine) dendrimer complexes and nanocomposites, *Macromolecules,* **35**, pp. 5105–5115.

73. Appelhans, D., Oertel, U., Mazzeo, R., Komber, H., Hoffmann, J., Weidner, S., Brutschy, B., Voit, B., and Ottaviani, M. F. (2010). Dense-shell

glycodendrimers: UV/Vis and electron paramagnetic resonance study of metal ion complexation, *Proc. R. Soc. A*, **466**, pp. 1489–1513.

74. Garcia-Gallego, S., Serramia, M. J., Arnaiz, E., Diaz L., Munoz-Fernandez, M. A., Gomez-Sal, P., Ottaviani, M. F., Gomez, R., and de la Mata, F. J. (2011). Transition-metal complexes based on a sulfonate-containing N-donor ligand and their use as HIV antiviral agents, *Eur. J. Inorg. Chem.*, pp. 1657–1665.

75. García-Gallego, S., Rodríguez, J. S., Jiménez, J. L., Cangiotti, M., Ottaviani, M. F., Muñoz-Fernandez, M., Gomez, R., and de la Mata, F. J. (2012). Polyanionic N-donor ligands as chelating agents in transition metal complexes: Synthesis, structural characterization and antiviral properties against HIV, *Dalton Trans.*, **41**, pp. 6488–6499.

76. Ottaviani, M. F., Cangiotti, M., Fiorani, L., Barnard, A., Jones, S. P., and Smith, D. K. (2012). Probing dendron structure and nanoscale self-assembly using computer-aided analysis of EPR spectra, *New J. Chem.*, **36**, pp. 469–476.

77. Galán, M., Sánchez-Rodríguez, J., Cangiotti, M., García-Gallego, S., Jiménez, J. L., Gómez, R., Ottaviani, M. F., Muñoz-Fernández, M. Á., and de la Mata, F. J. (2012). Antiviral properties against HIV of water soluble copper carbosilane dendrimers and their EPR characterization, *Curr. Med. Chem.*, **19**, pp. 4984–4994.

78. Garcia-Gallego, S., Cangiotti, M., Fiorani, L., Fattori, A., Munoz-Fernandez, M. A., Gomez, R., Ottaviani, M. F., and De la Mata, F. J. (2013). Anionic sulfonated and carboxylated PPI dendrimers with the EDA core: Synthesis and characterization of selective metal complexing agents, *Dalton Trans.*, **42**, pp. 5874–5889.

79. Ottaviani, M. F., Cangiotti, M., Fattori, A., Coppola, C., Lucchi, S., Ficker, M., Petersen, J. F., and Christensen, J. B. (2013). Copper(II) complexes with 4-carbomethoxypyrrolidone functionalized PAMAM-dendrimers: An EPR study, *J. Phys. Chem. B*, **117**, pp. 14163–14172.

80. Ottaviani, M. F., Cangiotti, M., Fattori, A., Coppola, C., Posocco, P., Laurini, E., Liu, Z., Liu, C., Fermeglia, M., Peng, L., and Pricl, S. (2014). Copper(II) binding to flexible triethanolamine-core PAMAM dendrimers: A combined experimental/in silico approach, *Phys. Chem. Chem. Phys.*, **16**, pp. 685–694.

81. Furlan, S., La Penna, G., Appelhans, D., Cangiotti, M., Ottaviani, M. F., and Danani, A. (2014). Combined EPR and molecular modeling study of PPI dendrimers interacting with copper ions: Effect of generation and maltose decoration, *J. Phys. Chem. B*, **118**, pp. 12098–12111.

82. Rossi, J. C., Maret, B., Vidot, K., Francoia, J. P., Cangiotti, M., Lucchi, S., Coppola, C., and Ottaviani, M. F. (2015). Multi-technique characterization of poly-L-lysine dendrigrafts–Cu(II) complexes for biocatalysis, *Macromol. Biosci.*, **15**, pp. 275–290.

83. Moreno, S., Ortega, P., de la Mata, F. J., Ottaviani, M. F., Cangiotti, M., Fattori, A., Munoz-Fernandez, M. A., and Gomez, R. (2015). Bifunctional chelating agents based on ionic carbosilane dendrons with DO3A at the focal point and their complexation behavior with copper(II), *Inorg. Chem.*, **54**, pp. 8943–8956.

84. Peña-González, C. E., Sánchez-Nieves, J., García-Broncano, P., Ottaviani, M. F., Cangiotti, M., Fattori, A., Hierro-Oliva, M., González-Martín, M. L, Pérez-Serrano, J., Muñoz-Fernández, M. Á., Gómez, R., and de la Mata, F. J. (2016). Dendronized anionic gold nanoparticles: Synthesis, characterization and antiviral activity, *Chem. Eur. J.*, **22**, pp. 2987–2999.

85. Ottaviani, M. F., Yordanova, S., Cangiotti, M., Vasileva-Tonkova, E., Fattori, A., Stoyanov, S., and Grabchev, I. (2016). Spectral characterization and *in vitro* microbiological activity of new bis-1,8-naphthalimides and their Cu(II) complexes, *J. Mol. Struct.*, **1110**, pp. 72–82.

86. Grabchev, I., Yordanova, S., Vasileva-Tonkova, E., Cangiotti, M., Fattori, A., Alexandrova, R., Stoyanov, S., and Ottaviani, M. F. (2016). A novel benzofurazan-cyclam conjugate and its Cu(II) complex: Synthesis, characterization and *in vitro* cytotoxicity and antimicrobial activity, *Dyes Pigments*, **129**, pp. 71–79.

87. Budil, D. E., Lee, S., Saxena, S., and Freed, J. H. (1996). Nonlinear-least-squares analysis of slow-motion EPR spectra in one and two dimensions using a modified Levenberg–Marquardt algorithm, *J. Magn. Reson. Ser. A.*, **120**, pp. 155–189.

Chapter 4

Fluorescent (Phosphorus) Dendrimers and Their Use in Biology

Anne-Marie Caminade and Aurélien Hameau
Laboratoire de Chimie de Coordination, CNRS, 205 Route de Narbonne, BP 44099,
31077 Toulouse Cedex 4, France
anne-marie.caminade@lcc-toulouse.fr

4.1 Introduction

Fluorescence is an emission in the UV, visible, or IR domains, due to electronic transitions. After the absorption of one quantum of energy (or two in the case of two-photon absorption [1]), leading to a molecule in an excited singlet state, the return to the ground state can occur in three different ways, as shown in Fig. 4.1: (i) a non-radiative decay (no emission); (ii) fluorescence occurring rapidly from a singlet state; or (iii) intersystem crossing from a singlet state to a triplet state, then inducing phosphorescence.

Energy transfer can also occur between molecules. Förster/fluorescence resonance energy transfer (FRET) is particularly important in biology. It concerns non-radiative energy transfer due to long range dipole–dipole interactions between two fluorophores: one donor of energy and the other one acceptor. The wavelengths

Phosphorus Dendrimers in Biology and Nanomedicine: Synthesis, Characterization, and Properties
Edited by Anne-Marie Caminade, Cédric-Olivier Turrin, and Jean-Pierre Majoral
Copyright © 2018 Pan Stanford Publishing Pte. Ltd.
ISBN 978-981-4774-33-8 (Hardcover), 978-1-315-11085-1 (eBook)
www.panstanford.com

of absorption and emission have to be chosen to induce a good overlap, as shown in Fig. 4.2. This phenomenon can occur only if the two fluorophores are in close proximity between 10 and 100 Å. The efficiency of transfer (Φ_T) is extremely sensitive to the separation distance between fluorophores, because it varies in proportion to the inverse sixth power of the distance (R) separating the donor and acceptor molecules: $\Phi_T = 1/[1+(R/R_0)^6]$ where R_0 is the Förster radius at which half of the excitation energy of donor is transferred to the acceptor. FRET is a very efficient tool for studying protein–protein or protein–DNA interactions, or changes in the conformation of proteins.

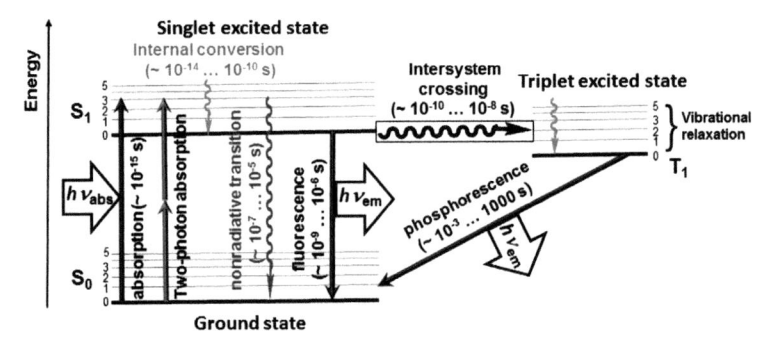

Figure 4.1 Jablonski-type diagram displaying one- and two-photon absorption (TPA), and the origin of the emission by fluorescence or phosphorescence.

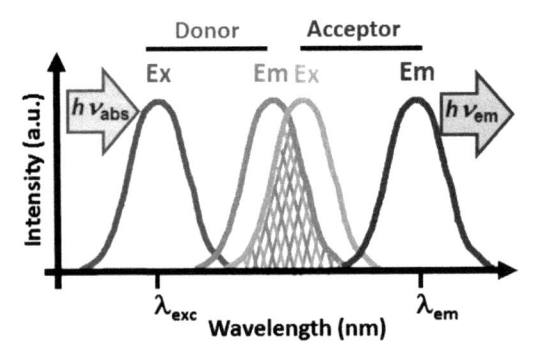

Figure 4.2 Schematic representation of FRET experiment. The hachured part corresponds to the emission of the donor and the excitation of the acceptor.

Several hundreds of publications have reported the synthesis, photo-physical properties, and several uses of fluorescent dendrimers bearing at least one luminescent group in their structure, and several reviews have gathered many of these papers [2–6]. The position of the chromophore(s) is generally dictated by the desired aim. In fact, a large variety of types and locations of fluorescent groups exists and both parameters have a tremendous influence on the luminescence properties. Fluorescence is a very powerful technique for many purposes, in particular for biological imaging. This chapter will give selected examples of fluorescent phosphorus dendrimers, organized depending on the location of the fluorophore (surface, core, or internal structure). It will end with an emerging topic concerning fluorescence induced by two-photon absorption. In both cases, the use of these dendrimers for biological experiments will be highlighted.

4.2 Dendrimers with Fluorophores as Terminal Groups

The easiest way to introduce fluorescent entities consists in grafting them to the terminal functions of dendrimers. However, in this case, non-negligible electronic interaction between adjacent chromophoric units may happen, both in the ground state and in the excited state. Another problem that is frequently encountered is an important decrease in the solubility, particularly in water, which precludes in many cases their use in the field of biology. This problem is often overcome by grafting a reduced number of fluorophores as terminal groups, particularly in a stochastic way.

4.2.1 Full Substitution on the Surface of Dendrimers by Fluorescent Groups

The poly(phosphorhydrazone) (PPH) dendrimers have as terminal functions either aldehydes or $P(S)Cl_2$ groups. For grafting fluorophores to these terminal groups, the fluorophores have to be modified with a suitable function for the grafting. In general, primary amines or hydrazines are used for the condensation with terminal aldehydes, whereas phenols are used for the substitution on terminal $P(S)Cl_2$ groups. Figure 4.3 displays three examples of amino derivatives of pyrene [7, 8] or anthracene [7] to be reacted with aldehydes (case A), and four examples of phenol derivatives of naphthalene [7], rhodamine B [9], maleimide [10], or dansyl [11,12], to be reacted with P(S)Cl$_2$ terminal functions (case B). An example of a fluorescent dendrimer (generation 4) obtained by condensation with 1-pyrenemethylamine is also shown (case C), as well as an example of a fluorescent Janus dendrimer with dansyl derivatives on one side (Fig. 4.3, case D).

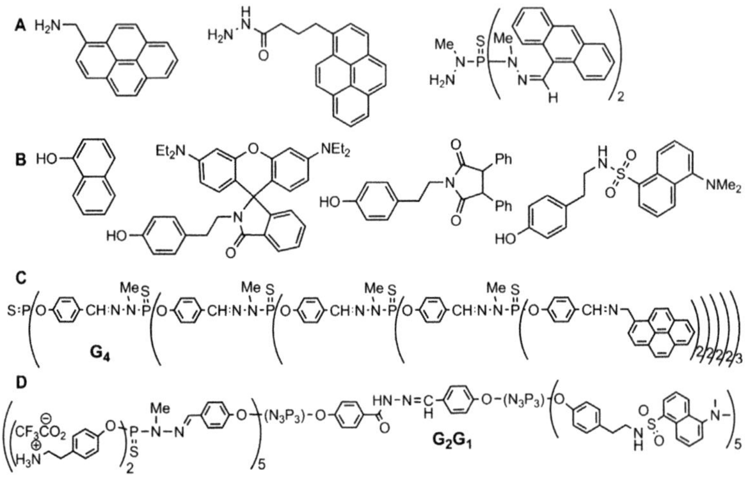

Figure 4.3 Types of fluorophores linked to the surface of poly(phosphorhydrazone) dendrimers. **A**: for reaction with aldehyde terminal groups; **B**: for reaction with P(S)Cl$_2$ terminal functions; **C**: example of a fluorescent generation 4 PPH dendrimer with pyrene as terminal groups; **D**: example of a Janus dendrimer with Dansyl fluorescent terminal groups on one side, and ammonium terminal groups on the other side.

Most of these fluorescent entities were grafted to the surface of PPH dendrimers for specific purposes. The hydrazinopyrene was grafted to PPH dendrons (dendritic wedges), which were then incorporated inside silica, but the fluorescence was not measured [8]. The fluorescence of Rhodamine B derivatives depends on the opening or not of the spirolactam ring: the open form is fluorescent, while the ring-closed form (shown in Fig. 4.2) is not. The functionalization of Rhodamine B by tyramine (the phenol) induced a ring closure. The spirolactam (closed) form is kept when grafted to the first-generation PPH dendrimers. Addition of HCl to try to open the spirolactam ring in fact induced the protonation of the NEt$_2$ groups but did not induce the ring opening; thus, the dendrimer was not fluorescent [9].

The 1-pyrenemethylamine, anthracene, and naphthalene were used as terminal groups of PPH dendrimers in view of elaborating organic light-emitting diodes (OLEDs) [7], but several difficulties were encountered. The second-generation PPH dendrimer covered by naphthalene derivatives was not fluorescent, as well as when covered by anthracene, presumably due to a non-radiative decay induced by the close proximity of heteroatoms. In the case of the 1-pyrenemethylamine, the CH_2 linker may preclude this decay, and the generations 2, 3, and 4 of PPH dendrimers (case C in Fig. 4.3) are indeed fluorescent. These compounds are even electroluminescent as expected, but the threshold voltage inducing the emission of light is too high (18–20 V) to use them for OLEDs [7]. The maleimide derivative was grafted as terminal groups of PPH dendrimers from generations 0 to 3. All compounds are fluorescent in solution in THF or dichloromethane, but the fluorescence quantum yield decreased when the generation of the dendrimer increased [10].

4.2.2 Fluorescent Groups Linked to Part of the Surface of Dendrimers

In view of the difficulties encountered to obtain brightly fluorescent fully substituted PPH dendrimers, it was tempting to decrease the number of fluorophores. In the first attempt, Janus dendrimers, *i.e.,* dendrimers constituted of two different dendritic wedges associated through their core, were synthesized [13]. A small dendron bearing dansyl derivatives was synthesized and its fluorescence properties were assayed. The fluorescence quantum yield (Φ) of this dendron was 0.51 in dioxane, but only 0.17 in water [12]. This dendron was linked to other dendrons bearing either Boc-protected amines or protonated primary amines as terminal groups. The fluorescence quantum yields of the corresponding Janus dendrimers measured in dioxane depended on the type of terminal functions: between 0.42 and 0.56 with the Boc-protected amines, and between 0.30 and 0.46 with the protonated primary amines (case D in Fig. 4.3). This decrease might be related to a partial protonation of the dansyl groups [11].

Another way to decrease the number of fluorophores on the surface of dendrimers consists in their stochastic functionalization. Such work has been generally carried out for biological purposes, to track the behavior of water-soluble and biologically active dendrimers in biological media. The first example for PPH dendrimers concerned a first generation having azabisphosphonic acid salts as terminal functions, and approximately one fluoresceine isothiocyanate (FITC) per dendrimer (G1 in Fig. 4.4). This compound was used for confocal video microscopy, which showed that this fluorescent dendrimer binds to human monocytes (immune white blood cells) and gets internalized in a few seconds [14]. This fluorescent dendrimer pertains to a family of dendrimers having as terminal functions azabisphosphonic acid salts, which have a lot of biological properties, toward the human immune system, and against inflammatory diseases [15–17]. These properties are emphasized in Chapter 12.

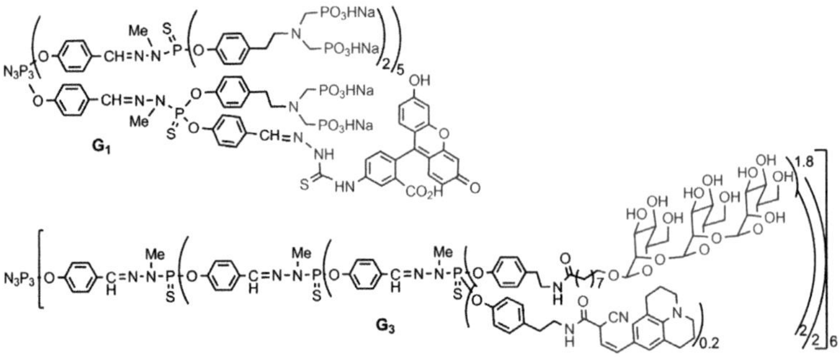

Figure 4.4 Two examples of fluorescent dendrimers stochastically functionalized by a few fluorophores and having biological properties.

The second example of stochastic functionalization concerns a G3 PPH dendrimer having as terminal functions three mannose entities on each terminal group, and ca. 10% of a julolidine derivative (G3 in Fig. 4.4). This fluorescent dendrimer pertains to a family of dendrimers having as terminal functions one, two, or three mannose entities in series, which are able to prevent *in vivo* acute lung inflammation [18]. The fluorescent derivatives were used to demonstrate the direct interaction of this dendrimer with human DC-SIGN receptors and mannose receptor. The properties of this family of dendrimers are emphasized in Chapter 10.

The stochastic functionalization is interesting for research purposes, but it is not fully satisfactory, since it might induce batch-to-batch inconsistencies, and thus irreproducible biological results, as shown for another type of dendrimers (PAMAM) [19]. To avoid these problems, while having a reduced number of fluorophores, the fluorophores can be introduced at different levels in the internal structure of dendrimers, as will be shown in the following section.

4.3 Dendrimers with Fluorophores inside the Structure

Different locations have been used to include fluorophores inside the structure of poly(phosphorhydrazone) PPH dendrimers: linked to the branching points, being the core, or linked to the core. This latter location is also called "off-center."

4.3.1 Fluorescent Groups Linked to the Internal Branching Units

Two ways have been used for the grafting of fluorophores to the branching units, inside the structure of PPH dendrimers. The first example is based on the selectivity of the functionalization of each Cl independently on P(X)Cl$_2$ functions (X = S or O) [20]. A first-generation dendrimer with 3 P(O)Cl$_2$ terminal functions was first functionalized with amino or hydrazido pyrene using a single Cl of each end group. Then, the growing of the dendrimer was carried out by reaction of hydroxybenzaldehyde on the remaining Cl, followed by the condensation with H$_2$NNMeP(S)Cl$_2$ (see Chapter 1) to afford the dendrimers shown in Fig. 4.5 (case A) [21].

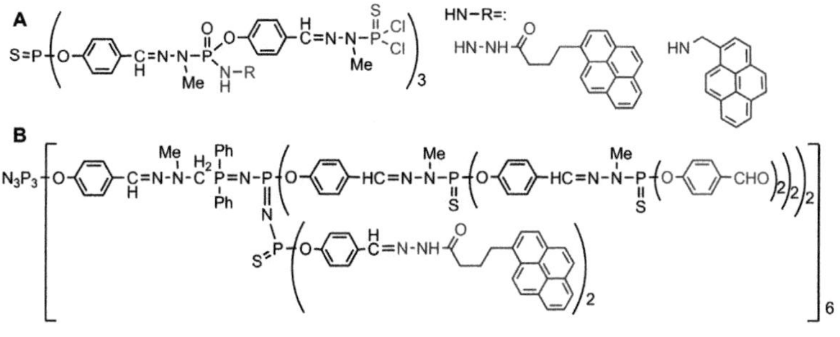

Figure 4.5 Fluorophore inside the structure of PPH dendrimers. **A**: grafting of fluorophores during the synthesis of the dendrimer. **B**: grafting of the fluorophores after the synthesis of the dendrimer (post-functionalization).

The second example is based on the possibility to create P=N–P=S linkages at selected levels inside the structure, during the synthesis of the dendrimers (see Chapter 1) [22–24]. These linkages are stable but can be activated using strong electrophiles such as alkyl triflates [25, 26]. Indeed, alkylation occurs exclusively on the sulfur atoms included in these linkages and not on the other P=S groups inside the structure. This alkylation induces a weakening of the P=S bond, which is easily cleaved using a nucleophilic phosphine such as $P(NMe_2)_3$, generating phosphines (PIII) inside the structure [27]. These phosphines can be used for Staudinger reactions with azides, in particular with phosphorus azides, to create P=N–P=N–P=S linkages. If the phosphorus azide bears, for instance, two aldehydes, they are suitable to introduce new functions inside the dendrimers [28]. These functions can be hydrazidopyrene, as shown in Fig. 4.5 (case B). Steady-state fluorescence spectra and decays of excitation of this dendrimer dissolved in various solvents (acetonitrile, diglyme, dioxane, triethyleneglycol, and cyclohexanol) revealed that the movements of the internal pyrenes were not reduced by interactions with the structure of the dendrimer. Indeed, the ratio of emission intensities of pyrene–pyrene excimer and of pyrene monomer was very close for the dendrimer and for a small model, and depended only on the viscosity of the solvents [29].

4.3.2 Fluorescent Phthalocyanine as Core of Dendrimers

In the case of poly(phosphorhydrazone) dendrimers, only an octa-substituted phthalocyanine was used as fluorescent core. The synthesis was carried out up to generation 5, functionalized with ammonium terminal groups (Fig. 4.6) [30]. The core was used first as a sensor for analyzing the properties of the internal structure. It was shown that the dendritic shell mimics a highly polar solvent, that the core is more isolated when the generation of the dendrimer increases, and consequently, the fluorescence quantum yield increased also. Furthermore, the phthalocyanine core of higher generations of dendrimers (from G3) is a highly sensitive optical sensor for H_3O^+ and OH^- [31]. These experiments were carried out with a free phthalocyanine, as no fluorescence was observed with the corresponding cobalt complexes, presumably due to the coupling of the unfilled d-orbitals of cobalt with the π-orbital system of the phthalocyanine, which provided very efficient channels for π^* deactivation [32].

The fifth generation of the phthalocyanine-cored PPH dendrimers ended by ammonium groups is water soluble. It was used for some preliminary biological studies. This dendrimer showed a rather moderate cytotoxicity toward HeLa (human epitheloid cervical carcinoma cell line), HEK 293 (human embryonic kidney cells), and HUVEC cells (human umbilical vein endothelial cell) in serum-containing medium. The cytotoxicity was generally lower than that of lipofectin. This dendrimer efficiently delivered in HeLa cells a fluorescein-labelled oligodeoxyribonucleotide and a DNA plasmid containing the functional gene of enhanced green fluorescent protein (EGFP) [33].

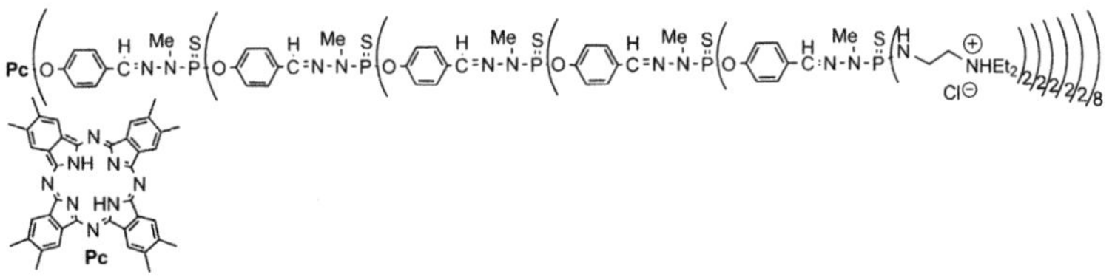

Figure 4.6 Structure of a generation 5 PPH dendrimer built from an octafunctional and fluorescent phthalocyanine core and used for transfection experiments.

4.3.3 Fluorescent Groups Linked to the Core (Off-Center)

Hexachlorocyclotriphosphazene is a versatile tool to synthesize specially engineered dendrimers, as it is possible to specifically react one Cl among six [34, 35]. It has been used, in particular, to obtain off-center dendrimers, *i.e.*, dendrimers in which one function emanating from the core is different from all the other functions. Such property has been in particular exploited for grafting one fluorophore to the core of PPH dendrimers with various terminal functions, as shown in Fig. 4.7.

A pyrene derivative was grafted off-center to the core of a small PPH dendrimer having phosphine terminal groups (case A in Fig. 4.7). The fluorescence of this compound was not measured, as the pyrene was used for the deposit of this dendrimer by π-stacking onto cobalt nanoparticles covered by graphene layers. This assembly was used for catalytic experiments after complexation of the phosphines with palladium. Thanks to the interaction of the pyrene with the magnetic cobalt nanoparticles, this dendritic catalyst could be recovered and reused at least 12 times, with no decrease in catalytic efficiency [36].

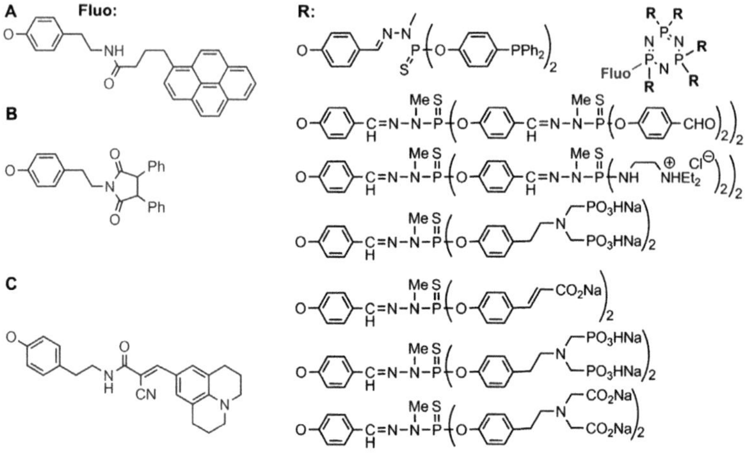

Figure 4.7 Three types of fluorophores linked off-center to the cyclotriphosphazene core of PPH dendrimers having different types of terminal functions. **A**: pyrene; **B**: maleimide; **C**: julolidine.

The maleimide derivative that was grafted to the surface of dendrimers was also used as fluorescent off-center entity. The synthesis was carried out up to the second generation of PPH dendrimers, with aldehyde terminal functions (Fig. 4.7, case B). The quantum yield of generation zero (one maleimide, five aldehydes) is high (0.77) in organic solvents (dichloromethane or THF), but a dramatic drop is observed for generations 1 and 2 (0.22 and 0.20, respectively), presumably due to interactions with the branches of the dendrimer [10].

Grafting *N,N*-diethylethylenediamine in the last step of the synthesis, instead of hydroxybenzaldehyde afforded a dendrimer with ammonium terminal functions. This dendrimer was brightly fluorescent in dichloromethane, but poorly fluorescent in water. However, a few biological experiments could be carried out with it. The cytotoxicity was measured toward HeLa cells and A549 cells (human lung cancer); it was found relatively low, and surprisingly less toxic after 48 h than after 24 h. The interaction of this dendrimer with plasmid DNA (BACE-GFP) was analyzed by circular dichroism (CD), which indicated a possible disturbing of the helical B-type structure of DNA [37].

Another type of fluorescent off-center dendrimer was also synthesized by grafting five maleimide derivatives to the hexa-chloro cyclotriphosphazene core, whereas the single remaining Cl was used for the growing of a small dendrimer, ended by two hy-droxyphosphonate terminal functions. This compound was grafted to a nanocrystalline mesoporous titania thin film through the phos-phonates, affording a brilliantly fluorescent film. This film was used as a sensitive sensor for the detection of phenolic compounds, which quenched the fluorescence. The quenching was by far more efficient for the dendrimer linked to the film than for the dendrimer in solu-tion, especially for the detection of resorcinol and 2-nitroresorcinol (see Chapter 5) [38].

The julolidine derivative (Fig. 4.7, case C) was linked off-center to afford a first-generation dendrimer having azabisphosphonic acid salts as terminal groups [14, 39]. As indicated previously for the stochastic functionalization of the surface with FITC (see Section 4.2.2), this family of dendrimers has a lot of biological properties toward the human immune system [15–17] (see Chapter 12). This compound has been used, in particular, to study the activation of hu-man monocytes [14, 39], and also for FRET experiments (see Fig. 4.2), with phycoerythrin-coupled antibodies against various typi-cal monocytes receptors. Fluorescence emission of phycoerythrin induced by FRET was observed only for the antibody against the innate receptor TLR2, indicating a close proximity of the julolidine-dendrimer to this receptor [14]. This dendrimer was used also to study the inhibition of the proliferation of CD4$^+$ T lymphocytes [40]. The analogous compound bearing azabiscarboxylic acid salts in-stead of the azabisphosphonic acid salts as terminal functions was also synthesized [41], as well as a dendrimer having a single carbox-ylic acid salt for each terminal function instead of two [42]. Study of the biological properties demonstrated that both compounds bear-ing carboxylic acid salts have no influence on human monocytes, contrarily to the azabisphosphonate salt analog.

4.4 Two-Photon Absorption Properties of Fluorophores Linked to Dendrimers

All the previous examples concerned classical fluorophores excited with one-photon. An emerging topic concerns multiphoton absorption, most generally two-photon absorption [1]. The simultaneous absorption of two photons (TPA) (see Fig. 4.1) is a third-order non-linear process to excite a molecule. TPA is generally used for two-photon-excited fluorescence, with a laser as source of excitation. The excitation of a dye having good TPA properties occurs approximately at two times the wavelength at which one-photon excitation occurs, for instance in the near-infrared instead of the ultraviolet region. This property is particularly appealing for biological studies, as it induces a better preservation of cells and of living tissues. Two reviews have gathered examples of dendrimers having TPA properties [43, 44]. This section will be organized in three parts, depending on the location of the TPA fluorophores: as terminal groups, at the core, or as branches of poly(phosphorhydrazone) dendrimers.

4.4.1 TPA Fluorescent Groups Linked to the Surface of Dendrimers

As for classical fluorophores, the easiest way to obtain dendrimers bearing TPA fluorophores is their grafting as terminal functions. The first example of PPH dendrimers with TPA properties was obtained with specifically engineered fluorene derivatives conjugated with two triple bonds (Fig. 4.8). Generations 1 to 4 of PPH dendrimers were synthesized (12 to 96 TPA blue emitting fluorophores, respectively). The TPA cross section σ^2 of the fourth generation is 55,900 GM (Goeppert-Mayer: 10^{-50} cm^4 s photon^{-1}) at 705 nm. This value for this "organic nanodot" is comparable to that of inorganic quantum dots, without any problem of blinking [45]. Another example of TPA dendrimer was also elaborated from fluorene, but conjugated with two double bonds, affording a second-generation green emitting dendrimer (Fig. 4.8). The TPA cross section of this dendrimer was 35,000 GM at 740 nm [46].

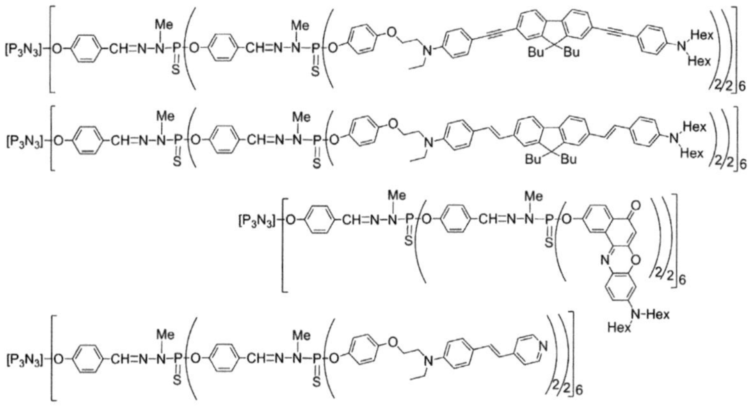

Figure 4.8 Examples of poly(phosphorhydrazone) dendrimers bearing TPA fluorophores as terminal functions.

Another family of PPH dendrimers was functionalized by derivatives of Nile Red (generations 1 and 2, with 12 and 24 red emitting fluorophores, respectively), but the fluorescence quantum yield (Φ) for this family was too low for practical purposes (Fig. 4.8) [47].

The pyridinyl ethenyl phenylamino derivative shown in the lower part of Fig. 4.8 was grafted to generations 1 and 2 of PPH dendrimers, but also to other organic derivatives. Comparison of the TPA cross section values of all these compounds demonstrated a TPA cooperative enhancement, as a consequence of purely electrostatic through-space interchromophoric interactions. The TPA enhancement depended on the number and distribution of chromophores and increased when the chromophores were in closest proximity [48].

4.4.2 TPA Fluorescent Groups at the Core of Dendrimers

The previous examples have afforded important fundamental results, but none of these dendrimers are soluble in water; thus, none of them could be used for bioimaging. For such purpose, a TPA fluorophore was placed at the core of dendrimers, linked to two cyclotriphosphazene units, and functionalized with water solubilizing terminal functions (Fig. 4.9, case A). The dendritic branches efficiently prevented the deleterious influence of water on the fluorescence of the fluorene derivative conjugated with two double bonds, as shown by the quantum yield in water (Φ = 0.22 for the monomeric fluorophore, 0.71 for the second-generation dendrimer).

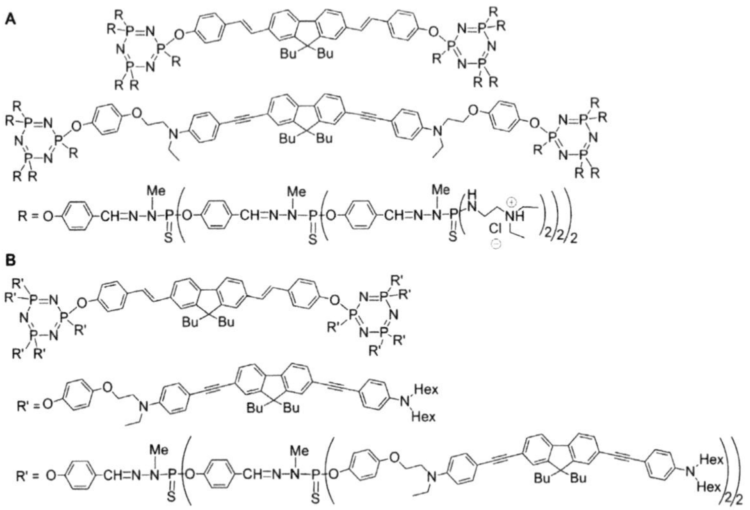

Figure 4.9   A: TPA fluorophores used as core of water-soluble dendrimers. **B**: TPA fluorophores used both as core and as terminal functions of dendrimers (dumbbell-like dendrimers).

The second generation has been used for *in vivo* imaging. This dendrimer in solution in water was injected intravenously to a rat. Two-photon imaging of the rat olfactory bulb was obtained, with no obvious toxic effect observed during the experiment [49]. The same compound was used as contrast agent for *in vivo* three-dimensional two-photon excited fluorescence of blood vessels of living Xenopus tadpole, after intracardiac injection [50].

In the case of the fluorene derivative conjugated with two triple bonds, the distance between the two cyclotriphosphazenes is longer (Fig. 4.9, case A), and the branches of the dendrimer are not large enough to prevent the quenching of fluorescence by water. Indeed, the fluorescence quantum yield of the second generation having the expanded chromophoric linker at the core is 0.42 in DMSO, but only 0.075 in water [51].

The core functionalized by the fluorene derivative conjugated with two double bonds was also used to have two layers of fluorophores (generations 0 to 2). These compounds were synthesized to study possible interactions between chromophores, depending on their relative location. The photo-physical properties of these "dumbbell-like" dendrimers (Fig. 4.9, case B) were compared to that of the "spherical" dendrimers (Fig. 4.8) bearing the same terminal functions. It was shown that the global TPA efficiency is different for the two series. The photo-luminescence efficiency of the "dumbbell-like" dendrimers is much poorer than that of the "spherical" dendrimers, presumably due to direct interaction of the core with the proximal fluorophores [52].

4.4.3 TPA Fluorescent Groups as Branches of Dendrimers

Having TPA fluorophores as terminal groups necessitates one function suitable for the grafting; having a TPA fluorophore at the core necessitates two identical functions for growing the branches of the dendrimers. Having TPA fluorophores in the branches of dendrimers necessitates two different functions, one for the grafting to the dendrimer, and another one for continuing the growing of the dendrimer. Furthermore, these non-symmetrical fluorophores should have ideally as functions one phenol and one aldehyde, to be used as substitutes of hydroxybenzaldehyde, classically used for the synthesis of PPH dendrimers [53]. This goal has been achieved in the case of the TPA fluorophore based on the fluorene derivative conjugated with two triple bonds. This fluorophore was integrated at the level of the first generation of PPH dendrimers, bearing water solubilizing terminal functions such as cationic groups (ammoniums) or neutral poly(ethylene glycol) (PEG) (Fig. 4.10, case A). The PEGylated dendrimer displayed both a higher quantum yield (0.39 *versus* 0.24) and a higher TPA cross section (13,600 *versus* 8,400 GM) than the corresponding cationic derivative, in water [46].

The same fluorophore was also used for obtaining a dendrimer composed of two consecutive layers of fluorophores (Fig. 4.10, case B). An additive behavior was expected but was not observed. Indeed, a decrease in both the quantum yield (0.43 *versus* 0.75) and the TPA cross section per chromophore (472 *versus* 733 GM) was observed by comparison with the dendrimer having a single layer of chromophores (only the terminal chromophores) [50].

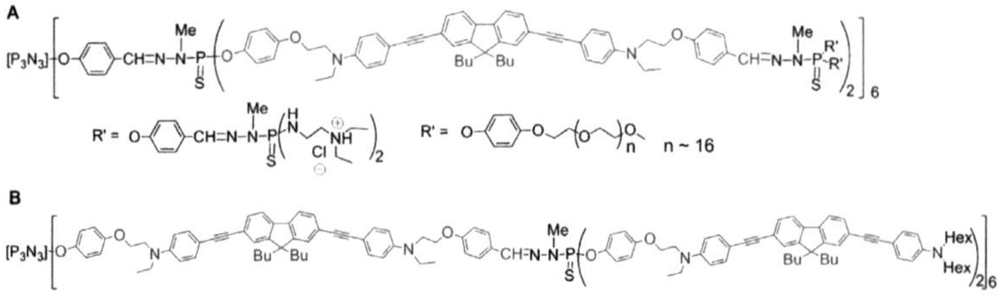

Figure 4.10 A: Water-soluble PPH dendrimers having one layer of TPA fluorophores used as branches at the level of the first generation. **B**: Example of PPH dendrimer having two layers of TPA fluorophores.

4.5 Conclusion

The versatility of the synthesis of poly(phosphorhydrazone) dendrimers has already permitted the synthesis of a large variety of fluorescent dendrimers, as symbolized in Fig. 4.11 (the circles correspond to classical fluorophores, the ovals to fluorophores having two-photon absorption properties). The diversity of these dendritic structures is correlated to the diversity of the fluorescent entities. Indeed, the location of fluorophores depends on the number and type of anchoring point they possess. With a single anchoring point, the fluorophore can be placed on the surface (in full, in part, or stochastically) of the dendrimer, or off-center to the core. With two (or more) identical anchoring points, the fluorophore can be used as core of dendrimers. With two different anchoring points, the fluorophore can be used as branches of dendrimers. Playing with these fluorescent entities, highly sophisticated structures, such as two layers of fluorophores could be obtained.

At the beginning, most of these compounds were synthesized for photo-physical studies, for determining the influence of the dendritic structure upon the fluorescence, or the influence of the close proximity of several fluorophores. Later on, several of these compounds were synthesized with the aim of using them as nanotools for biology. Among the properties that have been already demonstrated with fluorescent phosphorus dendrimers, one can cite the partial elucidation of the mechanism of interaction of polyanionic dendrimers with human immune cells, and of polycationic dendrimers for transfection experiments. Of interest also is the imaging of the blood vessels in the olfactory bulb of a living rat and of the blood vessels of a tadpole, in two- and three-dimensional, with dendrimers having TPA properties. In view of these results, the use of fluorescent dendrimers for biology holds great promises for the future.

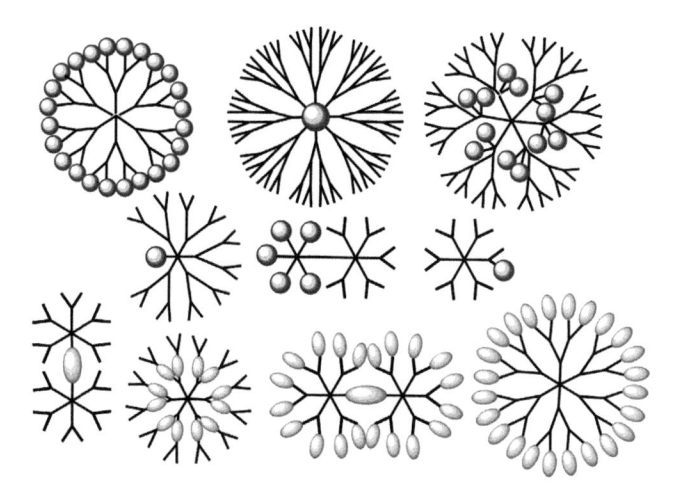

Figure 4.11 Types of fluorescent phosphorus dendrimers already synthesized. Circles: classical fluorophores; ovals: TPA fluorophores.

References

1. Terenziani, F., Katan, C., Badaeva, E., Tretiak, S., and Blanchard-Desce, M. (2008). Enhanced two-photon absorption of organic chromophores: Theoretical and experimental assessments, *Adv. Mater.*, **20**, pp. 4641–4678.

2. Balzani, V., Ceroni, P., Maestri, M., and Vicinelli, V. (2003). Light-harvesting dendrimers, *Curr. Opin. Chem. Biol.*, **7**, pp. 657–665.

3. De Schryver, F. C., Vosch, T., Cotlet, M., Van der Auweraer, M., Mullen, K., and Hofkens, J. (2005). Energy dissipation in multichromophoric single dendrimers, *Acc. Chem. Res.*, **38**, pp. 514–522.

4. Lo, S. C. and Burn, P. L. (2007). Development of dendrimers: Macromolecules for use in organic light-emitting diodes and solar cells, *Chem. Rev.*, **107**, pp. 1097–1116.

5. Hwang, S. H., Moorefield, C. N., and Newkome, G. R. (2008). Dendritic macromolecules for organic light-emitting diodes, *Chem. Soc. Rev.*, **37**, pp. 2543–2557.

6. Caminade, A. M., Hameau, A., and Majoral, J. P. (2009). Multicharged and/or water-soluble fluorescent dendrimers: Properties and uses, *Chem. Eur. J.*, **15**, pp. 9270–9285.

7. Brauge, L., Veriot, G., Franc, G., Deloncle, R., Caminade, A. M., and Majoral, J. P. (2006). Synthesis of phosphorus dendrimers bearing chromophoric end groups: Toward organic blue light-emitting diodes, *Tetrahedron*, **62**, pp. 11891–11899.

8. Turrin, C. O., Maraval, V., Caminade, A. M., Majoral, J. P., Mehdi, A., and Reye, C. (2000). Organic–inorganic hybrid materials incorporating phosphorus-containing dendrimers, *Chem. Mater.*, **12**, pp. 3848–3856.

9. Wei, Y.Q., Laurent, R., Majoral, J. P., and Caminade, A. M. (2010). Synthesis and characterization of phosphorus-containing dendrimers bearing rhodamine derivatives as terminal groups, *ARKIVOC: Online J. Organic Chem.*, pp. 318–327.

10. Franc, G., Mazeres, S., Turrin, C. O., Vendier, L., Duhayon, C., Caminade, A. M., and Majoral, J. P. (2007). Synthesis and properties of dendrimers possessing the same fluorophore(s) located either peripherally or off-center, *J. Org. Chem.*, **72**, pp. 8707–8715.

11. Fuchs, S., Pla-Quintana, A., Mazeres, S., Caminade, A. M., and Majoral, J. P. (2008). Cationic and fluorescent "Janus" dendrimers, *Org. Lett.*, **10**, pp. 4751–4754.

12. Hameau, A., Fuchs, S., Laurent, R., Majoral, J. P., and Caminade, A. M. (2011). Synthesis of dye/fluorescent functionalized dendrons based on cyclotriphosphazene, *Beilstein J. Org. Chem.*, **7**, pp. 1577–1583.

13. Caminade, A. M., Laurent, R., Delavaux-Nicot, B., and Majoral, J. P. (2012). "Janus" dendrimers: Syntheses and properties, *New J. Chem.*, **36**, pp. 217–226.

14. Poupot, M., Griffe, L., Marchand, P., Maraval, A., Rolland, O., Martinet, L., L'Faqihi-Olive, F. E., Turrin, C. O., Caminade, A. M., Fournie, J. J., Majoral, J. P., and Poupot, R. (2006). Design of phosphorylated dendritic architectures to promote human monocyte activation, *FASEB J.*, **20**, pp. 2339–2351.

15. Griffe, L., Poupot, M., Marchand, P., Maraval, A., Turrin, C. O., Rolland, O., Metivier, P., Bacquet, G., Fournie, J. J., Caminade, A. M., Poupot, R., and Majoral, J. P. (2007). Multiplication of human natural killer cells by nanosized phosphonate-capped dendrimers, *Angew. Chem. Int. Ed.*, **46**, pp. 2523–2526.

16. Hayder, M., Poupot, M., Baron, M., Nigon, D., Turrin, C. O., Caminade, A. M., Majoral, J. P., Eisenberg, R. A., Fournie, J. J., Cantagrel, A., Poupot, R., and Davignon, J. L. (2011). A phosphorus-based dendrimer targets inflammation and osteoclastogenesis in experimental arthritis, *Science Transl. Med.*, **3**, 11.

17. Caminade, A. M., Fruchon, S., Turrin, C. O., Poupot, M., Ouali, A., Maraval, A., Garzoni, M., Maly, M., Furer, V., Kovalenko, V., Majoral, J. P., Pavan, G. M., and Poupot, R. (2015). The key role of the scaffold on the efficiency of dendrimer nanodrugs, *Nature Comm.*, **6**, 7722.

18. Blattes, E., Vercellone, A., Eutamene, H., Turrin, C. O., Theodorou, V., Majoral, J. P., Caminade, A. M., Prandi, J., Nigou, J., and Puzo, G. (2013). Mannodendrimers prevent acute lung inflammation by inhibiting neutrophil recruitment, *Proc. Natl. Acad. Sci. USA*, **110**, pp. 8795–8800.

19. Mullen, D. G., Fang, M., Desai, A., Baker, J. R., Orr, B. G., and Holl, M. M. B. (2010). A quantitative assessment of nanoparticle-ligand distributions: Implications for targeted drug and imaging delivery in dendrimer conjugates, *ACS Nano*, **4**, pp. 657–670.

20. Lartigue, M. L., Slany, M., Caminade, A. M., and Majoral, J. P. (1996). Phosphorus-containing dendrimers: Synthesis of macromolecules with multiple tri- and tetrafunctionalization, *Chem. Eur. J.*, **2**, pp. 1417–1426.

21. Severac, M., Leclaire, J., Sutra, P., Caminade, A. M., and Majoral, J. P. (2004). A new way for the internal functionalization of dendrimers, *Tetrahedron Lett.*, **45**, pp. 3019–3022.

22. Galliot, C., Prevote, D., Caminade, A. M., and Majoral, J. P. (1995). Polyaminophosphines containing dendrimers: Syntheses and characterizations, *J. Am. Chem. Soc.*, **117**, pp. 5470–5476.

23. Brauge, L., Magro, G., Caminade, A. M., and Majoral, J. P. (2001). First divergent strategy using two AB2 unprotected monomers for the rapid synthesis of dendrimers, *J. Am. Chem. Soc.*, **123**, pp. 6698–6699.

24. Maraval, V., Caminade, A. M., Majoral, J. P., and Blais, J. C. (2003). Dendrimer design: How to circumvent the dilemma of a reduction of steps or an increase of function multiplicity? *Angew. Chem. Int. Ed.*, **42**, pp. 1822–1826.

25. Larre, C., Caminade, A. M., and Majoral, J. P. (1997). Chemoselective polyalkylations of phosphorus-containing dendrimers, *Angew. Chem. Int. Ed. Engl.*, **36**, pp. 596–599.

26. Larre, C., Donnadieu, B., Caminade, A. M., and Majoral, J. P. (1998). Phosphorus-containing dendrimers: Chemoselective functionalization of internal layers, *J. Am. Chem. Soc.*, **120**, pp. 4029–4030.

27. Larre, C., Bressolles, D., Turrin, C., Donnadieu, B., Caminade, A. M., and Majoral, J. P. (1998). Chemistry within megamolecules: Regiospecific functionalization after construction of phosphorus dendrimers, *J. Am. Chem. Soc.*, **120**, pp. 13070–13082.

28. Galliot, C., Larre, C., Caminade, A. M., and Majoral, J. P. (1997). Regioselective stepwise growth of dendrimer units in the internal voids of a main dendrimer, *Science*, **277**, pp. 1981–1984.

29. Brauge, L., Caminade, A. M., Majoral, J. P., Slomkowski, S., and Wolszczak, M. (2001). Segmental mobility in phosphorus-containing dendrimers. Studies by fluorescent spectroscopy, *Macromolecules*, **34**, pp. 5599–5606.

30. Leclaire, J., Coppel, Y., Caminade, A. M., and Majoral, J. P. (2004). Nanometric sponges made of water-soluble hydrophobic dendrimers, *J. Am. Chem. Soc.*, **126**, pp. 2304–2305.

31. Leclaire, J., Dagiral, R., Fery-Forgues, S., Coppel, Y., Donnadieu, B., Caminade, A. M., and Majoral, J. P. (2005). Octasubstituted metal-free phthalocyanine as core of phosphorus dendrimers: A probe for the properties of the internal structure, *J. Am. Chem. Soc.*, **127**, pp. 15762–15770.

32. Leclaire, J., Dagiral, R., Pla-Quintana, A., Caminade, A. M., and Majoral, J. P. (2007). Metallated phthalocyanines as the core of dendrimers: Synthesis and spectroscopic studies, *Eur. J. Inorg. Chem.*, pp. 2890–2896.

33. Maszewska, M., Leclaire, J., Cieslak, M., Nawrot, B., Okruszek, A., Caminade, A. M., and Majoral, J. P. (2003). Water-soluble polycationic dendrimers with a phosphoramidothioate backbone: Preliminary studies of cytotoxicity and oligonucleotide/plasmid delivery in human cell culture, *Oligonucleotides*, **13**, pp. 193–205.

34. Caminade, A. M., Hameau, A., and Majoral, J. P. (2016). The specific functionalization of cyclotriphosphazene for the synthesis of smart dendrimers, *Dalton Trans.*, **45**, pp. 1810–1822.

35. Caminade, A. M., Ouali, A., Hameau, A., Laurent, R., Rebout, C., Delavaux-Nicot, B., Turrin, C. O., Moineau Chane-Ching, K., and Majoral, J. P. (2016). Cyclotriphosphazene, an old compound applied to the synthesis of smart dendrimers with tailored properties, *Pure Appl. Chem.*, **88**, pp. 919–929.

36. Keller, M., Colliere, V., Reiser, O., Caminade, A. M., Majoral, J. P., and Ouali, A. (2013). Pyrene-tagged dendritic catalysts noncovalently grafted onto magnetic Co/C nanoparticles: An efficient and recyclable system for drug synthesis, *Angew. Chem. Int. Ed.*, **52**, pp. 3626–3629.

37. Kazmierczak-Baranska, J., Pietkiewicz, A., Janicka, M., Wei, Y. Q., Turrin, C. O., Majoral, J. P., Nawrot, B., and Caminade, A. M. (2010). Synthesis of a fluorescent cationic phosphorus dendrimer and preliminary biological studies of its interaction with DNA, *Nucleosides Nucleotides Nucleic Acids*, **29**, pp. 155–167.

38. Martinez-Ferrero, E., Franc, G., Mazeres, S., Turrin, C. O., Boissiere, U., Caminade, A. M., Majoral, J. P., and Sanchez, C. (2008). Optical properties of hybrid dendritic-mesoporous titania nanocomposite films, *Chem. Eur. J.*, **14**, pp. 7658–7669.

39. Rolland, O., Griffe, L., Poupot, M., Maraval, A., Ouali, A., Coppel, Y., Fournie, J. J., Bacquet, G., Turrin, C. O., Caminade, A. M., Majoral, J. P., and Poupot, R. (2008). Tailored control and optimisation of the number of phosphonic acid termini on phosphorus-containing dendrimers for the ex-vivo activation of human monocytes, *Chem. Eur. J.*, **14**, pp. 4836–4850.

40. Portevin, D., Poupot, M., Rolland, O., Turrin, C. O., Fournie, J. J., Majoral, J. P., Caminade, A. M., and Poupot, R. (2009). Regulatory activity of azabisphosphonate-capped dendrimers on human CD4(+) T cell proliferation enhances ex-vivo expansion of NK cells from PBMCs for immunotherapy, *J. Transl. Med.*, **7**, 13.

41. Ledall, J., Fruchon, S., Garzoni, M., Pavan, G. M., Caminade, A. M., Turrin, C. O., Blanzat, M., and Poupot, R. (2015). Interaction studies reveal specific recognition of an anti-inflammatory polyphosphorhydrazone dendrimer by human monocytes, *Nanoscale*, **7**, pp. 17672–17684.

42. Ielasi, F., Ledall, J., Anes, A. P., Fruchon, S., Caminade, A. M., Poupot, R., Turrin, C. O., and Blanzat, M. (2016). Influence of PPH dendrimers' surface functions on the activation of human monocytes: A study of their interactions with pure lipid model systems, *Phys. Chem. Chem. Phys.*, **18**, pp. 21871–21880.

43. Ma, H. and Jen, A. K. Y. (2001). Functional dendrimers for nonlinear optics, *Adv. Mater.*, **13**, pp. 1201–1205.

44. Andraud, C., Fortrie, R., Barsu, C., Stephan, O., Chermette, H., and Baldeck, P. L. (2008). Excitonically coupled oligomers and dendrimers for two-photon absorption, photoresponsive polymers II, *Adv. Polym. Sci.*, **214**, pp. 149–203.

45. Mongin, O., Krishna, T. R., Werts, M. H. V., Caminade, A. M., Majoral, J. P., and Blanchard-Desce, M. (2006). A modular approach to two-photon absorbing organic nanodots: Brilliant dendrimers as an alternative to semiconductor quantum dots? *Chem. Commun.*, pp. 915–917.

46. Mongin, O., Rouxel, C., Vabre, J. M., Mir, Y., Pla-Quintana, A., Wei, Y. Q., Caminade, A. M., Majoral, J. P., and Blanchard-Desce, M. (2009). Customized multiphotonics nanotools for bioapplications: Soft organic nanodots as an eco-friendly alternative to quantum dots, in: N. Kobayashi, F. Ouchen, and I. Rau (Eds.), *Nanobiosystems: Processing, Characterization, and Applications II*, SPIE -Int Soc Optical Engineering, Bellingham, WA, USA, 7403.

47. Robin, A. C., Parthasarathy, V., Pla-Quintana, A., Mongin, O., Terenziani, F., Caminade, A. M., Majoral, J. P., and Blanchard-Desce, M. (2010). Cooperative TPA enhancement via through-space interactions in organic nanodots built from dipolar chromophores, in: M. Eich, J. M. Nunzi, R. Jakubiak, and T. G. Goodson III (Eds.), *Linear and Nonlinear Optics of Organic Materials X.* SPIE 7774.

48. Terenziani, F., Parthasarathy, V., Pla-Quintana, A., Maishal, T., Caminade, A. M., Majoral, J. P., and Blanchard-Desce, M. (2009). Cooperative two-photon absorption enhancement by through-space interactions in multichromophoric compounds, *Angew. Chem. Int. Ed.*, **48**, pp. 8691–8694.

49. Krishna, T. R., Parent, M., Werts, M. H. V., Moreaux, L., Gmouh, S., Charpak, S., Caminade, A. M., Majoral, J. P., and Blanchard-Desce, M. (2006). Water-soluble dendrimeric two-photon tracers for *in vivo* imaging, *Angew. Chem. Int. Ed.*, **45**, pp. 4645–4648.

50. Mongin, O., Rouxel, C., Robin, A. C., Pla-Quintana, A., Krishna, T. R., Recher, G., Tiaho, F., Caminade, A. M., Majoral, J. P., and Blanchard-Desce, M. (2008). Brilliant organic nanodots: Novel nano-objects for bionanophotonics, in: E. M. Heckman, T. B. Singh, and J. Yoshida (Eds.), *Nanobiosystems: Processing, Characterization, and Applications*, SPIE -Int Soc Optical Engineering, Bellingham, 7040.

51. Rouxel, C., Charlot, M., Mongin, O., Krishna, T. R., Caminade, A. M., Majoral, J. P., and Blanchard-Desce, M. (2012). From graftable biphotonic chromophores to water-soluble organic nanodots for biophotonics: The importance of environmental effects, *Chem. Eur. J.*, **18**, pp. 16450–16462.

52. Mongin, O., Pla-Quintana, A., Terenziani, F., Drouin, D., Le Droumaguet, C., Caminade, A. M., Majoral, J. P., and Blanchard-Desce, M. (2007). Organic nanodots for multiphotonics: Synthesis and photophysical studies, *New J. Chem.*, **31**, pp. 1354–1367.

53. Launay, N., Caminade, A. M., Lahana, R., and Majoral, J. P. (1994). A general synthetic strategy for neutral phosphorus-containing dendrimers, *Angew. Chem. Int. Ed. Engl.*, **33**, pp. 1589–1592.

Chapter 5

Biomaterials Made of Phosphorus Dendrimers: Toward Diagnosis Tools

Anne-Marie Caminade and Béatrice Delavaux-Nicot
Laboratoire de Chimie de Coordination, CNRS, 205 Route de Narbonne, BP 44099, 31077 Toulouse Cedex 4, France
anne-marie.caminade@lcc-toulouse.fr

5.1   Introduction

The functionalization of solid surfaces is a particularly important area of research, not only for materials sciences, but also for many different practical uses such as catalysis, sensors, or optoelectronic devices, to name a few. It is known that the properties of many materials are critically influenced by the nature of their surface constitution [1]. A large variety of chemical entities has already been used for the functionalization of the surface of materials, including polymers [2], through covalent or non-covalent interactions.

Dendrimers pertain to the field of polymers, due to their repetitive structure, made of branched monomers. However, they are never synthesized by polymerization reactions, but step-by-step, to ensure a perfectly controlled structure. The main advantage of using

Phosphorus Dendrimers in Biology and Nanomedicine: Synthesis, Characterization, and Properties
Edited by Anne-Marie Caminade, Cédric-Olivier Turrin, and Jean-Pierre Majoral
Copyright © 2018 Pan Stanford Publishing Pte. Ltd.
ISBN 978-981-4774-33-8 (Hardcover), 978-1-315-11085-1 (eBook)
www.panstanford.com

dendrimers compared to monomers for the functionalization of solid surfaces is the large number of anchoring points, which should enhance the stability. Compared to polymers, dendrimers induce a high reproducibility, due to their precisely controlled structure.

In this chapter, we will display the use of poly(phosphorhydrazone) (PPH) dendrimers for the functionalization of solid surfaces, either by non-covalent or covalent interactions, and the use of some of the obtained devices as nano-tools for biology, particularly as biosensors.

5.2 Non-covalent Functionalization of Solid Surfaces by Phosphorus Dendrimers

5.2.1 Non-covalent Functionalization by Neutral Dendrimers

There are different ways to functionalize surfaces by non-covalent interactions, depending on whether the functional entities are neutral or charged. A generation 4 PPH dendrimer ended by thiols was deposited by spin coating onto a silicon wafer, to form a monolayer. A flattening of the dendrimer was observed, with a loss of height of almost 70%. The modified surface was brought in contact with a solution of gold clusters $Au_{55}(PPh_3)_{12}Cl_6$. Partial removal of the ligands of the clusters during the interaction with the thiols induced the formation of a gold cluster monolayer on thiol-functionalized dendrimers, as expected. However, these hybrid systems were subject to dramatic changes when stored under an atmosphere of dichloromethane for about one week. Nanosized crystals of the naked cluster Au_{55} of about 20 nm were obtained on the dendrimer surface, indicating a total loss of the ligands of the clusters, while preserving the structure [3]. The full process is shown in Fig. 5.1.

The crystal of a quartz crystal microbalance coated by gold was functionalized by a thick layer (ca 90 nm) of PPH dendrimers having aldehyde terminal functions (generations 1–4 and 9). These devices were used as chemical sensors for studying the adsorption of vapors of 30 volatile organic compounds (VOC), mainly vapors of solvents. The adsorption induced changes in the frequency of the quartz crystal (ΔF), depending on the quantity of the adsorbed VOC [4]. An excellent correlation was observed between the quantity of vapor adsorbed and the solubility of the dendrimer in the corresponding solvent, as shown in Fig. 5.2, for generations 1 and 4 of PPH dendrimers.

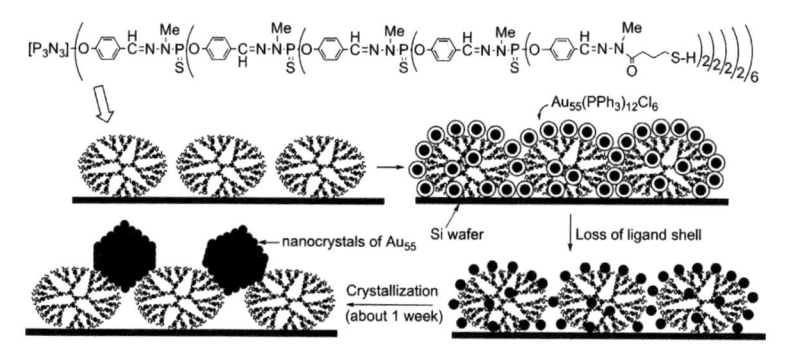

Figure 5.1 Monolayer of thiol-ended PPH dendrimers deposited on an Si wafer, used for growing nanocrystals of the naked gold cluster Au_{55}.

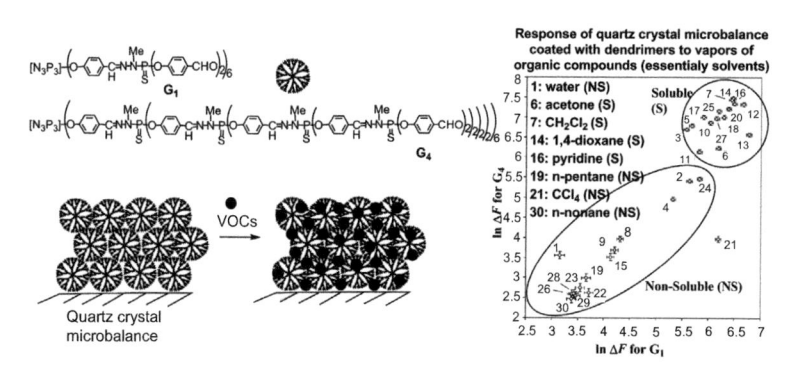

Figure 5.2 Chemical structure of G1 and G4 PPH dendrimers used for detecting the adsorption of volatile organic compounds (VOCs) by the modification of the frequency of the quartz crystal (right).

A more specific interaction was obtained with a small PPH dendrimer having a pyrene emanating from the core (off-center, see Chapter 4) and palladium complexes of phosphines as terminal functions. Interaction of the pyrene by π-stacking occurred at room temperature on cobalt nanoparticles covered by graphene. Heating at 60°C induced desorption of the dendrimers, which was fully reversible when cooling to room temperature. Such reversible behavior appeared as highly suitable for catalysis experiments. Suzuki couplings (catalyzed couplings of boronic acids with aryl bromides) were attempted at 60°C, in particular for the synthesis of Felbinac, a non-steroidal anti-inflammatory drug, which was obtained in quantitative yield. Interestingly, the Co nanoparticles covered by the dendrimers are magnetic; thus, they were easily recovered using a magnet and reused. Eleven recoveries and reuses were carried out, yielding in all cases 100% in Felbinac [5]. The process is schematized in Fig. 5.3.

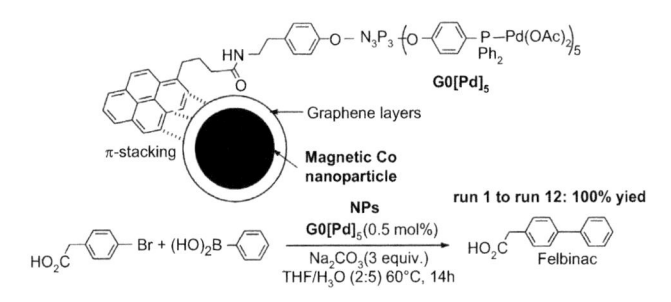

Figure 5.3 A small off-center PPH dendrimer (G0[Pd]$_5$) interacting by π-stacking with magnetic cobalt nanoparticles covered by graphene, and their use for catalyzing the synthesis of Felbinac. Recovery and re-use were carried out 11 times using a magnet.

5.2.2 Layer-by-Layer Functionalization of Solid Surfaces by Dendrimers

The previous paragraphs have displayed some examples of non-covalent interaction of neutral dendrimers with diverse surfaces. However, in most cases of non-covalent interactions, electrostatic interactions between negatively and positively charged entities are used. Such process can be applied to many different entities, in particular to positively and negatively charged polymers, which can be deposited onto solid surfaces layer-by-layer (LbL) [6]. Such a process has been largely applied to positively and negatively charged generation 4 PPH dendrimers, either alone, as illustrated in Fig. 5.4, or in combination with poly(allylamine hydrochloride) (PAH), poly(styrenesulfonate) (PSS) [7], carboxylated quantum dots [8], carboxylated hyperbranched polyglycerols [9], or DNA [10].

Such a process has been applied to flat surfaces, to convex surfaces (microspheres) [7, 10, 11], and to concave surfaces (nanopores) [8, 12], for the elaboration of nano-objects obtained by templating strategies [13], using PPH dendrimers. Some of these processes will be emphasized in the forthcoming paragraphs.

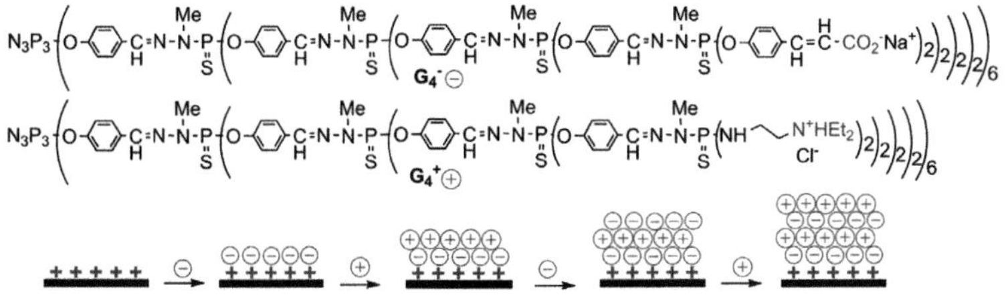

Figure 5.4 Chemical structure of generation 4 PPH dendrimers with negatively charged (CO_2^-; G4$^-$) or positively charged (N$^+$HEt$_2$; G4$^+$) terminal functions. Schematization of their use for layer-by-layer deposition on a flat charged surface.

The LbL process was carried out also using positively charged dendrimers and negatively charged gold nanoparticles (instead of the dendrimers). The thickness of the resulting multilayer was studied in different conditions. Addition of NaCl increased the ionic strength, which induced an expansion of the dendrimers and of the thickness of the layers (Fig. 5.5). On the contrary, upon UV exposure, a decrease in the thickness was observed due to the removal of the dendrimers, which were fragmented by UV light [14]. The resulting multilayer of gold was used as a sensor for five different alcohols (methanol, ethanol, propanol, butanol, and pentanol). A distinct red shift of the L-SPR (localized surface plasmon resonance) peak wavelength of the gold multilayer was observed, depending on the alcohol used (Fig. 5.5, right) [15].

Besides flat surfaces, the LbL process was also applied to ordered nanoporous alumina templates, first coated with 3-aminopropyl dimethylethoxysilane (APDMS). The positively charged template was then immerged in a water solution of negatively charged generation 4 PPH dendrimers (G4$^-$ in Fig. 5.4), to deposit a first layer of dendrimers inside the pores. After washing, the negatively charged template was immerged in a water solution of positively charged generation 4 PPH dendrimers (G4$^+$ in Fig. 5.4), to deposit a second layer of dendrimers inside the pores, and washed.

Additional dendrimer monolayers were deposited using the same process. Twenty bilayers of positively and negatively charged PPH dendrimers were deposited by this LbL process. Removal of the template was performed in hard conditions, using either KOH or H_3PO_4 + Chromium(III)oxide (Fig. 5.6). The dendrimer layers were not destroyed by this process, and an array of nanotubes of dendrimers was obtained, which were the replica of the pores. Individual nanotubes were also visualized by transmission electron microscopy (TEM). The length of the nanotubes was that of the template (80 µm), and the thickness of the wall was 40 nm, indicating a very important flattening of the dendrimers [12]. Contrarily to the well-known carbon nanotubes, these nanotubes of dendrimers have a perfectly defined and highly reproducible size and can be easily functionalized [16].

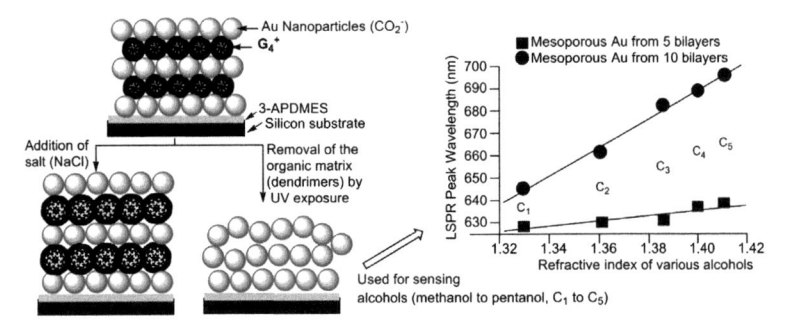

Figure 5.5 LbL process using the positively charged dendrimer G4+ and negatively charged gold nanoparticles. Removal of the dendrimers afforded a multilayer of gold nanoparticles, usable for sensing alcohols.

These experiments were carried out first with porous templates having nanopores of diameter 400 nm, then with smaller nanopores of diameters 30–116 nm, and the ionic strength was also varied. It was shown that deposition inside the nanopores can become inhibited, even if the diameter of the dendrimers is much smaller than the diameter of the nanopores. The dependence of the thickness of the deposited layers by LbL on ionic strength was significantly stronger in the case of the nanopores, compared to flat surfaces [17].

Nanoporous gold membranes prefunctionalized by 3-mer-captopropyl trimethoxysilane were also used for the LbL deposition of positively charged, then negatively charged, generation 4 poly(phosphorhydrazone) dendrimers, until the pores got clogged. The LbL deposition was analyzed by propagating surface plasmon resonance (P-SPR) and localized SPR (L-SPR). A very regular shift of the resonance angle of the P-SPR excitation was observed when the number of dendrimers increased. The L-SPR signal weakened after deposition of eight double layers of dendrimers. At this step, the dendrimers were no longer deposited inside the pores, but only on the surface of the membrane [18].

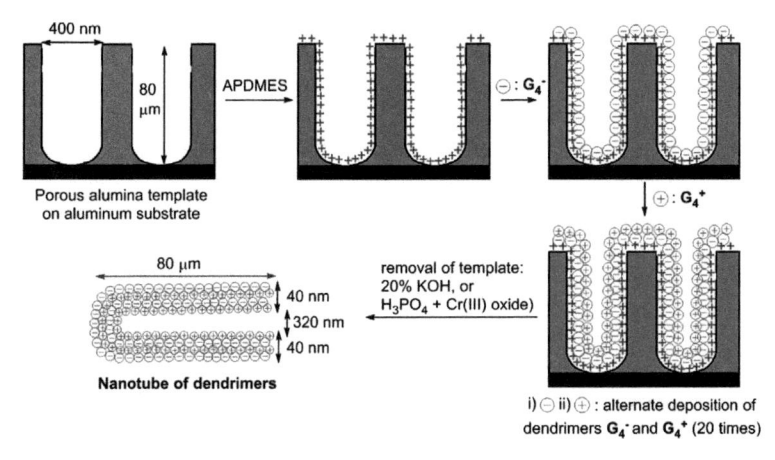

Figure 5.6 Layer-by-layer synthesis of nanotubes of dendrimers. The chemical structure of G4+ and G4- is shown in Fig. 5.4.

For all the previous examples, the LbL deposition necessitated the use of two different entities with opposite charges. A more original way to apply the LbL method would consist in using a single component instead of two. The flexibility of the synthesis of dendrimers allows the elaboration of dendrons, which are dendritic wedges with one function at the level of the core, different from the functions of the terminal groups. Dendrons are suitable for the synthesis of Janus dendrimers, most generally obtained by associating two different dendrons through their core [19]. Janus dendrimers composed of carboxylic acid functions on one side and amines on the other side are suitable candidates for LbL deposition with a single component, as these functions are precursors of carboxylate and ammonium terminal groups, used in the previous experiments [20]. In the first step, the Janus dendrimer was negatively charged and deposited on a positively charged surface, obtained from 3-aminopropyldimethyl-silane (Fig. 5.7, case A). The amines of the neutral surface were then quaternized using methyliodide, to afford a positively charged surface (Fig. 5.7, case B). The second layer of the negatively charged bis-dendrons was then deposited (Fig. 5.7, case C). Up to four layers of these Janus dendrimers could be deposited using the same process [21].

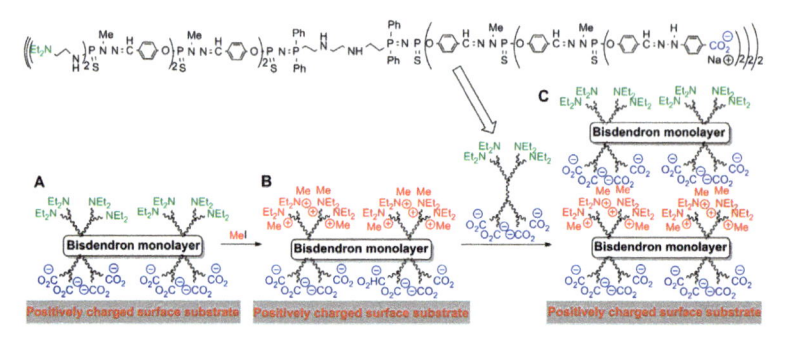

Figure 5.7 Use of bisdendrons (Janus dendrimers) for the synthesis of multilayers by LbL, using a single component.

5.2.3 Biomaterials and Sensors Issued from Non-covalent Functionalization by Dendrimers

Starting from silica or quartz surfaces, the LbL deposition of positively and negatively charged dendrimers, as shown in Fig. 5.4, was carried out in view of obtaining substrates for the culture of cells. The influence of the charge of the outermost layer of dendrimers on the adhesion and maturation of fetal cortical rat neurons was assessed. It was shown that the fetal rat neurons attached preferentially and matured slightly faster when the outermost layer was composed of positively charged PPH dendrimers, compared with the outermost layer composed of negatively charged PPH dendrimers [22].

However, the main property that has been shown for these LbL thin films and nano-objects is their use as biosensors, based on the specific recognition of DNA fragments. Biosensors are gaining an increasing importance in medicinal, forensic, and environmental analyses. They are based on the hybridization (supramolecular interaction) occurring between complementary oligonucleotides (single-stranded DNA; ss-DNA). The hybridization is based on hydrogen bonds, between adenine and thymine, and between cytosine and guanine. In most cases, one oligonucleotide is linked to a solid surface (the probe), and the target is in solution, and bears a fluorescent label. In this way, the hybridization is detected by fluorescence. The principle of the process is shown in Fig. 5.8. The nature of the linker between the probe and the solid surface is of special importance [23], and it is known that dendrimers can play a very important role as three-dimensional linkers to increase the efficiency of hybridization [24]. Hybridization is a very powerful process, which has been applied inside microcapsules and nanotubes composed of layers of poly(phosphorhydrazone) dendrimers, and also on flat multilayers.

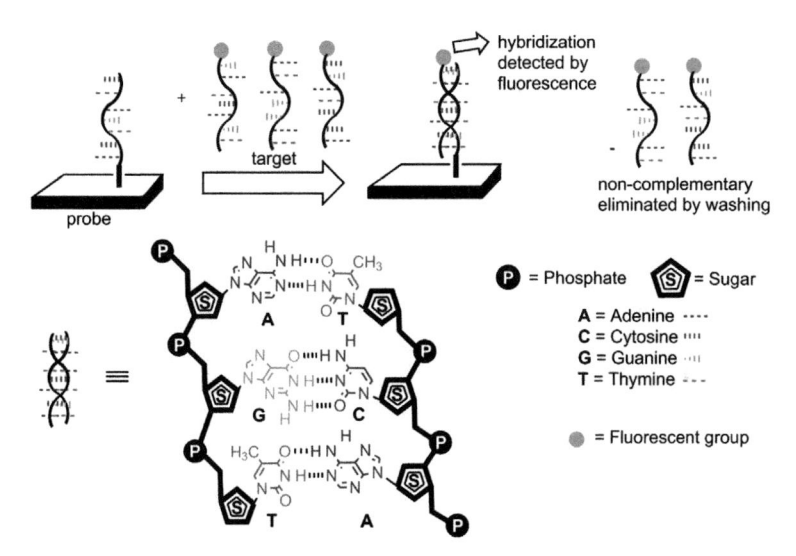

Figure 5.8 Principle of biosensors based on the hybridization between complementary oligonucleotides or fragments of ss-DNA. The hybridization is detected by fluorescence induced by the complementary fluorescently labeled oligonucleotide.

Microcapsules were obtained by using melamine/formaldehyde microspheres, covered by LbL deposition of positively charged dendrimers G4$^+$ and PSS (or negatively charged dendrimers and PAH), followed by the removal of the template through the multilayer, using HCl (pH 1.3) [7]. The same process was carried out with high–molecular weight ss-DNA used as the first layer, around the microsphere. After removal of the template to obtain the microcapsules, low–molecular weight ss-DNA labeled with Cy-5 were added to the solution containing the capsules. If the fluorescent ss-DNA was complementary (ss-DNA-Cy-5-match) to the high–molecular weight ss-DNA, the fluorescence was detected inside the microcapsule. The complementary ss-DNA-Cy-5-match diffused through the wall of the capsule "like a snake," and the hybridized DNA stayed inside the capsule [25]. On the contrary, if the low–molecular weight ss-DNA labeled with Cy-5 was not complementary (ss-DNA-Cy-5-mismatch) to the high–molecular weight ss-DNA, the fluorescence was detected only in the wall of the microcapsule, and the encapsulation of ss-DNA-Cy-5-mismatch was very weak, and it diffused easily outside the wall (Fig. 5.9) [26].

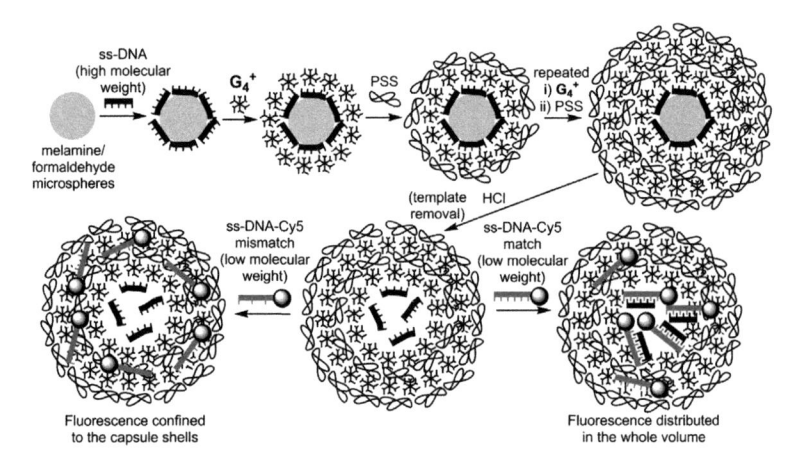

Figure 5.9 Synthesis of a microcapsule incorporating a high–molecular weight ss-DNA, and location of a short fluorescent ss-DNA, depending on whether it is complementary (match) or not (mismatch).

In the case of nanotubes, the LbL process was carried out using, at some layers, ZnCdSe alloys (quantum dots; QDs) coated with carboxylates, instead of negatively charged dendrimers. The wavelengths of absorption and emission of these QDs depended on the ratio of the three metals. The QDs were selected and precisely located to induce a cascade energy transfer [8]. In the last step, a single-stranded oligonucleotide was grafted to the last layer of quantum dots (inside the nanotubes), activated with *N*-hydroxysuccinimide (NHS) and 1-ethyl-3-(dimethylamino) propylcarbodiimide (EDC). Hybridization was carried out with a complementary oligonucleotide labeled with fluorescent Cy-5 (Fig. 5.10). The photoluminescence intensity of Cy-5 was enhanced by the cascade energy transfer induced by the selected quantum dots [27].

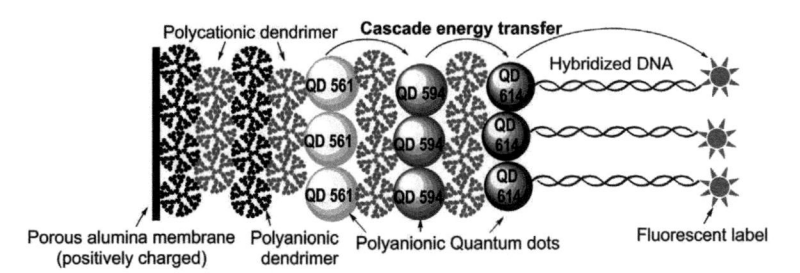

Figure 5.10 Wall of nanotubes of dendrimers and quantum dots, creating a cascade energy transfer for enhanced detection of DNA hybridization.

LbL deposition of positively and negatively charged PPH dendrimers G4$^+$ and G4$^-$ was also carried out on a gold substrate coated with 3-MPA (mercaptopropionic acid). As in the case of nanotubes, the probe DNA was grafted through activation of the terminal carboxylates with NHS/EDC. The hybridization with a fluorescent complementary oligonucleotide was detected by surface plasmon field-enhanced fluorescence spectroscopy (Fig. 5.11). The sensitivity of this DNA array depended on the number of layers of dendrimers: with one bilayer, the sensitivity was 5×10^{-11} M, and with four bilayers, it was 3×10^{-11} M [28].

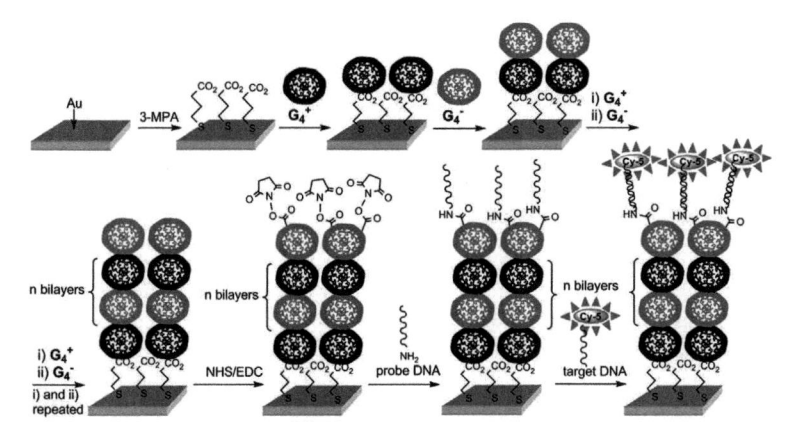

Figure 5.11 Gold-coated glass surfaces as support of multilayers of dendrimers obtained by the LbL process, and its use for the hybridization of target DNA.

In order to increase the sensitivity, a bilayer containing a negatively charged perylene diimide–cored fluorescent star polymer (FSP) and the positively charged PPH dendrimer G4$^+$ was constructed on a silver substrate. As in the previous cases, the probe oligonucleotide was grafted through the activation of the terminal carboxylates with NHS/EDC, and hybridization was carried out with a complementary Cy-5-labeled oligonucleotide. Energy transfer between FSP and Cy-5 resulted in an extraordinary efficient detection of the DNA hybridization, using surface plasmon field-enhanced fluorescence spectroscopy (SPFS) (Fig. 5.12). Detection limit as small as 10^{-18} M could be achieved [29]. This limit is by four orders of magnitude better than one of the best previously reported DNA detections [30] (see Fig. 5.18).

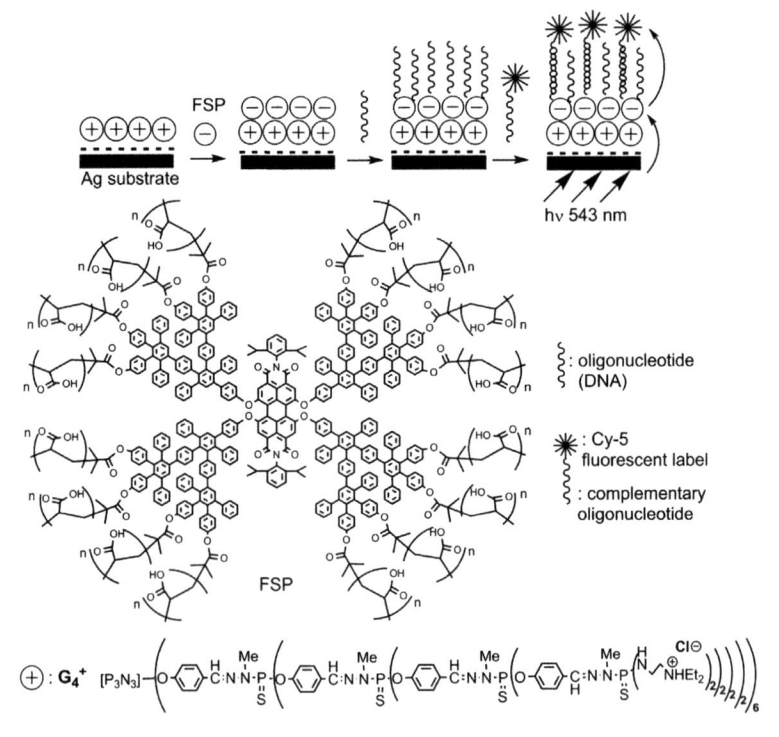

Figure 5.12 An ultrasensitive DNA array (detection limit 10^{-18} M) on a silver substrate, composed of a negatively charged fluorescent star polymer (FSP) and the positively charged PPH dendrimer G4$^+$.

5.3 Covalent Functionalization of Solid Surfaces by Phosphorus Dendrimers

In many cases (but not all), the covalent grafting of dendrimers to solid surfaces necessitates first the coating of the surface by a function suitable to react with the dendrimers. This is achieved, in particular, by using aminosilanes, as shown, for instance, in Figs. 5.6 and 5.7. In the case of the non-covalent association, the amine is protonated to afford a positively charged surface. In the case of covalent associations, the amine is neutral, thus suitable for condensation reactions, particularly with aldehydes.

5.3.1 Covalent Functionalization by Aldehyde-Ended Dendrimers

The very first examples of functionalization of solid surfaces were obtained with phosphorus dendrimers built from a trifunctional (PS) core, and bearing aldehydes as terminal functions. They were used for the coating of quartz slides pre-functionalized with aminopropyl triethoxysilane (APTES) (Fig. 5.13). Characterization of the morphology of the modified surface by AFM revealed that the surface was uniformly and densely covered by a single layer of dendrimers [31].

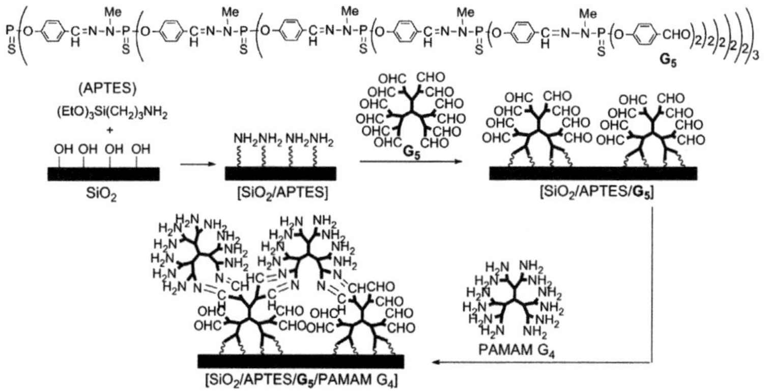

Figure 5.13 Covalent functionalization of a quartz surface using a generation 5 PPH dendrimer with aldehyde terminal functions (G5), followed by the condensation with generation 4 PAMAM dendrimers.

Several aldehyde functions of the PPH dendrimers were used for the condensation on the surface, but many aldehydes remained available for further reactions. Polyamidoamide (PAMAM, generation 4) dendrimers having NH_2 terminal functions were condensed with the aldehyde layer (Fig. 5.13), resulting in an almost complete coverage of the surface. In a further step, the remaining amino groups of the PAMAM dendrimers were used for immobilization of poly(styrene-divinylbenzene-acroleine) microspheres (diameter 310 nm) covered by aldehydes [31]. The degree of coverage was 0.61, very close to the theoretical value for the rapid immobilization of particles (0.62) [32]. The quartz or glass slides covered by aldehydes were used for the covalent immobilization of a protein, human serum albumin (HSA). AFM studies revealed that HSA formed clusters of more than 50 proteins on the layer of PPH dendrimers [33].

A related process was recently applied to silica nanoparticles (diameter 12 nm), modified with APTES and first-generation PPH dendrimers. In the next step, the remaining aldehydes were condensed with an amino-poly(ethylene glycol) (PEG); then the imine functions were reacted with dimethylphosphite used as solvent. Diverse analytical techniques (solid state NMR, UV-Vis., FTIR, HRTEM, STEM, EDX, TGA, etc., see Chapter 2) indicated that in average, among 12 aldehydes, one did not react, 6 were used for the grafting to the silica nanoparticles, and 5 reacted with PEG (Fig. 5.14). Addition of silver acetate to the suspensions in water of the functionalized silica nanoparticles induced the formation of silver nanoparticles, composed of various silver oxides (AgO, Ag_2O, Ag_3O, etc.). The same process was carried out in the presence of sodium borohydride as reducing agent, leading to Ag^0 nanoparticles. The antibacterial activity of all these materials, including silver, was tested. The smaller nanoparticles displayed the highest activity, and Ag^{II} was found slightly more efficient than Ag^0 [34].

In the previous examples, the full solid surface was covered by the dendrimers. If a micro-imprinted surface is used, which possess APTES only in specific areas, the dendrimers with aldehyde terminal functions interact only with the areas coated with APTES. However, AFM images revealed that the dendrimers agglomerated inside the APTES patterns with typical heights of 100 nM (±40 nm), showing that the interaction was not exclusively covalent [35]. Another way to obtain a partial coverage of the solid surface by dendrimers involved use of micro-contact printing. A solution of dendrimer G4 (N_3P_3 core, aldehyde terminal functions) was deposited on the stamp, then dried under nitrogen flow, and the final step was the printing of the PPH dendrimers on a silicon wafer treated with APTES. A high-fidelity printing was observed, affording well-resolved dendrimer lines [36]. The full process is shown in Fig. 5.15.

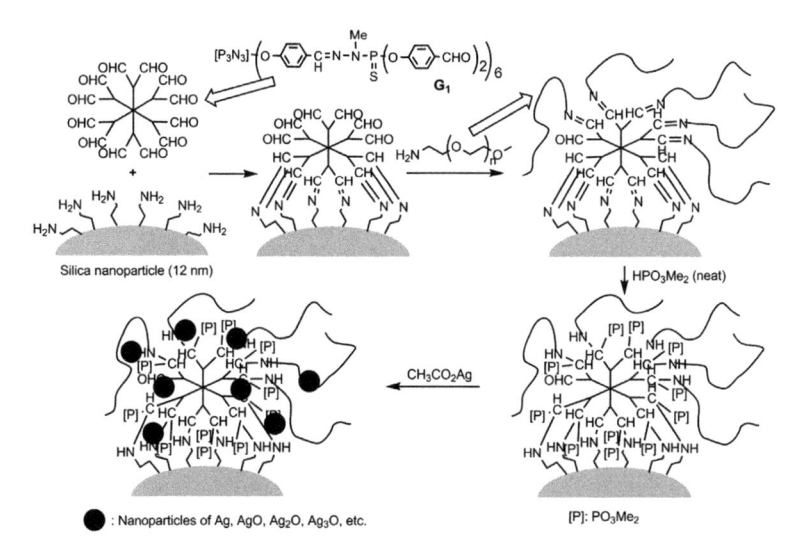

Figure 5.14 Covalent functionalization of silica nanoparticles with first generation PPH dendrimer G1, and further reactivity.

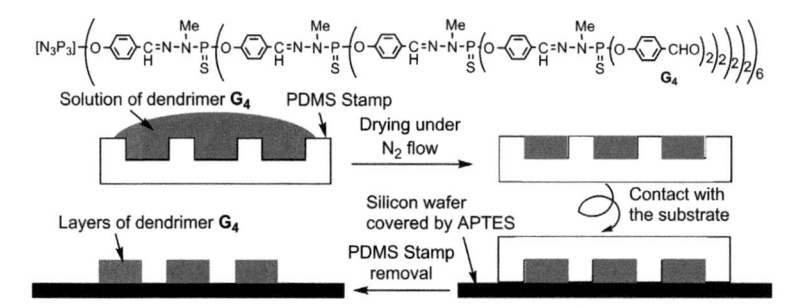

Figure 5.15 Chemical structure of PPH dendrimer G4, and its use for the partial coverage of a silicon wafer covered by APTES, using micro-contact printing.

5.3.2 Biomaterials and Sensors Issued of Direct Covalent Functionalization of Surfaces

In all the previous examples of covalent functionalization of solid surfaces by dendrimers, a linker was used between the dendrimer and the solid surface. Such process has found diverse applications for the elaboration of biosensors, as will be emphasized at the end of this chapter. However, direct grafting of some dendrimers has also been carried out, and has also led to sensors and biomaterials.

The covalent modification of a nano-crystalline TiO_2 mesostructured film was carried out with a small Janus dendrimer having five fluorescent maleimide groups on one side, and two phosphonates on the other side, for grafting to TiO_2. The resulting functionalized film was brightly fluorescent and was used as chemical sensor. Indeed, the fluorescence of the maleimide groups is quenched by hydrogen bonds with the carbonyl groups, in particular with phenols. High quenching efficiency toward phenolic OH moieties was observed with most phenols, especially with resorcinol and 2-nitroresorcinol, for which less than 1% of fluorescence of the film remained. Comparison of the quenching efficiency of the dendrimer in solution or grafted to the film indicated in almost all cases a better efficiency of the quenching in the solid state (Fig. 5.16) [37].

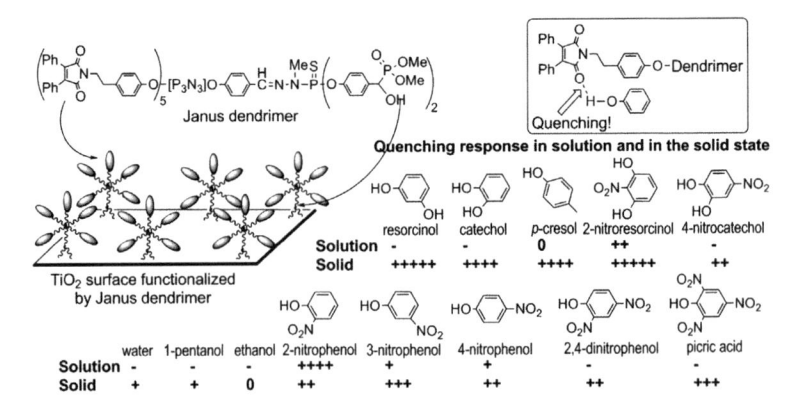

Figure 5.16 A chemical sensor for phenols, based on a small Janus fluorescent dendrimer. Indication of the detection efficiency for the phenols (10 mM). +++++ corresponds to a total disappearance of the fluorescence.

The PPH dendrimer ended by thiols, shown in Fig. 5.1, was tentatively used for the direct coating of gold surfaces, but produced only a disordered layer [38]. To overcome this problem, a masked thiol was used (a cyclic dithiolane). This function was grafted off-center (Chapter 4) to generations 1 and 2 of PPH dendrimers having either positively or negatively charged terminal functions. The reaction with glass slides covered by gold was only efficient in the case of generation 1 (Fig. 5.17). The dithiolane group was presumably too buried inside the dendritic structure of generation 2 to be anchored to the gold surface. The functionalized slides were then used for the culture of human osteoblasts. A very different behavior was observed, depending on the surface charges. The positively charged surfaces induced a dramatic decrease in the number of cells and of their viability (black bars in Fig. 5.17), accompanied by a dramatic increase in the caspase 3/7 activity (these enzymes are only active when a cell undergoes apoptosis) measured by fluorescence (grey bars in Fig. 5.17). On the contrary, adhesion and proliferation of osteoblasts were observed on the negatively charged surface, and these cells were not apoptotic (Fig. 5.17) [39]. The opposite behavior was observed previously in the case of multilayers of dendrimers, for the culture of cortical rat neurons, which matured slightly faster on the positively charged outermost layer [22]. This difference is a clear illustration of the known influence of the nano-topography [40] and of charges [41] on the adhesion and viability of cells.

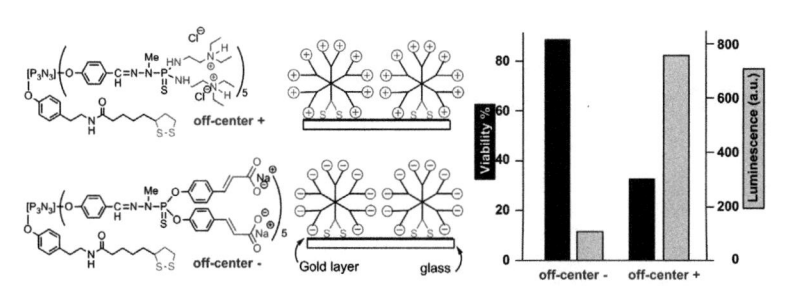

Figure 5.17 Off-center dendrimers having an off-center dithiolane group for grafting to gold surfaces, and positively or negatively charged terminal functions. Viability of human osteoblasts (black bars) and luminescence (grey bars) indicating the caspase 3/7 activity, as a marker of apoptosis.

5.3.3 DNA Chips Issued of Covalent Functionalization of Surfaces

The method shown in the upper part of Fig. 5.13 has been applied to glass slides, using several generations of PPH dendrimers ended by aldehydes, to obtain "dendrislides." On the remaining aldehydes, amino-modified oligonucleotides were then grafted, and all the imine functions, as well as the unreacted aldehydes, were reduced to increase the stability of this DNA chip. Then fluorescent complementary oligonucleotides were added to induce the hybridization (Fig. 5.8), which was detected by fluorescence. The best signal-to-noise ratios were obtained with generations 4 to 7 of PPH dendrimers. G4 was chosen because it is more easily synthesized, than higher generations. Comparison of the efficiency of detection using this dendrislide with 11 commercially available functionalized slides showed that at target concentrations 0.001 nM (10^{-12} M) of DNA, a fluorescence signal was still quantifiable only using the dendrislides (Fig. 5.18) [42] (see also Chapter 14). This sensitivity is better than the one obtained for the experiment shown in Fig. 5.11 (3×10^{-11} M) [28], but less good than for the experiment shown in Fig. 5.12 (10^{-18} M) [29].

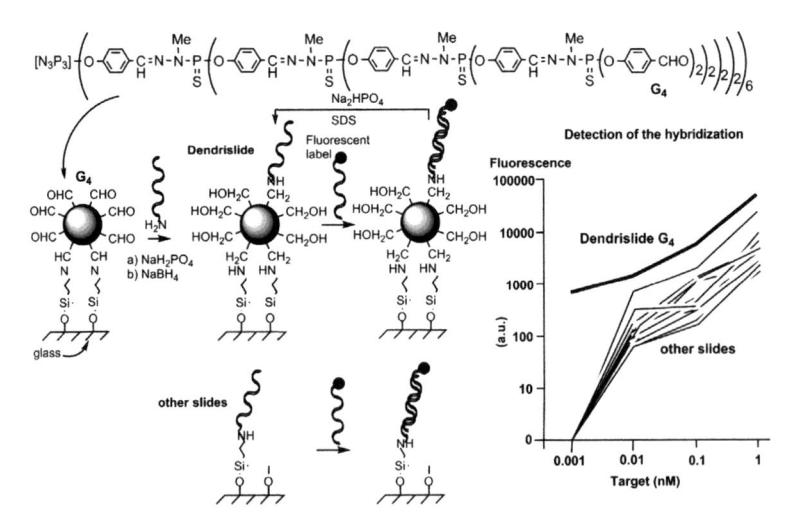

Figure 5.18 Elaboration of DNA chips with dendrimer G4 (dendrislide), and proof of their sensitivity compared to 11 other slides, not functionalized by dendrimers.

However, these DNA chips are very robust, easy to prepare and handle, and the detection of the hybridization is easier, compared to the case shown in Fig. 5.12. The reusability of these DNA chips was tested using $NaHPO_4$ and SDS, to induce the release of the target (Fig. 5.18) and was found excellent even after 10 hybridization/stripping cycles [43]. The probe oligonucleotides are generally deposited by a spotter, but they can also be deposited onto the dendrislide by micro-contact printing, using a method analogous to the one shown in Fig. 5.15, but with oligonucleotides on the stamp instead of dendrimers [44].

Besides the DNA chips, the dendrislides have been used for different purposes. The first example concerned the detection of specially engineered liposomes. Three types of probe oligonucleotides were spotted on the dendrislides (one complementary to one series of liposomes, another complementary to the other series of liposomes, and a third one not complementary). Oligonucleotides complementary, or not, to the oligonucleotides bound to the dendrislides were grafted to liposomes, including fluorescent dyes, either green (rhodamine), in the wall of the liposomes, or red (Cy5), inside the liposome. Both series of liposomes were then mixed and deposited on a dendrislide spotted with three different oligonucleotides. Each kind of liposome binded specifically to the spot corresponding to the complementary oligonucleotide on the dendrislide; thus, green fluorescence was detected on some spots, red fluorescence on others, and no fluorescence for others, depending on the probe oligonucleotides initially spotted (Fig. 5.19) [45].

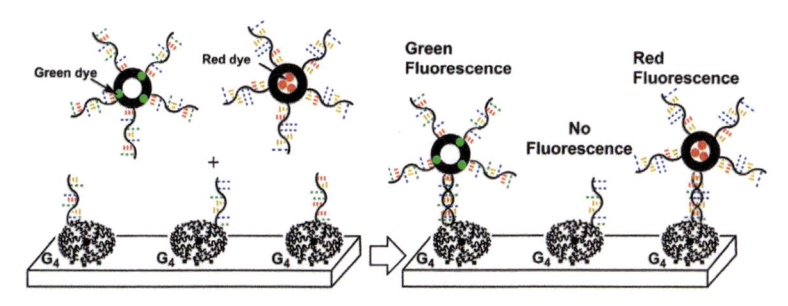

Figure 5.19   Dendrislide used as liposome chip. The hybridization induces a specific fluorescence on specific spots.

Recently, dendrislides were used for the measurement of the strength of the interaction between glutathione-*S*-transferase (GST) and its cognate antibody, by AFM. For this purpose, the GST was grafted to the dendrislide, and the GST antibody was linked to the AFM tip, using the G4 dendrimer also as linker. The single-molecule force interaction between the GST and its cognate antibody could be measured using this device (67 ± 11 pN) (Fig. 5.20, left). A blank experiment was carried out with the GST already interacting with its antibody; no interaction was detected, as expected (Fig. 5.20, right) [46].

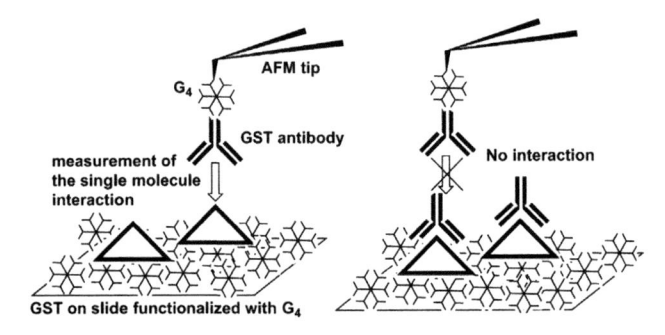

Figure 5.20 Measurement by AFM of single-molecule interaction between GST (glutathione-*S*-transferase) and its cognate antibody. The G4 dendrimer was used as a linker both between the GST and the glass slide, and between the GST antibody and the AFM tip.

The same G4 dendrimer was also linked to other supports than glass, for instance to a piezoelectric membrane. A probe oligonucleotide was first linked to the PPH dendrimers; then a complementary oligonucleotide bearing biotin on one end was hybridized. In the last step, gold colloids coated with streptavidin were added. Due to the strong interaction between biotin and streptavidin, the gold colloids were linked to the membrane (Fig. 5.21). The mass loading induced by the interaction between streptavidin and biotin was detected by a modification of the resonant frequency of the membrane. The mass sensitivity has been estimated to −3.6 Hz/pg, which was by a factor of several hundred better than state-of-the-art values for piezoelectric mass-sensing devices [47]. This experiment confirmed the potential of PPH dendrimers for biosensors.

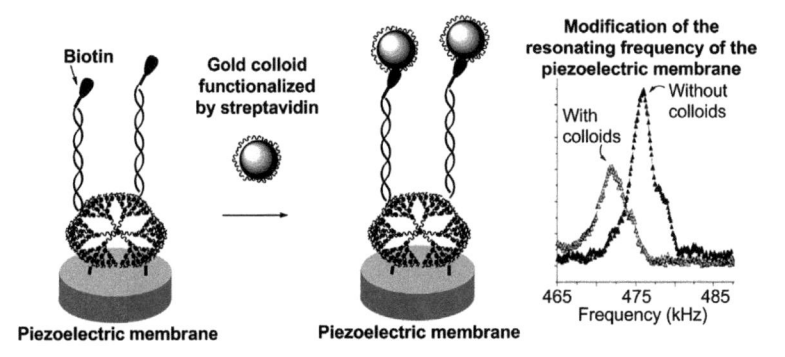

Figure 5.21 Piezoelectric membrane functionalized with G4 dendrimers, then with probe and target oligonucleotide bearing biotin, for the capture of gold colloids coated with streptavidin. The graph displays the modification of the resonating frequency of the piezoelectric membrane induced by the capture of the colloids.

All this work inspired Archer *et al.* for using the same type of process (PPH dendrimers with aldehyde terminal functions as linkers) on super-paramagnetic beads functionalized by NH_2 groups. The functionalized beads were first used for the capture of genomic DNA. Analyses of the target were performed in two different ways: by fluorescence if the target bears a fluorescent label, or by subtractive hybridization after the release of the targets, in a single step. The latter process necessitated heating at 95°C for 10 min in salt conditions to denature the double-stranded DNA fragments, and to release the target to be analyzed/quantified (Fig. 5.22). The single-step subtractive hybridization with the device composed of dendrimers afforded better performances over the conventional two-step method using streptavidin-coated magnetic beads [48].

An analogous process was used by the same group for identifying low-abundance target nucleic acids in a complex matrix. The simultaneous capturing of two low-abundance pathogenic nucleic acids in a complex matrix (800-fold excess of background nucleic acid) was successfully carried out. Recovery of the targets was also performed by heat denaturation, thanks to the stability of the device [49]. The coated magnetic beads were also used for the selective removal of host nucleic acids, in view of increasing the detection sensitivity of low-abundance pathogenic species by PCR (polymerase chain reaction). Under optimal conditions, 90–95% of human genomic DNA could be subtracted [50]. A recent sequel of this work consisted in the capture of RNA, to increase the detection sensitivity of bacterial or viral agents in complex host–pathogen mixtures. The concept was tested using rat thymus RNA with *Escherichia coli* RNA as a model system. The capture efficiency was comparable with commercially available enrichment kits [51].

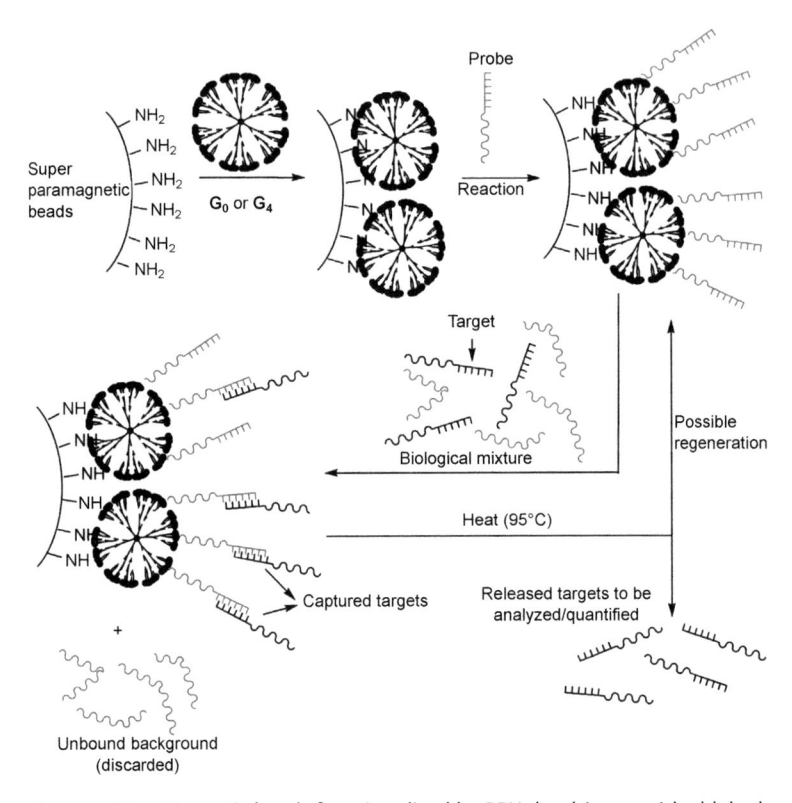

Figure 5.22 Magnetic beads functionalized by PPH dendrimers with aldehyde terminal functions and used for the selective extraction of DNA (or RNA) fragments.

5.4 Conclusion

The first examples of interactions between materials and dendrimers date back to the 1990s and were carried out with the aim of providing fundamental knowledge at the nanoscale. However, the utility of these researches has been identified very early, in particular with the elaboration of a cardiac diagnostic system used in hospitals since 1998 [52]. The dendrimers increase both the sensitivity and the robustness of the devices. We have shown in this chapter that PPH dendrimers possess an important potential for the elaboration or modification of materials at the nanometric scale. Very original researches have been carried out first, such as the elaboration of nanotubes and microcapsules, exclusively composed of dendrimers, or the modification of diverse surfaces, such as silica, titania, gold, quartz, or glass by electrostatic or covalent interactions. These researches have led to the elaboration of diverse types of macro-devices, controlled at the nanometer scale, particularly stable, reusable, and highly sensitive DNA chips. Indeed, when used as linkers between the solid surface and the oligonucleotide probe, dendrimers allow a higher loading in oligonucleotide, and their remoteness from the solid favors hybridization with the target, which occurs as easily as in solution. This system is very versatile and is usable for the control of food-processing industry (detection of bacteria in meat and dairy) or for detecting various diseases (respiratory and sexual diseases, cancers), as proposed by the start-up Dendris [53], using a technology based on PPH dendrimers (see Chapter 14). The dramatic increase in sensitivity observed with these devices justifies the use of dendrimers for commercial applications, despite their cost.

References

1. Nebhani, L. and Barner-Kowollik, C. (2009). Orthogonal transformations on solid substrates: Efficient avenues to surface modification, *Adv. Mater.*, **21**, pp. 3442–3468.

2. Grainger, D. W. (1997). Synthetic polymer ultrathin films for modifying surface properties, *Prog. Colloid Polym. Sci.*, **103**, pp. 243–250.

3. Schmid, G., Emmrich, E., Majoral, J. P., and Caminade, A. M. (2005). The behavior of Au-55 nanoclusters on and in thiol-terminated dendrimer monolayers, *Small*, **1**, pp. 73–75.

4. Gerasimov, A. V., Ziganshin, M. A., Vandyukov, A. E., Kovalenko, V. I., Gorbatchuk, V. V., Caminade, A. M., and Majoral, J. P. (2011). Specific vapor sorption properties of phosphorus-containing dendrimers, *J. Colloid Interface Sci.*, **360**, pp. 204–210.

5. Keller, M., Colliere, V., Reiser, O., Caminade, A. M., Majoral, J. P., and Ouali, A. (2013). Pyrene-tagged dendritic catalysts noncovalently grafted onto magnetic Co/C nanoparticles: An efficient and recyclable system for drug synthesis, *Angew. Chem. Int. Ed.*, **52**, pp. 3626–3629.

6. Decher, G. (1997). Fuzzy nanoassemblies: Toward layered polymeric multicomposites, *Science*, **277**, pp. 1232–1237.

7. Kim, B. S., Lebedeva, O. V., Kim, D. H., Caminade, A. M., Majoral, J. P., Knoll, W., and Vinogradova, O. I. (2005). Assembly and mechanical properties of phosphorus dendrimer/polyelectrolyte multilayer microcapsules, *Langmuir*, **21**, pp. 7200–7206.

8. Feng, C. L., Zhong, X. H., Steinhart, M., Caminade, A. M., Majoral, J. P., and Knoll, W. (2007). Graded-bandgap quantum-dot-modified nanotubes: A sensitive biosensor for enhanced detection of DNA hybridization, *Adv. Mater.*, **19**, pp. 1933–1936.

9. Kim, D. H., Lee, O. J., Barriau, E., Li, X., Caminade, A. M., Majoral, J. P., Frey, H., and Knoll, W. (2006). Hybrid organic–inorganic nanostructures fabricated from layer-by-layer self-assembled multilayers of hyperbranched polyglycerols and phosphorus dendrimers, *J. Nanosci. Nanotechnol.*, **6**, pp. 3871–3876.

10. Kim, B. S., Lebedeva, O. V., Koynov, K., Gong, H. F., Caminade, A. M., Majoral, J. P., and Vinogradova, O. I. (2006). Effect of dendrimer generation on the assembly and mechanical properties of DNA/phosphorus dendrimer multilayer microcapsules, *Macromolecules*, **39**, pp. 5479–5483.

11. Kim, B. S., Lebedeva, O. V., Park, M. K., Knoll, W., Caminade, A. M., Majoral, J. P., and Vinogradova, O. I. (2010). THF-induced stiffening of polyelectrolyte/phosphorus dendrimer multilayer microcapsules, *Polymer*, **51**, pp. 4525–4529.

12. Kim, D. H., Karan, P., Goring, P., Leclaire, J., Caminade, A. M., Majoral, J. P., Gosele, U., Steinhart, M., and Knoll, W. (2005). Formation of dendrimer nanotubes by layer-by-layer deposition, *Small*, **1**, pp. 99–102.

13. Knoll, W., Caminade, A. M., Char, K., Duran, H., Feng, C. L., Gitsas, A., Kim, D. H., Lau, A., Lazzara, T. D., Majoral, J. P., Steinhart, M., Yameen, B., and Zhong, X. H. (2011). Nanostructuring polymeric materials by templating strategies, *Small*, **7**, pp. 1384–1391.

14. Blais, J. C., Turrin, C. O., Caminade, A. M., and Majoral, J. P. (2000). MALDI TOF mass spectrometry for the characterization of phosphorus-containing dendrimers. Scope and limitations, *Anal. Chem.*, **72**, pp. 5097–5105.

15. Zhao, W. B., Park, J., Caminade, A. M., Jeong, S. J., Jang, Y. H., Kim, S. O., Majoral, J. P., Cho, J., and Kim, D. H. (2009). Localized surface plasmon resonance coupling in Au nanoparticles/phosphorus dendrimer multilayer thin films fabricated by layer-by-layer self-assembly method, *J. Mater. Chem.*, **19**, pp. 2006–2012.

16. Caminade, A. M. and Majoral, J. P. (2010). Dendrimers and nanotubes: A fruitful association, *Chem. Soc. Rev.*, **39**, pp. 2034–2047.

17. Lazzara, T. D., Lau, K. H. A., Abou-Kandil, A. I., Caminade, A. M., Majoral, J. P., and Knoll, W. (2010). Polyelectrolyte layer-by-layer deposition in cylindrical nanopores, *ACS Nano*, **4**, pp. 3909–3920.

18. Yu, F., Ahl, S., Caminade, A. M., Majoral, J. P., Knoll, W., and Erlebacher, J. (2006). Simultaneous excitation of propagating and localized surface plasmon resonance in nanoporous gold membranes, *Anal. Chem.*, **78**, pp. 7346–7350.

19. Caminade, A. M., Laurent, R., Delavaux-Nicot, B., and Majoral, J. P. (2012). "Janus" dendrimers: Syntheses and properties, *New J. Chem.*, **36**, pp. 217–226.

20. Maraval, V., Maraval, A., Spataro, G., Caminade, A. M., Majoral, J. P., Kim, D. H., and Knoll, W. (2006). Design of tailored multi-charged phosphorus surface-block dendrimers, *New J. Chem.*, **30**, pp. 1731–1736.

21. Lee, O. J., Maraval, V., Caminade, A. M., Chung, K., Lau, K. H. A., Shin, K., Majoral, J. P., Knoll, W., and Kim, D. H. (2016). Layer-by-layer self-assembly of bisdendrons: An unprecedented route to multilayer thin films, *Macromol. Res.*, **24**, pp. 851–855.

22. Hernandez-Lopez, J. L., Khor, H. L., Caminade, A. M., Majoral, J. P., Mittler, S., Knoll, W., and Kim, D. H. (2008). Bioactive multilayer thin films of charged N,N-disubstituted hydrazine phosphorus dendrimers fabricated by layer-by-layer self-assembly, *Thin Solid Films*, **516**, pp. 1256–1264.

23. Dandy, D. S., Wu, P., and Grainger, D. W. (2007). Array feature size influences nucleic acid surface capture in DNA microarrays, *Proc. Natl. Acad. Sci. USA*, **104**, pp. 8223–8228.

24. Caminade, A. M., Padie, C., Laurent, R., Maraval, A., and Majoral, J. P. (2006). Uses of dendrimers for DNA microarrays, *Sensors*, **6**, pp. 901–914.

25. Feng, C. L., Caminade, A. M., Majoral, J. P., and Zhang, D. (2010). Selective encapsulation of dye molecules in dendrimer/polymer multilayer microcapsules by DNA hybridization, *J. Mater. Chem.*, **20**, pp. 1438–1441.

26. Feng, C. L., Caminade, A. M., Majoral, J. P., Gu, J. J., Zhu, S. M., Su, H. L., Hu, X. B., and Zhang, D. (2010). DNA hybridization induced selective encapsulation of small dye molecules in dendrimer based microcapsules, *Analyst*, **135**, pp. 2939–2944.

27. Feng, C. L., Zhong, X. H., Steinhart, M., Caminade, A. M., Majoral, J. P., and Knoll, W. (2008). Functional quantum-dot/dendrimer nanotubes for sensitive detection of DNA hybridization, *Small*, **4**, pp. 566–571.

28. Yu, Y. M., Feng, C. L., Caminade, A. M., Majoral, J. P., and Knoll, W. (2009). The detection of DNA hybridization on phosphorus dendrimer multilayer films by surface plasmon field-enhanced fluorescence spectroscopy, *Langmuir*, **25**, pp. 13680–13684.

29. Feng, C. L., Yin, M. Z., Zhang, D., Zhu, S. M., Caminade, A. M., Majoral, J. P., and Mullen, K. (2011). Fluorescent core-shell star polymers based bioassays for ultrasensitive DNA detection by surface plasmon fluorescence spectroscopy, *Macromol. Rapid Commun.*, **32**, pp. 679–683.

30. Cao, Y. C., Jin, R., and Mirkin, C. A. (2002). Nanoparticles with Raman spectroscopic fingerprints for DNA and RNA detection, *Science*, **297**, pp. 1536–1540.

31. Miksa, B., Slomkowski, S., Chehimi, M. M., Delamar, M., Majoral, J. P., and Caminade, A. M. (1999). Tailored modification of quartz surfaces by covalent immobilization of small molecules (gamma-aminopropyl-triethoxysilane), monodisperse macromolecules (dendrimers), and poly(styrene/acrolein/divinylbenzene) microspheres with narrow diameter distribution, *Colloid Polym. Sci.*, **277**, pp. 58–65.

32. Trznadel, M. and Slomkowski, S. (1996). Formation and morphology of latex monolayers. Computer simulation studies, *Colloid Polym. Sci.*, **274**, pp. 1109–1118.

33. Slomkowski, S., Miksa, B., Chehimi, M. M., Delamar, M., Cabet-Deliry, E., Majoral, J. P., and Caminade, A. M. (1999). Inorganic-organic systems with tailored properties controlled on molecular, macromolecular and microscopic level, *React. Funct. Polym.*, **41**, pp. 45–57.

34. Hameau, A., Colliere, V., Grimoud, J., Fau, P., Roques, C., Caminade, A. M., and Turrin, C. O. (2013). PPH dendrimers grafted on silica nanoparticles: Surface chemistry, characterization, silver colloids hosting and antibacterial activity, *RSC Adv.*, **3**, pp. 19015–19026.

35. Cau, J. C., Cerf, A., Thibault, C., Genevieve, M., Severac, C., Peyrade, J. P., and Vieu, C. (2008). Chemical engineering of silicon oxide surfaces using micro-contact printing for localizing adsorption events of

nanoparticles, dendrimers and bacteria, *Microelectron. Eng.*, **85**, pp. 1143–1146.

36. Thibault, C., Severac, C., Trevisiol, E., and Vieu, C. (2006). Microtransfer molding of hydrophobic dendrimer, *Microelectron. Eng.*, **83**, pp. 1513–1516.

37. Martinez-Ferrero, E., Franc, G., Mazeres, S., Turrin, C. O., Boissiere, U., Caminade, A. M., Majoral, J. P., and Sanchez, C. (2008). Optical properties of hybrid dendritic-mesoporous titania nanocomposite films, *Chem. Eur. J.*, **14**, pp. 7658–7669.

38. Emmrich, E., Franzka, S., Schmid, G., and Majoral, J. P. (2002). Monolayers of a fourth-generation thiol-terminated dendrimer, *Nano Lett.*, **2**, pp. 1239–1242.

39. de Jong, E. R., Deloch, N., Knoll, W., Turrin, C. O., Majoral, J. P., Caminade, A. M., and Koper, I. (2015). Synthesis and characterization of bifunctional dendrimers: Preliminary use for the coating of gold surfaces and the proliferation of human osteoblasts (HOB), *New J. Chem.*, **39**, pp. 7194–7205.

40. Aktas, C., Dorrschuck, E., Schuh, C., Miro, M. M., Lee, J., Putz, N., Wennemuth, G., Metzger, W., Oberringer, M., Veith, M., and Abdul-Khaliq, H. (2012). Micro- and nanostructured Al_2O_3 surfaces for controlled vascular endothelial and smooth muscle cell adhesion and proliferation, *Mater. Sci. Eng. C*, **32**, pp. 1017–1024.

41. Ohgaki, M., Kizuki, T., Katsura, M., and Yamashita, K. (2001). Manipulation of selective cell adhesion and growth by surface charges of electrically polarized hydroxyapatite, *J. Biomed. Mater. Res.*, **57**, pp. 366–373.

42. Le Berre, V., Trevisiol, E., Dagkessamanskaia, A., Sokol, S., Caminade, A. M., Majoral, J. P., Meunier, B., and Francois, J. (2003). Dendrimeric coating of glass slides for sensitive DNA microarrays analysis, *Nucleic Acids Res.*, **31**, p. 8.

43. Trevisiol, E., Le Berre-Anton, V., Leclaire, J., Pratviel, G., Caminade, A. M., Majoral, J. P., Francois, J. M., and Meunier, B. (2003). Dendrislides, dendrichips: A simple chemical functionalization of glass slides with phosphorus dendrimers as an effective means for the preparation of biochips, *New J. Chem.*, **27**, pp. 1713–1719.

44. Thibault, C., Le Berre, V., Casimirius, S., Trevisiol, E., Francois, J., and Vieu, C. (2005). Direct microcontact printing of oligonucleotides for biochip applications, *J. Nanobiotechnol.*, **3**, p. 7.

45. Chaize, B., Nguyen, M., Ruysschaert, T., Le Berre, V., Trevisiol, E., Caminade, A. M., Majoral, J. P., Pratviel, G., Meunier, B., Winterhalter, M.,

and Fournier, D. (2006). Microstructured liposome array, *Bioconjugate Chem.*, **17**, pp. 245–247.

46. Jauvert, E., Dague, E., Severac, M., Ressier, L., Caminade, A. M., Majoral, J. P., and Trevisiol, E. (2012). Probing single molecule interactions by AFM using bio-functionalized dendritips, *Sensors Actuators B Chem.*, **168**, pp. 436–441.

47. Nicu, L., Guirardel, M., Chambosse, F., Rougerie, P., Hinh, S., Trevisiol, E., Francois, J. M., Majoral, J. P., Caminade, A. M., Cattan, E., and Bergaud, C. (2005). Resonating piezoelectric membranes for microelectromechanically based bioassay: Detection of streptavidin-gold nanoparticles interaction with biotinylated DNA, *Sensors Actuators B Chem.*, **110**, pp. 125–136.

48. Archer, M. J., Lin, B. C., Wang, Z., and Stenger, D. A. (2006). Magnetic bead-based solid phase for selective extraction of genomic DNA, *Anal. Biochem.*, **355**, pp. 285–297.

49. Archer, M. J., Stenger, D. A., and Lin, B. C. (2008). Development and characterization of a solid phase for single-step enrichment of pathogenic targets, *Open Anal. Chem. J.*, **2**, pp. 47–54

50. Archer, M. J., Long, N., and Lin, B. C. (2010). Effect of probe characteristics on the subtractive hybridization efficiency of human genomic DNA, *BMC Research Notes*, **3**, 109.

51. Archer, M. J. and Lin, B. C. (2011). Development of a single-step subtraction method for eukaryotic 18S and 28S ribonucleic acids, *J. Biomed. Biotech.*, **7**. ID 910369.

52. Stratus® CS acute careTM Diagnostic Systems. https://usa.healthcare.siemens.com/point-of-care/cardiac/stratus-cs-urgent-care/technical-specifications.

53. http://www.dendris.fr

Chapter 6

PPH-Based Dendrimers as HIV Entry Inhibitors

Cédric-Olivier Turrin[a] and Muriel Blanzat[b]

[a]CNRS, LCC (Laboratoire de Chimie de Coordination) 205, route de Narbonne
F-31077 Toulouse, France. Université de Toulouse, UPS, INPT, LCC,
F-31077 Toulouse, France
[b]Laboratoire des IMRCP, Université de Toulouse, CNRS UMR 5623,
Université Toulouse III - Paul Sabatier, 118, route de Narbonne,
F-31062 Toulouse Cedex 9, France
cedric-olivier.turrin@lcc-toulouse.fr, blanzat@chimie.ups-tlse.fr

In 2014, new HIV infections were estimated at 2.0 million and the number of deaths due to HIV-related causes were estimated at 1.2 million, which is about 40% lower than the peak in the late 1990s and early 2000s. These encouraging figures are mostly due to the result of an increased access to antiretroviral therapy. Despite major progresses, HIV epidemic continues, and so the international community decided to tackle the problem and put an end to the AIDS epidemic as a public health threat by 2030.

After a brief introduction to the HIV replication cycle and the main strategies developed to block the HIV infection, this chapter reviews the different antiviral approaches with dendrimers with a

Phosphorus Dendrimers in Biology and Nanomedicine: Synthesis, Characterization, and Properties
Edited by Anne-Marie Caminade, Cédric-Olivier Turrin, and Jean-Pierre Majoral
Copyright © 2018 Pan Stanford Publishing Pte. Ltd.
ISBN 978-981-4774-33-8 (Hardcover), 978-1-315-11085-1 (eBook)
www.panstanford.com

particular focus on the strategy based on multivalent non-covalent HIV entry inhibitors.

6.1 Introduction

The human immunodeficiency virus (HIV) is responsible for the acquired immunodeficiency syndrome (AIDS) [1], a major health concern taking into account the spreading of the epidemic over the last four decades [2], which has killed more than 20 million people. As other lentiviruses, HIV is characterized by a long time of incubation. It can deliver a significant amount of viral RNA into the DNA of host cells, and it can infect non-dividing cells, a unique feature among retroviruses, making it one of the most efficient gene transfer machinery. Its cycle of replication (Fig. 6.1) is a succession of key events that have been thoroughly explored to develop antiviral strategies aiming at interrupting the cycle.

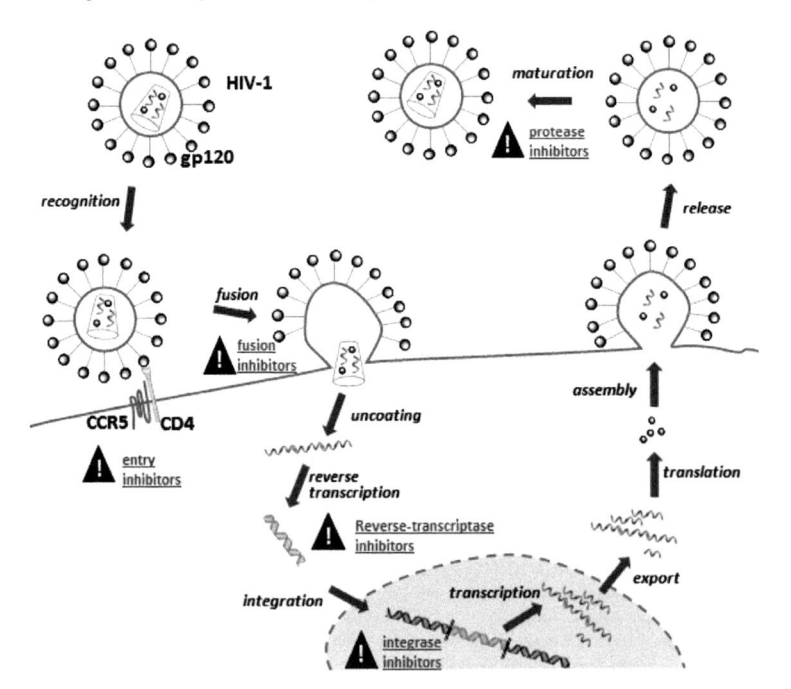

Figure 6.1   HIV-1 life cycle.

According to a very simplistic description, the cycle of replication can be divided into five main steps. The first phase involves the recognition of viral membrane proteins gp120 to CD4, a glycoprotein found on the surface of immune cells such as monocytes, macrophages, T helper cells, and dendritic cells, or to galactosylceramide (Gal beta 1-1'Cer or GalCer), which is a sphingolipid found on some CD4 negative cells of neural and colonic origin. Following these specific host–guest interactions involving regions of the viral proteins, like the arginine-rich V3 loop of gp120, and human co-receptors of CD4 like CCR5, CXCR4, membrane fusion occurs, and the viral RNAs, along with enzymes and proteins necessary to replication machinery, are released into the host cells. Receptor inhibitors and fusion inhibitors target these early steps. The second phase is the reverse transcription of the viral RNA to DNA thanks to the viral reverse transcriptase (RT) enzyme. This translating step is highly error prone, accounting for a high mutation rate for HIV. Nucleoside analogs or non-nucleoside analogs of RT slow down or stop the action of the RT enzyme; these drugs are often used in pairs. The third phase is the integration of the viral DNA into the host cell's own DNA by means of the viral integrase enzyme. Integrase inhibitors are also commonly used in polytherapy strategies. HIV-infected cells can be inactive for a long time. Upon activation, the DNA machinery produces a long protein chain of viral proteins that are separated by the protease viral enzyme, allowing the assembly into new virus particles, which are released from the host cell and go on to infect other cells. Protease inhibitors (PIs) interfere with the action of the viral protease enzyme, leading to defective viruses that cannot infect new cells. New strategies also target the assembly of the viral proteins or the inactivation of the virus genes by gene transfection.

6.2 Anti-HIV Strategies with Dendrimers

As mentioned earlier, antiviral strategies are generally targeted toward (i) the mechanism of interaction between the virus and its cellular targets, (ii) the cycle of replication of the virus, and (iii) the inactivation of virus genes. Among the large variety of new molecules that are currently being developed, dendrimers are 10- to 100-fold smaller than HIV, and they can be designed to block the early virus–cell interactions, following three main strategies. Dendrimers can interact in a nonspecific manner with the virus envelope [3, 4]. They can also interact specifically with some receptors or components of the viral membrane [5–7], or they can block some receptors located on the surface of the cells that are specifically targeted by the virus [8]. Other strategies with dendrimers [9, 10] aim at delivering enzyme inhibitors [11, 12] or silencing genes within infected cells [13, 14]. This section is a brief, non-exhaustive overview of selected examples involving mostly non-phosphorus-containing dendrimers for anti-HIV strategies.

6.2.1 Dendrimers as Gene Carriers in Anti-HIV Therapy

This field of research is highly connected to the numerous studies that have been made to develop dendrimeric systems for the delivery of genetic material [15]. Its application to anti-HIV strategies using silencing RNA (siRNA) has recently opened new perspectives [16–18]. Small interfering RNAs or silencing RNAs are short double-strained RNA that are complementary to specific regions of the mRNA, leading to its degradation [19, 20]. This strategy can be applied to prevent the production of some proteins that are vital to HIV replication machinery [21, 22]. Two research groups from Madrid have been developing positively charged carbosilane dendrimers [23] for a decade in order to transfect siRNA that target a region related to the coding of p24 protein of the viral capsid, GAG genomic region coding for structural proteins of the virus and NEF genes coding for envelop proteins of the virus. The water-soluble dendrimers developed by the group of de la Mata and Gomez efficiently bind small nucleic acid chains [24, 25] and form dendriplexes [26] that are stable toward RNase digestion and present low cytotoxicity at therapeutic concentrations. Efficient transfection rates have been measured in human peripheral mononuclear cells (PBMCs), and the presence of water-sensitive siloxane linkages within the dendrimer structure is assumed to favor the release of the transfected material

[27–29]. The ability of these dendriplexes to cross the blood–brain barrier (BBB) by transcytosis [30] could open new perspectives, although carbosilane dendrimers as anti-HIV gene carriers are still in a non-clinical development phase. Indeed, the consortium has recently stepped in the footprints of Starpharma and published several reports on polyanionic carbosilane dendrimers [31, 32] showing encouraging *in vivo* [33] results as topical microbicides, alone or in combination with other drugs, including antiretroviral drugs or entry inhibitors [7, 34–36].

According to an analogous approach, commercially available PAMAM dendrimers have been used to transfect a cocktail of dicer substrate siRNAs (dsiRNAs) targeting both viral and cellular transcripts to humanized mouse model for HIV-1 infection [37]. Weekly injections over a 5-week period of the dendriplexes following viral rebound led to complete inhibition of HIV-1, and biodistribution studies showed that the dendriplexes preferentially accumulated in peripheral blood mononuclear cells (PBMCs) and liver without discernable toxicity. PPH dendrimers have also been identified as potential gene carriers for the delivery of HIV peptides [38, 39] and siRNA [40, 41].

6.2.2 Delivering RT Inhibitors with Dendrimers

The number of reports related to drug delivery with dendrimers is a good indication of the promises of these macromolecules as drug-delivery tools, and a significant number of studies have reached the preclinical phase [42]. Terminal groups actually offer a versatile platform for drug conjugation and the grafting of targeting moieties, allowing the design of tailor-made multivalent pro-drugs [43]. Alternatively, cargo loading dendrimers with drugs offer a straightforward strategy [44], but with a lesser control on the loading stability and release mechanisms. In addition, these peripheral functional groups can be employed to tailor-make the properties of dendrimers, enhancing their versatility. In this regard, diverse strategies have been explored over the last decades. An RT nucleosidic inhibitor has been grafted on the surface on PAMAM dendrimers through a phosphate or and ester linker, and their anti-HIV activity has been compared *in vitro* to analogous monovalent PEGylated systems [11]. In another study, lamivudine and efavirenz, two other RT inhibitors, have been formulated with poly(propylenimine) (PPI) dendrimers, glycine-capped PPI, or mannose-capped PPI [12, 45], in order to favor cellular uptake by myeloid lymphocytes that are targeted by HIV. This targeting is expected to reduce the side effects of these potent drugs, and it was found *in vitro* that the cellular uptake in monocyte/macrophage lineages was increased up to 12-fold with mannose-capped PPI. The selectivity of these systems among monocytes/macrophages toward infected cells (*versus* non-infected cells) was significantly improved by grafting Tuftsin residues on PPI scaffolds [46].

Anionic carbosilane dendrimers have also been formulated with tenofovir, a nucleosidic RT inhibitor, and maraviroc, an entry inhibitor, and topical applications of these formulations in mouse models validated this multi-drug encapsulation approach in terms of anti-HIV-1 activity, cytotoxicity, and vaginal irritation [35, 36].

6.2.3 Viral Protein-Targeting Dendrimers

Gene expression of HIV-1 could be inhibited by molecules targeting viral gene regulatory proteins that drastically enhances the efficiency of viral transcription, such as Tat or its molecular targets [47]. In this regard, it has been shown that PAMAM dendrimers can interact with TAR RNA [48]. The Tat–TAR interactions are crucial to ensure an efficient viral transcription [49]. PAMAM–TAR interactions are assumed to modify the structure of TAR RNA, which results in an efficient inhibition of the interactions between TAR RNA and Tat regulatory protein [50].

6.2.4 Inhibiting HIV Entry with Dendrimers

Most antiviral strategies target replication steps taking place within infected cells, as those mentioned here earlier. However, perturbing the early interactions of the virus with host cells is also a major field of investigation. According to a schematic view, cell binding and HIV entry begin with an adhesion step [51], in which nonspecific interactions can have significant importance. Further recognition processes involve the viral transmembrane protein gp120 and CD4 or GalCer, and also CCR5 and CXCR4, two co-receptors engaged in the recognition of the gp120 by target cells. These specific interactions may also be stabilized by nonspecific interactions resulting from electrostatic interaction or lipophilic affinities. It should also be noticed that DC-SIGN [52] (dendritic cell-specific ICAM 3-grabbing non-integrin), a C-type lectin receptor located on the surface of macrophages and dendritic cells, plays an important role in mediating the HIV-1 infection. This transmembrane protein presents a carbohydrate recognition domain involved in the recognition of several pathogens, including HIV [53, 54], in peripheral mucosal tissues where dendritic cells (DC) are more abundant. This early recognition with DC, which are antigen presenting cells, routes HIV-1 to lymph nodes where the infection of T cells takes place.

Taking into account the importance of multivalency in these early steps of the replication cycle, a significant number of studies have been conducted to demonstrate the potential of dendrimers to inhibit these steps.

6.2.4.1 Strategies involving nonspecific interactions

Despite the generalization of polychemotherapies, which have significantly increased the lifespan of seropositive patients, it is admitted that HIV cannot be eradicated with the currently used anti-retroviral drugs [55]. In the absence of efficient vaccine, one option to circumvent the epidemic is the use of condoms and self-applied microbicides. Microbicides based on polyanionic nonspecific entry inhibitors interact with an arginine-rich region of the V3 loop of the gp120 presenting a local concentration of positive charges [56, 57]. In this regard, all polyanionic compounds derived from polymer materials, such as PRO2000, Carraguard, or dextran sulfate (DxS) [58–61], have clinically failed during phase I or phase II clinical trials [62]. The lack of activity of these systems has opened perspectives for the design of nonspecific HIV entry inhibitors as topical microbicides relying on nanotechnology-based systems such as dendrimers [63]. In this regard, dendrimers are the only nanotechnology-based systems that have entered clinical trials as topical microbicide for HIV prevention [64, 65]. In the early 1990s,

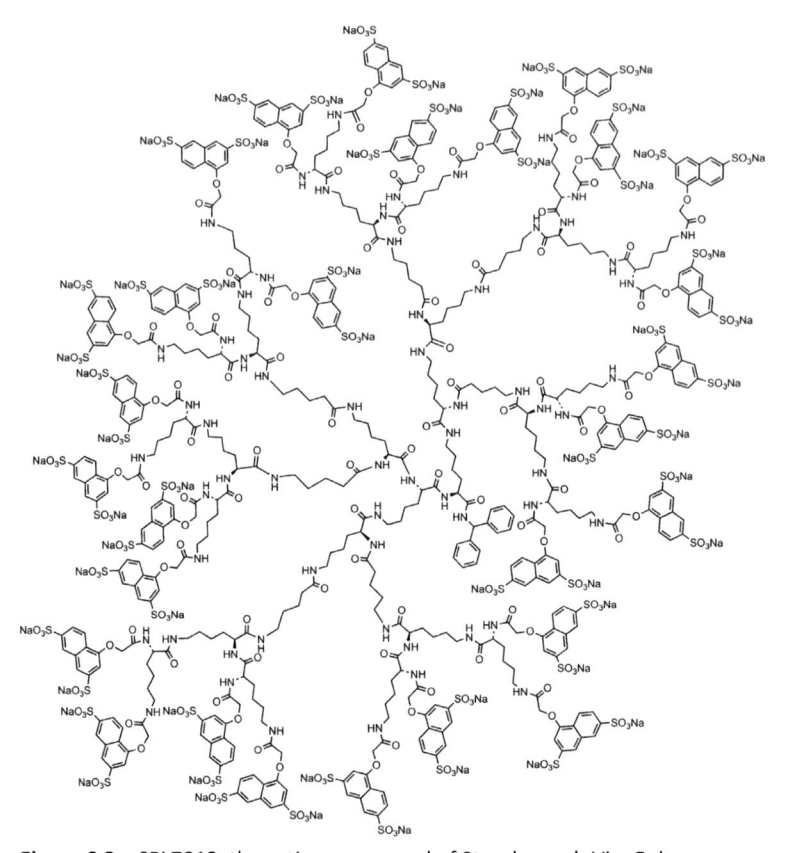

Figure 6.2 SPL7013, the active compound of Starpharma's VivaGel.

George Holan initiated at the Biomolecular Research Institute a research program dedicated to the use of dendrimers as drugs. Based on the dendrimer work and a set of antiviral and angiogenesis inhibition patents, the company Starpharma was founded in 1994. Translating his research to the company, he published with Barry Ross Matthews a patent on polyanionic and polycationic dendrimers with antiviral properties [66]. The latter was completed by eight patents that formed the intellectual property of Starpharma Ltd. Among a long series of dendrimers ended with anionic and cationic end groups having antiviral properties in the nanomolar and submacromolar range against HIV-1 and other viruses such as HIV-2, cytomegalovirus, and herpes simplex virus [67], dendrimer GH7013, a poly-L-lysine scaffold ended with naphtylsulfonate groups later renamed as SPL7013 (Fig. 6.2), was tested originally for antiviral HIV properties in 1998. VivaGel®, a water-based microbicide gel based on this active compound, successfully underwent phase I clinical trials [68]. However, although it was initially designed for anti-HIV-1 [69] purposes, its application latter was repositioned for topical treatment of bacterial vaginosis. This product has received EU approval for this application, and VivaGel-coated condoms are now commercially available in Australia.

Other polyanionic dendrimers have also shown interesting anti-HIV-1 properties *in vitro*. It is the case of a series of generation phosphorus-containing poly(phosphorhydrazone) (PPH) dendrimers capped with cinnamates [70], vinylphosphonates, or modified phosphonates. These compounds synthesized for anti-HIV application in the late 1990s [71] and later structurally optimized showed anti-HIV-1 properties in the submicromolar range [72, 73]. Interestingly, the presence of a lateral alkyl chain was found to fairly improve their activity, possibly by facilitating the interaction with lipophilic pockets of the V3 loop. As detailed in this chapter, these dendrimers were used as building blocks for the preparation of multivalent analogs of GalCer.

6.2.4.2 Strategies involving specific interactions

The recognition of HIV involves the viral protein gp120, and cellular receptors such as DC-SIGN, CD4, or GalCer, and co-receptors such as CXCR4 and CCR5. The recognition of DC-SIGN involves multivalent interaction with mannose-rich glycoproteins of pathogens [74]; dendrimers and other multivalent scaffolds have been successfully used to target these interactions [75–77]. Although some mannose-capped dendrons have been shown in microarray binding assays to inhibit the gp120 DC-SIGN interaction in the nanomolar range [78], these promising results have not been confirmed *in vitro*.

As mentioned in a previous section, several anionic carbosilane dendrimers have been recently synthesized and assayed as antiviral drug-delivery systems, *in vitro* and *in vivo*. Recent developments on this topic have been reviewed recently [7]. Noteworthy, promising synergistic effects have been measured *in vitro*, and some of these systems incorporating entry inhibitors targeting CXCR4 or CCR5 have been successfully assayed as topical microbicides on mice models, with encouraging inhibition profiles [32, 34, 35, 79]. Another strategy involving the grafting of cyclams on the surface of PAMAM dendrimers [67] as multivalent inhibitors of CXCR4 was inspired by the nanomolar inhibiting properties of AMD 11070 [80] and other cyclam-based compounds (Fig. 6.3). Although AMD 11070 was put in clinical hold during phase 1 clinical trials in 2006 because of hepatotoxicity and retinal changes observed during preclinical studies, it can be noticed that the multivalent presentation of cyclam-based inhibitors did show significant increase in the inhibiting properties of these compounds *in vitro*.

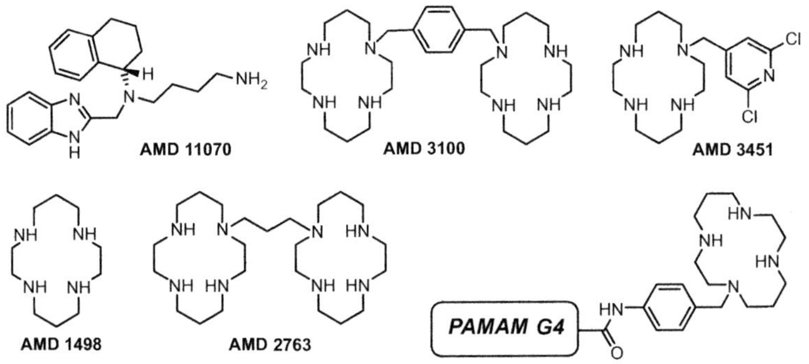

Figure 6.3 AMD 11070 and cyclams inhibiting CXCR4 co-receptor.

Another strategy based on multivalent analogs of GalCer is detailed here after.

6.3 Rational for the Design of GalCer Analogs

6.3.1 GalCer as an Alternative Receptor for HIV

Glycosphingolipids are a class of molecules composed of an *N*-acetylated sphingosine backbone linked to a carbohydrate through its terminal hydroxyl group. These carbohydrate presenting molecules, which are inserted in the lipid membrane of cells, are sometimes key molecular targets for pathogens such as viruses and bacteria [81]. It is the case of HIV for which GalCer and its sulfonated analog SGalCer have been identified as alternative receptors [82–88] for CD4 negative cells such as colonic [88, 89] or neuronal cells [87]. GalCer is a glycosphingolipid with a single D-galactose unit connected to a ceramide group composed of D-sphingosine and fatty acid with a hydroxyl group vicinal to the acyl group (Fig. 6.4), and it is not soluble in water.

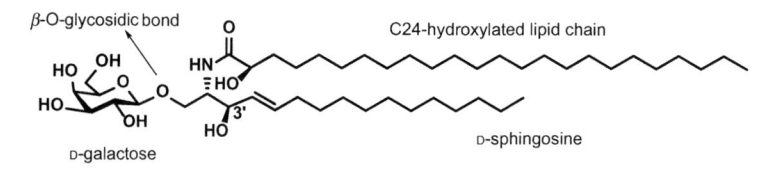

Figure 6.4 GalCer structure.

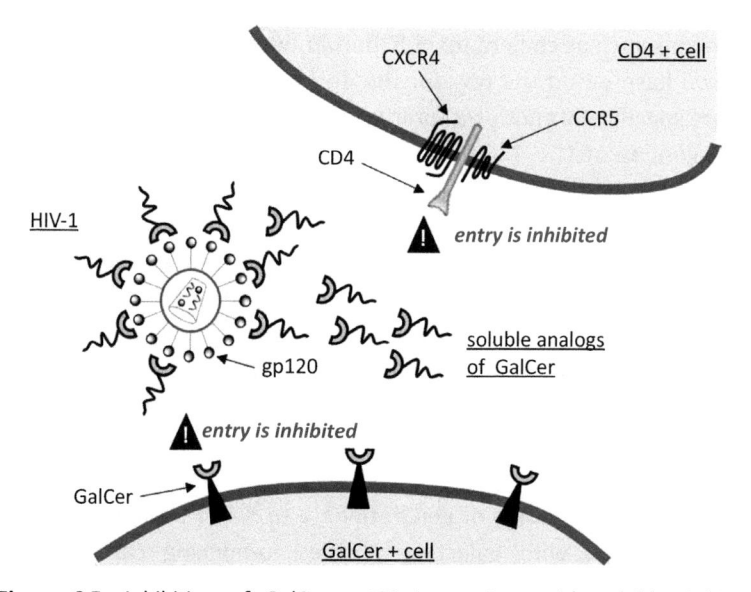

Figure 6.5 Inhibition of GalCer–gp120 interactions with soluble GalCer analogs.

The binding of HIV-1 to GalCer is mediated by the third variable (V3) loop of gp120, with an affinity close to 10 nM [83, 90], which is comparable to the affinity between gp120 and CD4, which has been measured between 2 and 5 nM [91–94]. Water-soluble synthetic analogs of GalCer targeting the gp120 V3 loop are then expected to prevent the infection of GalCer presenting cells and also the infection of CD4 positive cells (Fig. 6.5) [95, 96]. Additionally, it has been shown that GalCer–gp120 interactions are not affected by structural modifications on the ceramide junction [97], allowing a certain degree of liberty in the design of GalCer analogs, particularly in the design of multivalent analogs.

The design of multivalent inhibitors or ligands targeting cell receptors is directly inspired by the existence of polyvalent interactions in biological systems [98]. In this regard, dendrimers have obviously proved to present some key advantages [99], like their structural definition, in this field of research, although only a few studies have reached *in vivo* validation [77].

In the field of multivalent GalCer-based inhibitors, efforts of the group of C.-L. Schengrund on the design of PPI-based or PAMAM-based multivalent carbohydrates [100–103] to inhibit the adhesion of toxins such as cholera toxin B, botulinum toxin, or enterotoxin of *E. coli* have paved the way for the design of glycodendrimers, and more specifically multipresentation of glycosphingolipids as binding antagonists of HIV-1 infection. These PPI glycodendrimers were obtained by grafting a ganglioside isolated from bovine brain, namely phenylisothiocyanate derivatized (PITC) galb1-3galNAcb1-4[sialic acida2-3]-galb1-4glc residues, according to tedious procedures. These systems presented increased inhibition properties toward toxins in comparison with the free glycosphingolipid, which cannot be used alone because it may incorporate the cell's plasma membrane and become a non-desired functional component [102]. According to a first report by Schengrund *et al.* on multivalent HIV inhibitors mimicking GalCer or its 3′-sulfated derivative, sulfatide, or SGalCer, four series of generations 1 to 5 PPI dendrimers have been covered with galactose entities mimicking carbohydrate glycoclusters found in lipid rafts [104]. The first series was prepared from the ceramide saccharide derivative of purified natural GalCer. The grafting of synthons 3-(β-D-galactopyranosylthio)propionic acid and 3-(β-D-3-sulfogalactopyranosylthio)propionic acid afforded galactopyranosyl- and 3-sulfogalactopyranosyl-derivatized dendrimers, and the fourth series was obtained by random sulfation of the 3-(β-D-galactopyranosylthio)propionic acid functionalized dendrimers (Fig. 6.6) [105].

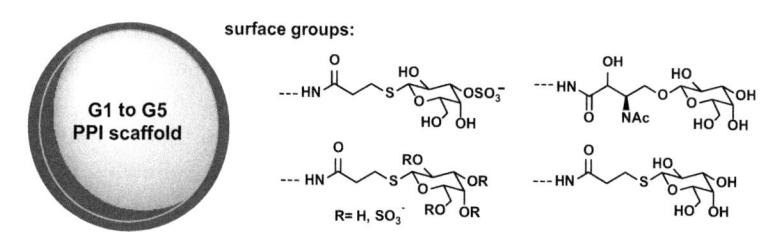

Figure 6.6 GalCer and SGalCer multivalent analogs prepared from generation 1 to generation 5 PPI scaffolds.

In vitro assessment of the anti-HIV-1 properties of these dendrimers revealed a better activity for the sulfated species (IC_{50} = 20–90 µM) in comparison with the non-sulfated ones (CI_{50} > 0.1 mM), and all compounds were found to be less active than dextran sulfate (DxS). These findings were correlated to a higher degree of sulfation for DxS (almost 2.3 sulfate group per glucosyl moiety) in comparison with less than 1 sulfate group per galactose residue for the glycodendrimers. These dendrimers were found to have a good safety profile *in vitro*, and in the case of generations 3, 4, and 5 PPI dendrimers terminated with SGalCer, the IC_{50} were found to be 90, 70, and 20 µM, respectively, whereas DxS was found to have an IC_{50} of 1.6 µM. In order to compare the activity of these multivalent systems and to evaluate the influence of multivalency effects, the relative IC_{50}, defined as $RIC_{50} = IC_{50} \times N$, with N being the number of interacting entities, is a practical parameter. DxS being approximately composed of 170 glucoside residues [105], its RIC_{50} is lower than the ones of SGalCer PPI dendrimers. Interestingly, the latter present nonlinear dendrimeric effect, the generation 4 being the less active one (Table 6.1).

Table 6.1 Activity of SGalCer-coated PPI dendrimers developed by Schengrund *et al.*

Compound	N^a	IC_{50} (µM)	RIC_{50} (µM)
G3 PPI (SGalCer)	16	90	1440
G4 PPI (SGalCer)	32	70	2240
G5 PPI (SGalCer)	64	20	1280
Dextran sulfate	170	1.6	272

[a]N is the number of functional groups.

The authors assumed that the lower inhibition induced by the nonsulfated glycodendrimers was related to their inability to block the interaction of the positively charged V3-loop of gp120 with sulfated tyrosine residues of the *N*-terminus of the CCR5 chemokine co-receptors, which are negatively charged [106]. Following these findings, another generation 5 PPI dendrimer presenting 64 SGalGer moieties with an average of two sulfate groups per galactose residue was prepared [107]. In the most favorable case, that is the inhibition of infection with an X4R5 HIV-1 strain on cell lines expressing CCR5, the IC_{50} of the dendrimer was measured at 0.6 nm (RIC_{50} = 38.4 nM), whereas DxS had an IC_{50} of 2.0 nm (RIC_{50} = 340 nM).

6.3.2 From Covalent GalCer Analogs to Catanionic GalCer Analogs

6.3.2.1 Synthesis and characterization of catanionic GalCer analogs

The design of multivalent analogs of GalCer was inspired by the pioneer research work, in the early 1990s, of Gonzalez-Scarano, who synthetized the first soluble analogs of GalCer. In order to enhance water solubility and avoid enzymatic degradation, this analog was designed lacking a fatty acid group and bearing a β-C-glycosidic. Although the IC_{50} obtained for this analog was not outstanding, the *in vitro* biological tests validated the approach of using these synthetic ligands as inhibitors of HIV infection [108]. Consequently, different synthetic strategies to prepare GalCer analogs have been developed, expanding the knowledge on the structural elements required for gp120 recognition [109]: a D-galactose moiety, a β-glycosidic linkage, and a controlled hydrophilic/hydrophobic balance. Nevertheless, among all these strategies, the major synthetic difficulty in preparing GalCer analogs lies in the grafting of second hydrophobic chain via the ceramide junction. In the late 1990s, Blanzat *et al.* developed an innovative strategy based on the non-covalent binding of the two parts of the analog, producing soluble ion-pair analogs of GalCer, the so-called catanionic analogs [110].

The concept of catanionic surfactants was introduced and defined in 1987 by Jokela *et al.*, as an equimolar mixture of two oppositely charged surfactants, from which the inorganic counterions have been removed [111]. Catanionic surfactants are then uncharged and can be considered ionocovalent equivalents of double-chain surfactants (Fig. 6.7). The electrostatic interaction as well as the hydrophobic effect between alkyl chains in water ensures the integrity of this "supramolecule." Since the introduction of this concept in the late 1980s, catanionic systems have received increasing attention partly because of their various aggregated microstructures (micelles, vesicles, nanodiscs, etc.) [112–114] and also for their enhanced surface active properties [115].

Considering the catanionic amphiphile preparation, four methods have been described in the literature [115]: the extraction method, the precipitation method, the often-employed ion-exchange method [116], and the proton exchange method developed by Blanzat *et al.* for the preparation of GalCer analogs [117].

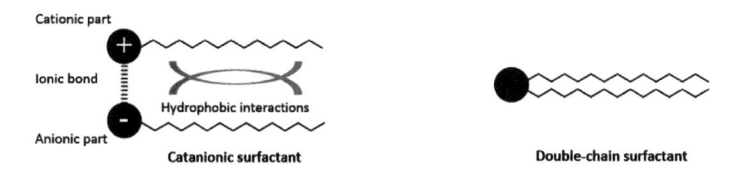

Figure 6.7 Schematic representations of a catanionic surfactant and the equivalent double-chain surfactant.

The first example of catanionic analog of GalCer was thus prepared by mixing equimolar quantities of *N*-alkylamino-1-deoxylactitol surfactant with a fatty acid in water. The completion of the acid–base reaction is driven by hydrophobic effects and van der Waals interactions and is accompanied by the total solubilization of the insoluble starting fatty acid. This supramolecular surfactant, perfectly stable for months as a white powder, was fully characterized by ^{1}H NMR, ^{13}C NMR, and electrospray mass spectrometry. Typically, clear evidence of catanionic formation could be found in the shifts observed for the carboxyl carbons in the ^{13}C NMR spectra: from about 175 ppm for the carboxylic acid neutral form to about 185 ppm for the negatively charged carboxylate forms observed in the catanionic analog of GalCer [110]. In mass spectrometry, observation of neutral non-covalent complexes requires its cationization, by adding low amounts of sodium iodide, as the sodium ion has a strong affinity for sugars [118]. For this catanionic analog of GalCer, a peak at m/z

622 was obtained for its sodium adduct [110], providing evidence for ionic association of the two-chain catanionic glycolipid.

6.3.2.2 Self-association properties of catanionic GalCer analogs

Among the large diversity of aggregates that catanionic surfactants can form in water, vesicles show good stability and dispersion properties in aqueous phase, which make them potential candidates for drug delivery [119].

During the extensive synthetic screening to prepare active catanionic GalCer analogs, a large diversity of catanionic vesicles bearing galactose moieties on their surface have been obtained [120–122]. Physicochemical studies performed on these nanovectors have proved their capacity to encapsulate whether hydrophilic compounds in their aqueous core [123], or hydrophobic drugs inside their bilayer [124], validating them as new candidates for drug delivery.

Considering HIV as a cellular pathology, rather than a viral pathology, the approach would consist in destroying or curing HIV-infected cells. Targeting HIV-infected cells can be performed by targeting gp120, expressed on the surface of HIV as well as HIV-infected cells. This strategy has been developed by Bronshtein *et al.* with CCR5-conjugated cell derived liposomes, which naturally bind viral glycoprotein gp120 [125]. The authors have proved that these CCR5-derived liposomes can specifically bind and fuse with their target cells and subsequently deliver their content into the infected cells leading to their destruction. First *in vitro* efficacy results of such system were obtained using EDTA as an encapsulated drug, which also significantly reduces the viability of controls. Although the selectivity of this drug could be improved, the *in vitro* biological tests validated the approach of using drug-delivery systems bearing CCR5 moieties to specifically target HIV-infected cells. With regard to the affinity of GalCer analogs with gp120, this strategy was also considered with catanionic vesicles bearing GalCer moieties on their surface [126]. As preliminary results in that direction, Mauroy *et al.* managed to form GalCer-derived catanionic vesicles capable of encapsulating active principles of various hydrophilicities and using different cellular uptake pathways to deliver them [123]. Especially, the authors could take advantage of the ability of these systems to fuse with cell membranes to specifically deliver anti-HIV drugs inside HIV-infected cells.

6.3.3 From Double-Chain to Multivalent Catanionic GalCer Analogs

Looking more specifically at the initial step of HIV-1 infection, cell adhesion occurs through the binding of the cell-surface receptor CD4 to the trimeric HIV-1 envelope glycoprotein gp120 [127]. To improve the affinity of the gp120/GalCer analogs and, therefore, their antiviral activities, different groups of research, as previously mentioned, have synthetized specific covalent multivalent analogs of GalCer. The resulting expected cooperative effects between the cell-surface proteins and the carbohydrate moieties validate the concept of multivalency for HIV entry inhibition [128–130].

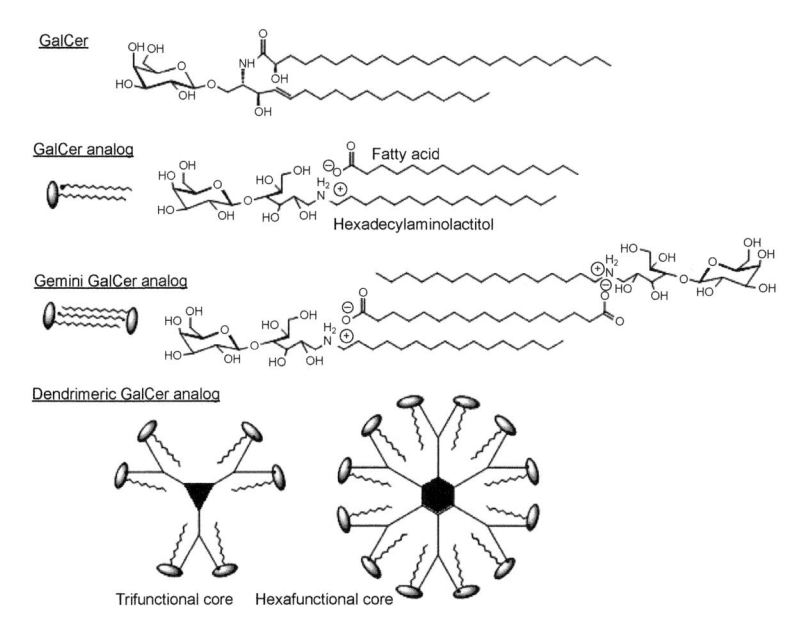

Figure 6.8 From monovalent catanionic GalCer analogs to multivalent GalCer analogs.

Concerning non-covalent multivalent analogs of GalCer, an extensive screening of the structural parameters influencing the anti-HIV activity has been performed. From preliminary information obtained from biological *in vitro* tests on two-chain catanionic analogs of GalCer, the authors showed that the cellular toxicity of these analogs, associated with an increased lipophilicity, reduces their efficacy. In order to counterbalance this lack of selectivity, Blanzat *et al.* proposed to improve the affinity of the gp120/GalCer analogs by doubling the number of GalCer moieties (gemini catanionic analog, Fig. 6.8) [110]. The first progress was achieved with a higher antiviral activity for this family of more complex catanionic systems. And these analogs were even more efficient as *in vitro* tests proved that the toxicity was not only governed by the hydrophobicity of the system. Indeed, a highly hydrophobic gemini displays both a high anti-HIV activity (IC_{50} = 0.5 μM) and a low cytotoxicity (CC50 > 100 μM), with an *in vitro* antiviral efficiency similar to that of DDI, a drug already used in anti-HIV polytherapies [131]. The supramolecular arrangement of the catanionic analog, namely the distribution of the hydrophilic and the hydrophobic parts, was proved to play a crucial role in the healthy cell disturbing functions of these analogs [126, 132, 133].

After the promising results obtained with doubling the number of GalCer moieties, the strategy was obviously to synthesize multivalent catanionic analogs of GalCer.

6.4 First Examples of Multivalent Catanionic Analogs of GalCer

As in the case of simple catanionic systems, the design of multivalent catanionic GalCer analogs is, to some extent, governed by two main features: peripheral acidic functions and a rather lipophilic scaffold. In addition, the acidic peripheral functions should be accessible to favor stable ion-pairing. In the case of PPH dendrimers, a rapid and simplified calculation of the peripheral surface per terminal group, applying de Gennes' [134] early theory on branched molecules indicates that each surface group of a Gn (n<5) PPH dendrimer with a trifunctional core has an average available surface of 600 A^2, whereas this value is lowered to approximately 300 A^2 in the case of Gc_n (n<5) dendrimers with a hexafunctional core. Taking in account the lipophilic character of PPH scaffolds, the absence of peripheral steric hindrance and the ability of PPH dendrimers to accommodate their interior to encapsulate large lipophilic molecules, PPH dendrimers are suitable candidates for the design of multivalent catanionic species.

6.4.1 Synthesis and Characterization

Carboxylic acid–capped PPH dendrimers can be readily obtained from aldehyde-terminated dendrimers following the Doebner modification to the Knoevenagel condensation (Fig. 6.9) [135].

The resulting cinnamic acid–capped dendrimers **1-Gn** are unambiguously characterized by NMR and FTIR. Typically, the singlet of the aldehyde proton at 9.9 ppm is replaced by a set of doublet at 6.6 and 7.7 ppm for the vinylic system ($^3J_{HHtrans}$ = 17.1 Hz), while the carboxylic acids are characterized on FTIR spectra by vibration bands at 1686, 1304, and 923 cm^{-1}. These compounds show good solubility in organic solvent, whereas they are insoluble in water [70]. The corresponding catanionic GalCer analogs **1-*Gal*-Gn** and **2-*Gal*-Gn** are obtained by proton exchange of the acidic dendrimers with a stoichiometric amount of *N*-hexadecylaminolactitol in water at room temperature (Fig. 6.10). The formation of the supramolecule is macroscopically traduced by the solubilization of both reactants, which are initially insoluble in water. The ion-pairing between carboxylate and ammonium entities can be monitored by NMR or FTIR spectroscopies.

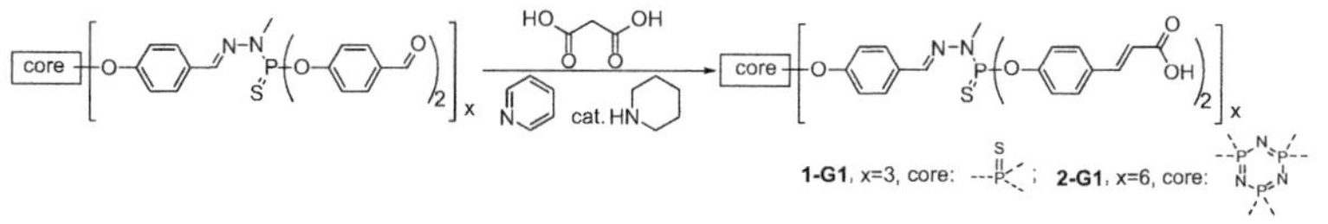

Figure 6.9 From aldehyde to cinnamic acid–terminated PPH dendrimers.

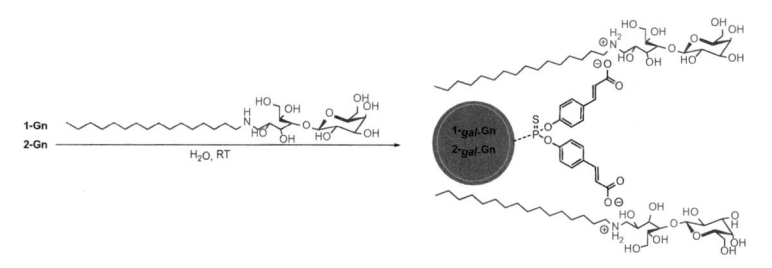

Figure 6.10 From aldehyde-terminated dendrimers to multivalent catanionic GalCer analogs.

6.4.2   First Biological Results

The HIV inhibition activities (IC_{50}) and cytotoxicities (CC_{50}) of both catanionic dendrimer families were evaluated *in vitro* on human T4-lymphoblastoid cell line [72]. These values as well as the *in vitro* therapeutic index (TI = CC_{50}/IC_{50}) are listed in Table 6.2, along with the results previously obtained for the free *N*-hexadecylaminolactitol moiety **L16** [136]. The RIC_{50} value, obtained by multiplying the IC_{50} values by the number of GalCer moieties N, allows the formal comparison of activities per active site.

Table 6.2   Classical HIV-1 inhibition and cytotoxicity results for free aminolactitol **L16** and dendrimers **1-*Gal*-Gn** and **2-*Gal*-Gn**

Compound	N^a	IC_{50}	$RIC_{50}{}^b$	CC_{50}	TI
L16	1	50	50	70	1.4
1-*Gal*-G1	6	2.1	12.6	3.5	1.7
1-*Gal*-G2	12	1.1	13.2	2.9	2.6
2-*Gal*-G0	6	0.37	2.22	9.3	25
2-*Gal*-G1	12	0.12	1.44	3.9	32

^{a}N is the number of terminal aminolactitol moieties. ^{b}RIC_{50} = N × IC_{50}, µM.

The inhibition activity is related to the number of GalCer moieties on the periphery of the dendrimers for both families of dendritic associations, **1-*Gal*-Gn** and **2-*Gal*-Gn**. The anti-HIV activity is actually doubled when growing one dendritic generation from the first to the second (IC_{50}(**1c-G2**) = 1.1 µM and IC_{50}(**1-*Gal*-G1**) = 2.1 µM) for the trifunctional cored assemblies, and at the same time the number of terminal sugar moieties is also doubled. This point is illustrated by identical RIC_{50} values for the **1-*Gal*-Gn** series. Likewise, the RIC_{50} values calculated for both compounds **2-*Gal*-G0** and **2-*Gal*-G1** having a cyclotriphosphazene core are in the same range, but they are significantly lower. Besides, all dendritic assemblies exhibit RIC_{50} values that are lower than the IC_{50} of the aminolactitol **L16**. According to these observations, the anti-HIV activity of multisite dendritic analogs was found to be better than the total sum of the activities of the equivalent monomeric analogs in the same stoichiometric ratios. On the one hand, these results confirmed the already reported and discussed multivalency effect [137] on the therapeutical activity of these dendritic inhibitors. On the other hand, the significant gap between the RIC_{50} calculated for both series **1-*Gal*-Gn** and **2-*Gal*-Gn** was attributed to the variability of shape of these dendritic assemblies, according to the type of core. Actually, the molecular models obtained after minimization in water indicated that thiophosphoryle-cored dendrimers **1-*Gal*-Gn** exhibited a cauliflower-like shape, whereas cyclotriphosphazene-cored dendrimers **2-*Gal*-Gn** were found to be more cylindrical (Fig. 6.11).

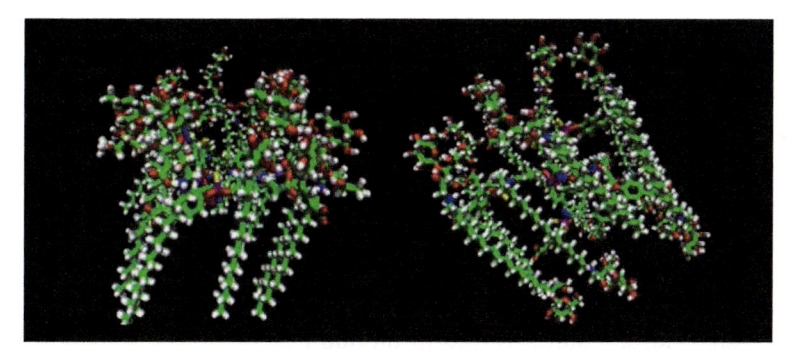

Figure 6.11 Molecular models obtained after minimization in water of the trifunctional cored assembly **1-*Gal*-G2** and the hexafunctional cored assembly **2-*Gal*-G1**.

The relative lack of activity observed for dendrimers **1-*Gal*-G2** and **2-*Gal*-G2** was associated to their non-globular structure, leading to different localization and distribution of the sugar heads, a topological feature that was assumed to be crucial for the accessibility of the active sites of the gp120.

6.4.3 The Question of Ion-Pair Stability

Even though the series of four catanionic dendrimers exhibited good anti-HIV activities, quite low therapeutic indexes were measured due to the relatively high CC_{50} values. In this first study, dendrimers **1-*Gal*-G1** and **1-*Gal*-G2** exhibited TI in the critical range, 1.5 and 3, respectively, whereas dendrimers **2-*Gal*-G0** and **2-*Gal*-G1** displayed TI significantly higher than 20. However, whatever the dendrimer core or the catanionic assembly shape, these compounds exhibited CC_{50} in the 1–10 μM range. This concentration is in the range of the CC_{50} of the free aminolactitol **L16** involved in the catanionic assemblies, which is known to have a detergent behavior [122]. Taking into account that for compounds with TI below 10, the antiviral activity can possibly be due to strong toxicity, and that the cinnamic-acid-terminated PPH dendrimers are non-cytotoxic, like many other anionic dendrimers [138–140], the cytotoxicity observed for these first series of dendrimers was assumed to be related to a possible release of free aminolactitol. In other words, a possible lack of stability of the non-covalent catanionic assembly was early identified as a cause for the low TIs.

6.5 Assessing the Ion-Pair Stability Hypothesis with Other Catanionic Dendrimers

6.5.1 Alternative Systems with Phosphonic Acids

In order to explore the influence of the chemical environment of the acid function involved in the ion-pairing on the activity of these catanionic systems, other phosphonic acid–terminated PPH dendrimers have been designed, some of them with lateral alkyl chains [73, 141, 142]. The presence of the alkyl chain was expected to increase the stability of the ion-pairing system by lipophilic interaction with the alkyl chains of the aminolactitol **L16**. The first **3-G1** series with vinyl-phosphonic acid surface functions (Fig. 6.12) was prepared from aldehyde-terminated PPH dendrimers using the Horner–Wadsworth–Emmons reaction with tetramethyl methylene bis(phosphonate). This procedure is somehow similar to the synthetic route to cinnamic acid–terminated dendrimers and afforded isosteric analogs after a demethylation procedure involving complete silylation of the phosphonates [143]. Another series (**4-G1** to **6-G1**) was obtained by grafting phosphonate derivatives [142] having a vicinal pendant alkyl chain and equipped with a suitable phenol function on $P(S)Cl_2$-terminated PPH dendrimers (Fig. 6.12). In all cases, NMR proved to be an efficient tool to monitor reactions and characterize the compounds [144].

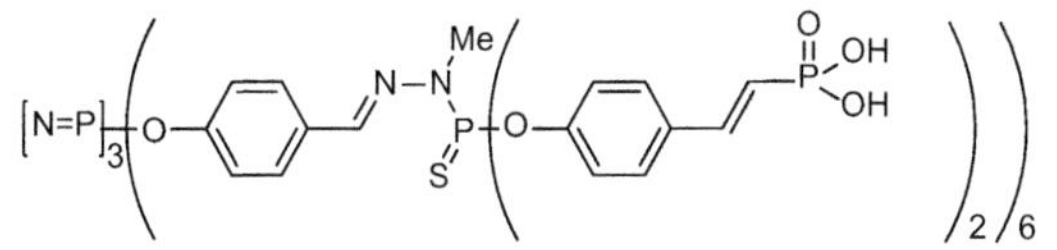

Figure 6.12 Phosphonic acid–terminated PPH dendrimers as alternative precursors for the preparation of multivalent GalCer analogs.

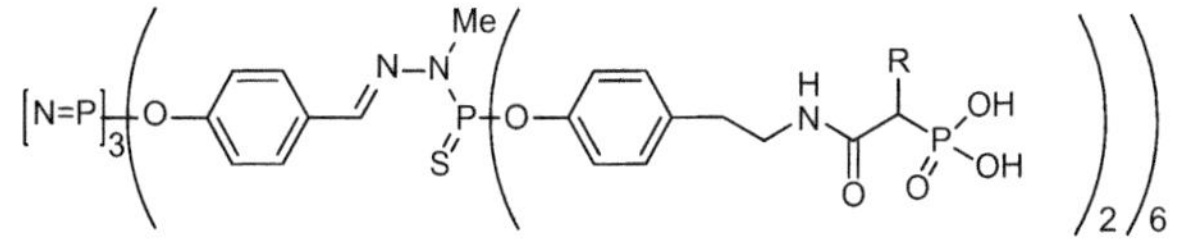

6.5.2 Biological Properties

6.5.2.1 Biological properties of polyanionic dendrimers involved in the catanionic systems

The sodium salts **X-*Na*-G1** of the corresponding **X-G1** acid–terminated dendrimers (X = 1 to 6) were assayed *in vitro* on human T4-lymphoblastoid cell line to assess their inhibitory effect against HIV-1 [142]. Interestingly, none of these compounds was found to be toxic in the whole range of concentrations (1×10^{-7} to 1×10^{-4} mol·L^{-1}). Consequently, the measured IC$_{50}$ could be correlated to an effective antiviral activity. Among this series, the IC$_{50}$ values were found to slightly depend on the chemical nature of phosphonate's vicinity. The influence of the alkyl chain (Table 6.3, entries 7–9) had already been evoked in other studies [142] and was assumed to be linked to its ability to interact with the lipophilic region of the V3 loop of gp120.

The vinyl phosphonate–terminated dendrimer (Table 6.3, entry 6) showed a good inhibitory activity (650 nmol·L^{-1}), typically in the range of activity of reference polyanion compounds [145], like PRO 2000 or DxS. Interestingly, the therapeutic index of **3-*Na*-G1** measured by default at 153 was found to be one order of magnitude lower than the target value of 1000 [146], whereas all other compounds had significantly lower TIs.

Table 6.3 HIV-1 inhibition and cytotoxicity of PPH dendrimers (sodium salts and catanionic GalCer analogs)

Entry	Compound	N^a	IC_{50}	CC_{50}	$RIC_{50}{}^b$	TI
1	**L$_{16}$**	1	50	70	50	1.4
2	**1-*Na*-G1**	6	7.5	>100	45	>13.4
3	**1-*Na*-G2**	12	–	–	–	–
4	**2-*Na*-G0**	6	–	–	–	–
5	**2-*Na*-G1**	12	–	–	–	–
6	**3-*Na*-G1**	12	0.65	>100	7.8	>153
7	**4-*Na*-G1**	12	25	>100	300	>4
8	**5-*Na*-G1**	12	1.5	>100	18	>67
9	**6-*Na*-G1**	12	16	>100	192	>6
10	**1-*Gal*-G1**	6	2.1	3.5	12.6	1.7
11	**1-*Gal*-G2**	12	1.1	2.9	13.2	2.6
12	**2-*Gal*-G0**	6	0.37	2.2	9.3	25
13	**2-*Gal*-G1**	12	0.12	1.4	1.4	32
14	**3-*Gal*-G1**	12	0.25	1.6	3.9	6.4
15	**4-*Gal*-G1**	12	0.40	1.9	4.8	4.8
16	**5-*Gal*-G1**	12	0.33	1.5	3.9	4.5
17	**6-*Gal*-G1**	12	0.31	6.1	3.7	19.7

[a]N is the number of terminal aminolactitol moieties
[b]$RIC_{50} = N \times IC_{50}$, μM

6.5.2.2 Biological properties of catanionic systems

The **X-*Gal*-Gn** (X = 1 to 6) series of catanionic multivalent GalCer analog compounds were assayed according to the same procedure (Table 6.3, entries 10 to 17). All compounds exhibited a relatively good anti-HIV-1 activity between 0.12 μM (Table 6.3, entry 13) and 0.40 μM (Table 6.3, entry 15), but their TIs were found to be dramatically affected by CC_{50} values. The most probable reason was assumed to be related to the possible lack of stability of the supramolecular assemblies in cell cultures, as stated earlier. As a result, the systems could eventually disassemble into dendrimeric phosphonates for which no cytotoxicity has been observed (Table 6.2, entries 1 to 6), and free *N*-hexadecylaminolactitol, which could be responsible for the relatively high CC_{50}. Assuming that a hypothetic complete disassembly of the catanionic systems would lead to 12 free *N*-hexadecylaminolactitol, the relative CC50 of the dissembled **X-*Gal*-G1** series should then be corrected by a factor of 12-fold, leading to CC50 that are in the range of *N*-hexadecylamino-lactitol, which is known to be cytotoxic on CEM-SS cells in the 10^{-4}–10^{-5} mol·L^{-1} range due to its detergent properties [72].

The results obtained *in vitro* clearly showed that the local environment of the negative charges, that is, the chemical nature of the phosphonate or the carboxylate neighboring groups, had a low impact on the biological activity of the corresponding catanionic multivalent analogs [5]. Actually, the GalCer analog series **1-*Gal*-G1** to **6-*Gal*-G1** showed good HIV-1 inhibitory properties in the submicromolar range, despite significant modifications of the nature of the acidic surface groups. These changes were implemented in order to increase the stability of the ion-pairing systems and subsequently modify their biological activities. Unfortunately, these systems were found to be all impaired by quite low therapeutic indexes originating from relatively high cytotoxicity values.

6.5.3 Self-Assembly Properties

The question addressed was to evaluate the contribution of the self-association properties of these catanionic systems upon their biological properties, in order to elucidate the origin of the fair, yet rather constant despite surface function modifications, IC$_{50}$ values, and the quite impairing CC$_{50}$ values.

The contribution of the lateral alkyl chains on the self-association properties of the catanionic dendrimers was evaluated by freeze-fracture experiments. For both **4-*Gal*-G1** and **5-*Gal*-G1**, spherical vesicles of 100–200 nm diameters were obtained, along with smaller aggregates (~50 nm) in the case of **5-*Gal*-G1** (Fig. 6.13). The small C3 chains were assumed to disturb the self-aggregation properties leading possibly to a partial segregation of the different partners of the catanionic entity, which were subsequently non-homogeneously distributed among the aggregates.

Concerning the particular case of catanionic dendrimer **6-*Gal*-G1**, less homogeneous samples were observed (Fig. 6.14), with a well-ordered set of fracturable and non-fracturable large multilamellar vesicles (few micrometers) coexisting with smaller fracturable unilamellar vesicles (Fig. 6.14). Based on these results, it was concluded that the long alkyl chains could possibly disturb the arrangement of the dendrimer with the aminosugar **L16** in the vesicular bilayer. The non-homogeneous distribution of both molecules in the bilayer, resulting from the steric hindrance generated by the additional C10 alkyl chains, could then lead to coexistence of dendrimer-rich areas and sugar-surfactant-rich areas.

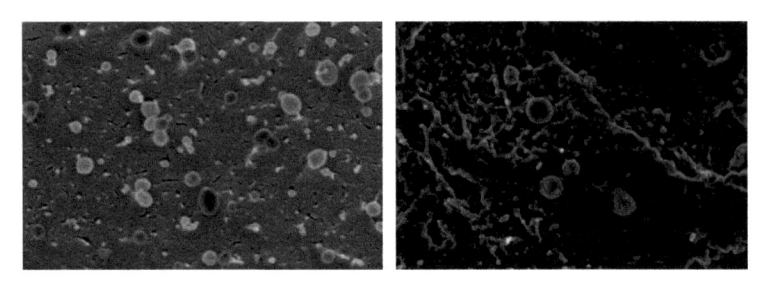

Figure 6.13 SEM images obtained after freeze-fracture of the samples for (left) **4-*Gal*-G1** and (right) **5-*Gal*-G1** at 1×10^{-3} M.

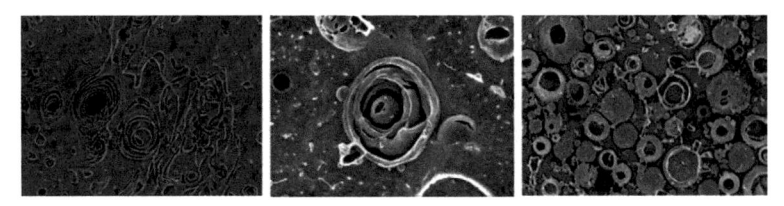

Figure 6.14 SEM images obtained after freeze-fracture of the samples for **6-*Gal*-G1** at 5×10^{-4} M.

From a biological point of view, the absence of correlation between the hydrophobic enhancement and the decrease in the cytotoxicity could find a possible explanation in this phenomenon. These physicochemical studies interestingly evidenced the fact that a partial segregation of the different partners of the catanionic entity occurs in aqueous solution for **6-*Gal*-G1** and also for **5-*Gal*-G1** to a lesser extent. In more diluted media such as in cell cultures in which concentrations are much lower that the CAC, it was anticipated that this tendency would also lead to partial dissociation of the ion-pairing system. These results strengthened the relevance of this hypothesis formulated earlier.

6.5.4 Confirming the Hypothesis with K_D Measurements

In order to shed light on the ion-pair disassembly issue, the K_D of representative anti-HIV-1 catanionic dendrimers were finally measured experimentally with model compound by fluorimetric titration. In this regard, a fluorescent analog of *N*-hexadecylaminolactitol **L16-FL** was designed, with suitable size parameters and hydrophilic–lipophilic balance (Fig. 6.15).

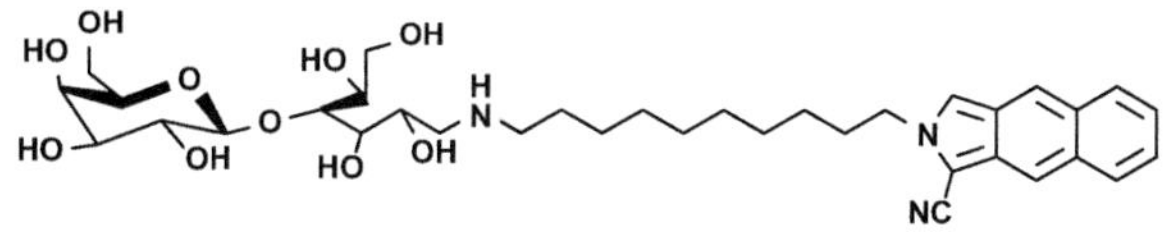

Figure 6.15   Fluorescent analog of *N*-hexadecylaminolactitol **L16-FL**.

The results highlighted the unexpected absence of influence of the dendrimeric scaffold, with K_D values all in the micromolar range, between 7.9 µM and 28.8 µM (Table 6.4). The lowest value associated to the most stable dendrimer-**L16-FL** stoichiometric assembly was obtained with dendrimer **2-G1**. This observation is counterintuitive considering the pK_a differences between acid dendrimers and the aminosugar, and it was due to steric demand issues. In this regard, the small, yet significant increase in K_D from **3-G1** to **6-G1** was related to the greater steric demand imposed by the presence of the alkyl chains.

Table 6.4 K_D values obtained by titration binding assay with **L16-FL**

Entry	Dendrimer	K_D (µM)
1	**2-G1**	7.9 ± 1.4
2	**3-G1**	28.8 ± 3.6
2	**4-G1**	12.5 ± 1.4
4	**5-G1**	16.5 ± 2.8
5	**6-G1**	24.8 ± 3.1

Although correlations between former biological results obtained with dendrimer-**L16** assemblies and this stability study involving a coumarin-modified derivative **L16-FL** required caution because of significant structural differences between both aminolactitols, it was concluded that these model study comforted the partial ion-pair disassembly hypothesis and subsequent release of free *N*-hexadecylaminolactitol. This disassembly was assumed to be responsible for the low TI measured for these dendrimer-based catanionic HIV-1 inhibitors. Actually, such systems are expected to compete in culture media with other ligands, which may show much stronger affinities for any of the two partners involved in the catanionic assembly, a competition that could lead to ion-pair redistribution. Taking into account that these inhibitors have a higher antiviral efficiency than the covalent dendrimeric analogs of GalCer [99], the catanionic approach could still be a relevant strategy provided that robust ion-pairing systems are involved.

6.6 Conclusion

Among the antiviral approaches to block the HIV infection, targeting the early interactions of the virus with host cells is a promising field of investigation for anti-HIV strategies. And among the large variety of molecules that are currently developed according to this approach, dendrimers have proved to be efficient multivalent inhibitors of early steps. In particular, a strategy that proposes to use the affinity of the virus for GalCer to inhibit HIV entry into cells has been widely discussed in this chapter. The strategy consists in simplifying the inhibitory systems to the key elements required for the virus–cell recognition, using a non-covalent approach with multivalent analogs of GalCer. This strategy confirmed the antiviral potential of such systems with a limitation due to their non-negligible toxicity attributed to a partial ion-pair disassembly in cell culture. One of the key issues for the design of multivalent GalCer catanionic analogs is thus to overcome this discrepancy. In this regard, the examples evoked earlier show that recent research on PPH-based catanionic dendrimer analogs of GalCer has allowed refining the design of such systems programmed to inhibit HIV entry and thus HIV infection.

References

1. Gallo, R. C. and Montagnier, L. (2003). The discovery of HIV as the cause of AIDS, *New Engl. J. Med.,* **349**, pp. 2283–2285.

2. http://kff.org/global-health-policy/fact-sheet/the-global-hivaids-epidemic/.

3. Bourne, N., Stanberry, L. R., Kern, E. R., Holan, G., Matthews, B., and Bernstein, D. I. (2000). Dendrimers, a new class of candidate topical microbicides with activity against herpes simplex virus infection, *Antimicrob. Agents Chemother.,* **44**, pp. 2471–2474.

4. Bernstein, D. I., Bourne, N., Ayisi, N. K., Ireland, J., Matthews, B., McCarthy, T., and Sacks, S. (2003). Evaluation of formulated dendrimer SPL7013 as a microbicide, *Antiviral Res.,* **57**, p. A66.

5. Perez-Anes, A., Stefaniu, C., Moog, C., Majoral, J.-P., Blanzat, M., Turrin, C.-O., Caminade, A.-M., and Rico-Lattes, I. (2010). Multivalent catanionic GalCer analogs derived from first generation dendrimeric phosphonic acids, *Bioorg. Med. Chem.,* **18**, pp. 242–248.

6. Borges, A. R., Wieczorek, L., Johnson, B., Benesi, A. J., Brown, B. K., Kensinger, R. D., Krebs, F. C., Wigdahl, B., Blumenthal, R., Puri, A., McCutchan, F. E., Birx, D. L., Polonis, V. R., and Schengrund, C.-L. (2010). Multivalent dendrimeric compounds containing carbohydrates expressed on immune cells inhibit infection by primary isolates of HIV-1, *Virology,* **408**, pp. 80–88.

7. Sepulveda-Crespo, D., Gomez, R., De La Mata, F. J., Jimenez, J. L., and Munoz-Fernandez, M. A. (2015). Polyanionic carbosilane dendrimer-conjugated antiviral drugs as efficient microbicides: Recent trends and developments in HIV treatment/therapy, *Nanomedicine,* **11**, pp. 1481–1498.

8. Yahi, N., Fantini, J., Baghdiguian, S., Mabrouk, K., Tamalet, C., Rochat, H., van Rietschoten, J., and Sabatier, J. M. (1995). SPC3, a synthetic peptide derived from the V3 domain of human immunodeficiency virus type 1 (HIV-1) gp120, inhibits HIV-1 entry into CD4+ and CD4- cells by two distinct mechanisms, *Proc. Natl. Acad. Sci. USA,* **92**, pp. 4867–4871.

9. Dzmitruk, V., Shcharbin, D., Pedziwiatr-Werbicka, E., and Bryszewska, M. (2011). Dendrimers in anti-HIV therapy, In: *Nanotechnology and Nanomaterials: Advances in Nanocomposite Technology* (InTech).

10. Peng, J., Wu, Z., Qi, X., Chen, Y., and Li, X. (2013). Dendrimers as potential therapeutic tools in HIV inhibition, *Molecules,* **18**, pp. 7912–7929.

11. Liang, Y., Narayanasamy, J., Rapp, K. L., Schinazi, R. F., and Chu, C. K. (2006). PAMAM dendrimers and branched polyethyleneglycol (nanoparticles) prodrugs of (-)-beta-D-(2R, 4R)-dioxolane-thymine (DOT) and their anti-HIV activity, *Antiviral Chem. Chemother.,* **17**, pp. 321–329.

12. Dutta, T. and Jain, N. K. (2007). Targeting potential and anti-HIV activity of lamivudine loaded mannosylated poly (propyleneimine) dendrimer, *Biochim. Biophys. Acta, Gen. Subj.,* **1770**, pp. 681–686.

13. Shcharbin, D., Dzmitruk, V., Shakhbazau, A., Goncharova, N., Seviaryn, I., Kosmacheva, S., Potapnev, M., Pedziwiatr-Werbicka, E., Bryszewska, M., Talabaev, M., Chernov, A., Kulchitsky, V., Caminade, A. M., and Majoral, J. P. (2011). Fourth generation phosphorus-containing dendrimers: Prospective drug and gene delivery carrier, *Pharmaceutics,* **3**, pp. 458–473.

14. Judith Perise-Barrios, A., Luis Jimenez, J., Dominguez-Soto, A., Javier de la Mata, F., Corbi, A. L., Gomez, R., and Angeles Munoz-Fernandez, M. (2014). Carbosilane dendrimers as gene delivery agents for the treatment of HIV infection, *J. Control. Release,* **184**, pp. 51–57.

15. Caminade, A. M., Turrin, C. O., and Majoral, J. P. (2008). Dendrimers and DNA: Combinations of two special topologies for nanomaterials and biology, *Chem. Eur. J.,* **14**, pp. 7422–7432.

16. Liu, X. and Peng, L. (2016). Dendrimer nanovectors for SiRNA delivery, *Methods Mol. Biol.,* **1364**, pp. 127–142.

17. Kang, H. M., DeLong, R., Fisher, M. H., and Juliano, R. L. (2005). Tat-conjugated PAMAM dendrimers as delivery agents for antisense and siRNA oligonucleotides, *Pharm. Res.,* **22**, pp. 2099–2106.

18. Wang, J., Lu, Z., Wientjes, M. G., and Au, J. L. S. (2010). Delivery of siRNA therapeutics: Barriers and carriers, *Aaps J.,* **12**, pp. 492–503.

19. Sharp, P. A. (2001). RNA interference—2001, *Genes Dev.,* **15**, pp. 485–490.

20. Coburn, G. A. and Cullen, B. R. (2003). siRNAs: A new wave of RNA-based therapeutics, *J. Antimicrob. Chemother.,* **51**, pp. 753–756.

21. Lee, M. T. M., Coburn, G. A., McClure, M. O., and Cullen, B. R. (2003). Inhibition of human immunodeficiency virus type 1 replication in primary macrophages by using Tat- or CCR5-specific small interfering RNAs expressed from a lentivirus vector, *J. Virol.,* **77**, pp. 11964–11972.

22. Han, W. L., Wind-Rotolo, M., Kirkman, R. L., and Morrow, C. D. (2004). Inhibition of human immunodeficiency virus type 1 replication by siRNA targeted to the highly conserved primer binding site, *Virology,* **330**, pp. 221–232.

23. DeVreese, K., KoflerMongold, V., Leutgeb, C., Weber, V., Vermeire, K., Schacht, S., Anne, J., DeClercq, E., Datema, R., and Werner, G. (1996). The molecular target of bicyclams, potent inhibitors of human immunodeficiency virus replication, *J. Virol.,* **70**, pp. 689–696.

24. Bermejo, J. F., Ortega, P., Chonco, L., Eritja, R., Samaniego, R., Mullner, M., de Jesus, E., de la Mata, F. J., Flores, J. C., Gomez, R., and Munoz-Fernandez, A. (2007). Water-soluble carbosilane dendrimers: Synthesis biocompatibility and complexation with oligonucleotides; Evaluation for medical applications, *Chem. Eur. J.*, **13**, pp. 483–495.

25. Chonco, L., Bermejo-Martin, J. F., Ortega, P., Shcharbin, D., Pedziwiatr, E., Klajnert, B., de la Mata, F. J., Eritja, R., Gomez, R., Bryszewska, M., and Munoz-Fernandez, M. A. (2007). Water-soluble carbosilane dendrimers protect phosphorothioate oligonucleotides from binding to serum proteins, *Org. Biomol. Chem.*, **5**, pp. 1886–1893.

26. Shcharbin, D., Pedziwiatr, E., Chonco, L., Bermejo-Martin, J., Ortega, P., de la Mata, F., Eritja, R., Gomez, R., Klajnert, B., and Munoz-Fernandez, M. (2007). Dendriplex of ODNs/carbosilane dendrimers does not interact with albumin, *Febs J.*, **274**, pp. 263–263.

27. Weber, N., Ortega, P., Clemente, M. I., Shcharbin, D., Bryszewska, M., de la Mata, F. J., Gomez, R., and Munoz-Fernandez, M. A. (2008). Characterization of carbosilane dendrimers as effective carriers of siRNA to HIV-infected lymphocytes, *J. Control. Release,* **132**, pp. 55–64.

28. Gonzalo, T., Isabel Clemente, M., Chonco, L., Weber, N. D., Diaz, L., Jesus Serramia, M., Gras, R., Ortega, P., Javier de la Mata, F., Gomez, R., Lopez-Fernandez, L. A., Angeles Munoz-Fernandez, M., and Luis Jimenez, J. (2010). Gene therapy in HIV-infected cells to decrease viral impact by using an alternative delivery method, *ChemMedChem,* **5**, pp. 921–929.

29. Chonco, L., Pion, M., Vacas, E., Rasines, B., Maly, M., Serramia, M. J., Lopez-Fernandez, L., De la Mata, J., Alvarez, S., Gomez, R., and Munoz-Fernandez, M. A. (2012). Carbosilane dendrimer nanotechnology outlines of the broad HIV blocker profile, *J. Control. Release,* **161**, pp. 949–958.

30. Jimenez, J. L., Clemente, M. I., Weber, N. D., Sanchez, J., Ortega, P., de la Mata, F. J., Gomez, R., Garcia, D., Lopez-Fernandez, L. A., and Munoz-Fernandez, M. A. (2010). Carbosilane dendrimers to transfect human astrocytes with small interfering RNA targeting human immunodeficiency virus, *BioDrugs,* **24**, pp. 331–343.

31. Vacas-Cordoba, E., Climent, N., De La Mata, F. J., Plana, M., Gomez, R., Pion, M., Garcia, F., and Angeles Munoz-Fernandez, M. (2014). Dendrimers as nonviral vectors in dendritic cell-based immunotherapies against human immunodeficiency virus: Steps toward their clinical evaluation, *Nanomedicine,* **9**, pp. 2683–2702.

32. Vacas-Cordoba, E., Galan, M., de la Mata, F. J., Gomez, R., Pion, M., and Angeles Munoz-Fernandez, M. (2014). Enhanced activity of

carbosilane dendrimers against HIV when combined with reverse transcriptase inhibitor drugs: Searching for more potent microbicides, *Int. J. Nanomed.,* **9**, pp. 3591–3600.

33. Sanchez-Rodriguez, J., Diaz, L., Galan, M., Maly, M., Gomez, R., Javier de la Mata, F., Jimenez, J. L., and Angeles Munoz-Fernandez, M. (2015). Anti-human immunodeficiency virus activity of thiol-ene carbosilane dendrimers and their potential development as a topical microbicide, *J. Biomed. Nanotechnol.,* **11**, pp. 1783–1798.

34. Sepulveda-Crespo, D., Serramia, M. J., Tager, A. M., Vrbanac, V., Gomez, R., De La Mata, F. J., Jimenez, J. L., and Munoz-Fernandez, M. A. (2015). Prevention vaginally of HIV-1 transmission in humanized BLT mice and mode of antiviral action of polyanionic carbosilane dendrimer G2-S16, *Nanomedicine,* **11**, pp. 1299–1308.

35. Sepulveda-Crespo, D., Lorente, R., Leal, M., Gomez, R., De la Mata, F. J., Luis Jimenez, J., and Angeles Munoz-Fernandez, M. (2014). Synergistic activity profile of carbosilane dendrimer G2-STE16 in combination with other dendrimers and antiretrovirals as topical anti-HIV-1 microbicide, *Nanomedicine,* **10**, pp. 609–618.

36. Sepulveda-Crespo, D., Sanchez-Rodriguez, J., Jesus Serramia, M., Gomez, R., Javier De La Mata, F., Luis Jimenez, J., and Angeles Munoz-Fernandez, M. (2015). Triple combination of carbosilane dendrimers, tenofovir and maraviroc as potential microbicide to prevent HIV-1 sexual transmission, *Nanomedicine,* **10**, pp. 899–914.

37. Zhou, J., Neff, C. P., Liu, X., Zhang, J., Li, H., Smith, D. D., Swiderski, P., Aboellail, T., Huang, Y., Du, Q., Liang, Z., Peng, L., Akkina, R., and Rossi, J. J. (2011). Systemic administration of combinatorial dsiRNAs via nanoparticles efficiently suppresses HIV-1 infection in humanized mice, *Mol. Ther.,* **19**, pp. 2228–2238

38. Vacas-Cordoba, E., Bastida, H., Pion, M., Hameau, A., Ionov, M., Bryszewska, M., Caminade, A. M., Majoral, J. P., and Munoz-Fernandez, M.-A. (2014). HIV-antigens charged on phosphorus dendrimers as tools for tolerogenic dendritic cells-based immunotherapy, *Curr. Med. Chem.,* **21**, pp. 1898–1909.

39. Ciepluch, K., Ionov, M., Majoral, J.-P., Muñoz-Fernández, M. A., and Bryszewska, M. (2014). Interaction of phosphorus dendrimers with HIV peptides: Fluorescence studies of nano-complexes formation, *J. Luminescence,* **148**, pp. 364–369.

40. Ferenc, M., Pedziwiatr-Werbicka, E., Nowak, K., Klajnert, B., Majoral, J.-P., and Bryszewska, M. (2013). Phosphorus dendrimers as carriers of siRNA: Characterisation of dendriplexes, *Molecules,* **18**, pp. 4451.

41. Briz, V., Serramia, M. J., Madrid, R., Hameau, A., Caminade, A. M., Majoral, J. P., and Munoz-Fernandez, M. A. (2012). Validation of a generation 4 phosphorus-containing polycationic dendrimer for gene delivery against HIV-1, *Curr. Med. Chem.,* **19**, pp. 5044–5051.

42. Kojima, C. (2015). Preclinical studies of dendrimer prodrugs, *Expert Opin. Drug Metab. Toxicol.,* **11**, pp. 1303–1315.

43. Turrin, C.-O. and Caminade, A.-M. (2011). Dendrimer conjugates for drug delivery. In: A. M. Caminade, C. O. Turrin, R. Laurent, A. Ouali, and B. Delavaux-Nicot (Eds.), *Dendrimers* (pp. 437–461): John Wiley & Sons, Ltd.

44. Turrin, C.-O. and Caminade, A.-M. (2011). Encapsulation of drugs inside dendrimers. In A. M. Caminade, C. O. Turrin, R. Laurent, A. Ouali, and B. Delavaux-Nicot (Eds.), *Dendrimers* (pp. 463–484): John Wiley & Sons, Ltd.

45. Dutta, T., Agashe, H. B., Garg, M., Balasubramanium, P., Kabra, M., and Jain, N. K. (2007). Poly (propyleneimine) dendrimer based nanocontainers for targeting of efavirenz to human monocytes/ macrophages *in vitro, J. Drug Target.,* **15**, pp. 89–98.

46. Dutta, T., Garg, M., and Jain, N. K. (2008). Targeting of efavirenz loaded tuftsin conjugated poly(propyleneimine) dendrimers to HIV infected macrophages *in vitro, Eur. J. Pharm. Sci.,* **34**, pp. 181–189.

47. Frankel, A. D. and Young, J. A. T. (1998). HIV-1: Fifteen proteins and an RNA, *Annu. Rev. Biochem.,* **67**, pp. 1–25.

48. Zhao, H., Li, J. R., Xi, F., and Jiang, L. (2004). Polyamidoamine dendrimers inhibit binding of Tat peptide to TAR RNA, *Febs Lett.,* **563**, pp. 241–245.

49. Bannwarth, S. and Gatignol, A. (2005). HIV-1 TAR RNA: The target of molecular interactions between the virus and its host, *Curr. HIV Res.,* **3**, pp. 61–71.

50. Wang, W., Guo, Z., Chen, Y., Liu, T., and Jiang, L. (2006). Influence of generation 2–5 of PAMAM dendrimer on the inhibition of Tat peptide/ TAR RNA binding in HIV-1 transcription, *Chem. Biol. Drug Design,* **68**, pp. 314–318.

51. Wilen, C. B., Tilton, J. C., and Doms, R. W. (2012). HIV: Cell binding and entry, *Cold Spring Harb. Perspect. Med.,* **2**, a006866.

52. van Kooyk, Y. and Geijtenbeek, T. B. H. (2003). DC-SIGN: Escape mechanism for pathogens, *Nat. Rev. Immunol.,* **3**, pp. 697–709.

53. Geijtenbeek, T. B. H., Torensma, R., van Vliet, S. J., van Duijnhoven, G. C. F., Adema, G. J., van Kooyk, Y., and Figdor, C. G. (2000). Identification of

DC-SIGN, a novel dendritic cell-specific ICAM-3 receptor that supports primary immune responses, *Cell,* **100**, pp. 575–585.

54. Geijtenbeek, T. B. H., Kwon, D. S., Torensma, R., van Vliet, S. J., van Duijnhoven, G. C. F., Middel, J., Cornelissen, I., Nottet, H., KewalRamani, V. N., Littman, D. R., Figdor, C. G., and van Kooyk, Y. (2000). DC-SIGN, a dendritic cell-specific HIV-1-binding protein that enhances trans-infection of T cells, *Cell,* **100**, pp. 587–597.

55. Mathers, C. D. and Loncar, D. (2006). Projections of global mortality and burden of disease from 2002 to 2030, *PLoS Med.,* **3**.

56. Gallaher, W. R., Ball, J. M., Garry, R. F., Martinamedee, A. M., and Montelaro, R. C. (1995). A general-model for the surface glycoproteins of HIV and other retroviruses, *AIDS Res. Hum. Retrovir.,* **11**, pp. 191–202.

57. Moulard, M., Lortat-Jacob, H., Mondor, I., Roca, G., Wyatt, R., Sodroski, J., Lu, Z., Olson, W., Kwong, P. D., and Sattentau, Q. J. (2000). Selective interactions of polyanions with basic surfaces on human immunodeficiency virus type 1 gp120, *J. Virol.,* **74**, pp. 1948–1960.

58. Santhosh, K. C., Paul, G. C., De Clercq, E., Pannecouque, C., Witvrouw, M., Loftus, T. L., Turpin, J. A., Buckheit, R. W., and Cushman, M. (2001). Correlation of anti-HIV activity with anion spacing in a series of cosalane analogues with extended polycarboxylate pharmacophores, *J. Med. Chem.,* **44**, pp. 703–714.

59. Mitsuya, H., Popovic, M., Yarchoan, R., Matsushita, S., Gallo, R. C., and Broder, S. (1984). Suramin protection of T-cells *in vitro* against infectivity and cytopathic effect of HTLV-III, *Science,* **226**, pp. 172–174.

60. Broder, S., Collins, J. M., Markham, P. D., Redfield, R. R., Hoth, D. F., Groopman, J. E., Gallo, R. C., Yarchoan, R., Lane, H. C., Klecker, R. W., Mitsuya, H., Gelmann, E., Resnick, L., Myers, C. E., and Fauci, A. S. (1985). Effects of Suramin on HTLV-III/Lav infection presenting as kaposis sarcoma or aids-related complex: Clinical-pharmacology and suppression of virus-replication *in vivo, Lancet,* **2**, pp. 627–630.

61. De Clercq, E. (1998). Recent developments in the chemotherapy of HIV infections, *Pure Appl. Chem.,* **70**, pp. 567–577.

62. Pirrone, V., Wigdahl, B., and Krebs, F. C. (2011). The rise and fall of polyanionic inhibitors of the human immunodeficiency virus type 1, *Antiviral Res.,* **90**, pp. 168–182.

63. Sánchez-Rodríguez, J., Vacas-Córdoba, E., Gómez, R., De La Mata, F. J., and Muñoz-Fernández, M. Á. (2015). Nanotech-derived topical

microbicides for HIV prevention: The road to clinical development, *Antiviral Res.,* **113**, pp. 33–48.

64. McCarthy, T. D., Karellas, P., Henderson, S. A., Giannis, M., O'Keefe, D. F., Heery, G., Paull, J. R. A., Matthews, B. R., and Holan, G. (2005). Dendrimers as drugs: Discovery and preclinical and clinical development of dendrimer-based microbicides for HIV and STI prevention, *Mol. Pharm.,* **2**, pp. 312–318.

65. Rupp, R., Rosenthal, S. L., and Stanberry, L. R. (2007). VivaGel (TM) (SPL7013 Gel): A candidate dendrimer microbicide for the prevention of HIV and HSV infection, *Int. J. Nanomed.,* **2**, pp. 561–566.

66. Matthews, B. R. and Holan, G. (2001). Antiviral dendrimers, US patent 6190650B1.

67. Gong, E., Matthews, B., McCarthy, T., Chu, J., Holan, G., Raff, J., Sacks, S. (2005). Evaluation of dendrimer SPL7013, a lead microbicide candidate against herpes simplex viruses, *Antiviral Res.,* **68**, pp. 139–146.

68. McGowan, I., Gomez, K., Bruder, K., Febo, I., Chen, B. A., Richardson, B. A., Husnik, M., Livant, E., Price, C., Jacobson, C., and Team, M. T. N. P. (2011). Phase 1 randomized trial of the vaginal safety and acceptability of SPL7013 gel (VivaGel) in sexually active young women (MTN-004), *Aids,* **25**, pp. 1057–1064.

69. Telwatte, S., Moore, K., Johnson, A., Tyssen, D., Sterjovski, J., Aldunate, M., Gorry, P. R., Ramsland, P. A., Lewis, G. R., Paull, J. R. A., Sonza, S., and Tachedjian, G. (2011). Virucidal activity of the dendrimer microbicide SPL7013 against HIV-1, *Antiviral Res.,* **90**, pp. 195–199.

70. Blanzat, M., Turrin, C. O., Perez, E., Rico-Lattes, I., Caminade, A. M., and Majoral, J. P. (2002). Phosphorus-containing dendrimers bearing galactosylceramide analogs: Self-assembly properties, *Chem. Commun.,* pp. 1864–1865.

71. Turrin, C. O. (2000). *Fonctionnalisation sur mesure de dendrimères phosphorés. De l'interface chimie-biologie aux matériaux hybrides.,* Université Paul Sabatier - Toulouse III, Toulouse.

72. Blanzat, M., Turrin, C. O., Aubertin, A. M., Couturier-Vidal, C., Caminade, A. M., Majoral, J. P., Rico-Lattes, I., and Lattes, A. (2005). Dendritic catanionic assemblies: In vitro anti-HIV activity of phosphorus-containing dendrimers bearing Gal beta(1)cer analogues, *ChemBioChem,* **6**, pp. 2207–2213.

73. Pérez-Anes, A., Spataro, G., Coppel, Y., Moog, C., Blanzat, M., Turrin, C. O., Caminade, A. M., Rico-Lattes, I., and Majoral, J. P. (2009). Phosphonate

terminated PPH dendrimers: Influence of pendant alkyl chains on the *in vitro* anti-HIV-1 properties, *Org. Biomol. Chem.,* **7**, pp. 3491–3498.

74. Bernardi, A., Jimenez-Barbero, J., Casnati, A., De Castro, C., Darbre, T., Fieschi, F., Finne, J., Funken, H., Jaeger, K.-E., Lahmann, M., Lindhorst, T. K., Marradi, M., Messner, P., Molinaro, A., Murphy, P. V., Nativi, C., Oscarson, S., Penades, S., Peri, F., Pieters, R. J., Renaudet, O., Reymond, J.-L., Richichi, B., Rojo, J., Sansone, F., Schaffer, C., Turnbull, W. B., Velasco-Torrijos, T., Vidal, S., Vincent, S., Wennekes, T., Zuilhof, H., and Imberty, A. (2013). Multivalent glycoconjugates as anti-pathogenic agents, *Chem. Soc. Rev.,* **42**, pp. 4709–4727.

75. Lasala, F., Arce, E., Otero, J. R., Rojo, J., and Delgado, R. (2003). Mannosyl glycodendritic structure inhibits DC-SIGN-mediated Ebola virus infection in cis and in trans, *Antimicrob. Agents Chemother.,* **47**, pp. 3970–3972.

76. Muñoz, A., Sigwalt, D., Illescas, B. M., Luczkowiak, J., Rodríguez-Pérez, L., Nierengarten, I., Holler, M., Remy, J.-S., Buffet, K., Vincent, S. P., Rojo, J., Delgado, R., Nierengarten, J.-F., and Martín, N. (2016). Synthesis of giant globular multivalent glycofullerenes as potent inhibitors in a model of Ebola virus infection, *Nat. Chem.,* **8**, pp. 50–57.

77. Blattes, E., Vercellone, A., Eutamene, H., Turrin, C. O., Theodorou, V., Majoral, J. P., Caminade, A. M., Prandi, J., Nigou, J., and Puzo, G. (2013). Mannodendrimers prevent acute lung inflammation by inhibiting neutrophil recruitment, *Proc. Natl. Acad. Sci. USA,* **110**, pp. 8795–8800.

78. Wang, S. K., Liang, P. H., Astronomo, R. D., Hsu, T. L., Hsieh, S. L., Burton, D. R., and Wong, C. H. (2008). Targeting the carbohydrates on HIV-1: Interaction of oligomannose dendrons with human monoclonal antibody 2G12 and DC-SIGN, *Proc. Natl. Acad. Sci. USA,* **105**, pp. 3690–3695.

79. Vacas Cordoba, E., Arnaiz, E., De La Mata, F. J., Gomez, R., Leal, M., Pion, M., and Angeles Munoz-Fernandez, M. (2013). Synergistic activity of carbosilane dendrimers in combination with maraviroc against HIV *in vitro*, *Aids,* **27**, pp. 2053–2058.

80. Schols, D., Claes, S., Hatse, S., Princen, K., Vermeire, K., De Clercq, E., Skerlj, R., Bridger, G., and Calandra, G. (2003). *Paper presented at the 10th Conference on Retroviruses and Opportunistic Infections*, Boston, USA.

81. Schnaar, R. L., Suzuki, A., and Stanley, P. (2009). Glycosphingolipids. In: A. Varki, R. D. Cummings, J. D. Esko, H. H. Freeze, P. Stanley, C. R.

Bertozzi, G. W. Hart, and M. E. Etzler (Eds.), *Essentials of Glycobiology*, 2nd edition, Cold Spring Harbor (NY): Cold Spring Harbor Laboratory Press.

82. Fantini, J., Cook, D. G., Nathanson, N., Spitalnik, S. L., and Gonzalez-Scarano, F. (1993). Infection of colonic epithelial-cell lines by type-1 human-immunodeficiency-virus is associated with cell-surface expression of galactosylceramide, a potential alternative gp120 receptor, *Proc. Natl. Acad. Sci. USA*, **90**, pp. 2700–2704.

83. Harouse, J. M., Bhat, S., Spitalnik, S. L., Laughlin, M., Stefano, K., Silberberg, D. H., and Gonzalezscarano, F. (1991). Inhibition of entry of HIV-1 in neural cell-lines by antibodies against galactosyl ceramide, *Science*, **253**, pp. 320–323.

84. Fantini, J., Cook, D. G., Nathanson, N., Spitalnik, S. L., and Gonzalez-Scarano, F. (1993). *Proc. Natl. Acad. Sci. USA*, **90**, pp. 2700–2704.

85. Furuta, Y., Eriksson, K., Svennerholm, B., Fredman, P., Horal, P., Jeansson, S., Vahlne, A., Holmgren, J., and Czerkinsky, C. (1994). Infection of vaginal and colonic epithelial cells by the human immunodeficiency virus type 1 is neutralized by antibodies raised against conserved epitopes in the envelope glycoprotein gp120, *Proc. Natl. Acad. Sci. USA*, **91**, pp. 12559–12563.

86. Hammache, D., Pieroni, G., Yahi, N., Delezay, O., Koch, N., Lafont, H., Tamalet, C., and Fantini, J. (1998). Specific interaction of HIV-1 and HIV-2 surface envelope glycoproteins with monolayers of galactosylceramide and ganglioside GM3, *J. Biol. Chem.*, **273**, pp. 7967–7971.

87. Harouse, J. M., Collman, R. G., and Gonzalezscarano, F. (1995). Human-immunodeficiency-virus type-1 infection of Sk-N-Mc cells: Domains of gp120 involved in entry into a CD4-negative, galactosyl-ceramide/3'-sulfo-galactosyl-ceramide-positive cell-line, *J. Virol.*, **69**, pp. 7383–7390.

88. Yahi, N., Baghdiguian, S., Moreau, H., and Fantini, J. (1992). Galactosyl ceramide (or a closely related molecule) is the receptor for human-immunodeficiency-virus type-1 on human colon epithelial Ht29 cells, *J. Virol.*, **66**, pp. 4848–4854.

89. Fantini, J., Yahi, N., Baghdiguian, S., and Chermann, J. C. (1992). Human colon epithelial-cells productively infected with human-immunodeficiency-virus show impaired differentiation and altered secretion, *J. Virol.*, **66**, pp. 580–585.

90. Conboy, J. C., McReynolds, K. D., Gervay-Hague, J., and Saavedra, S. S. (2002). Quantitative measurements of recombinant HIV surface

glycoprotein 120 binding to several glycosphingolipids expressed in planar supported lipid bilayers, *J. Am. Chem. Soc.,* **124**, pp. 968–977.

91. Lundin, K., Nygren, A., Arthur, L. O., Robey, W. G., Morein, B., Ramstedt, U., Gidlund, M., and Wigzell, H. (1987). A specific assay measuring binding of I-125 Gp 120 from HIV to T4+/CD4+ cells, *J. Immunol. Methods,* **97**, pp. 93–100.

92. Lasky, L. A., Nakamura, G., Smith, D. H., Fennie, C., Shimasaki, C., Patzer, E., Berman, P., Gregory, T., and Capon, D. J. (1987). Delineation of a region of the human-immunodeficiency-virus type-1 gp120 glycoprotein critical for interaction with the CD4 receptor, *Cell,* **50**, pp. 975–985.

93. Smith, D. H., Byrn, R. A., Marsters, S. A., Gregory, T., Groopman, J. E., and Capon, D. J. (1987). Blocking of HIV-1 infectivity by a soluble, secreted form of the CD4 antigen, *Science,* **238**, pp. 1704–1707.

94. Bhat, S., Spitalnik, S. L., Gonzalez-Scarano, F., and Silberberg, D. H. (1991). Galactosyl ceramide or a derivative is an essential component of the neural receptor for human immunodeficiency virus type 1 envelope glycoprotein gp120, *Proc. Natl. Acad. Sci. USA,* **88**, pp. 7131–7134.

95. Rico-Lattes, I., Gouzy, M. F., Andre-Barres, C., Guidetti, B., and Lattes, A. (1998). Synthetic bolaamphiphilic analogs of galactosylceramide (GalCer) potentially binding to the V3 domain of HIV-1 gp 120: Key role of their hydrophobicity, *New J. Chem.,* **22**, pp. 451–457.

96. Fantini, J., Hammache, D., Delezay, O., Yahi, N., AndreBarres, C., RicoLattes, I., and Lattes, A. (1997). Synthetic soluble analogs of galactosylceramide (GalCer) bind to the V3 domain of HIV-1 gp120 and inhibit HIV-1-induced fusion and entry, *J. Biol. Chem.,* **272**, pp. 7245–7252.

97. Fantini, J. and Yahi, N. (1993). *Medecine/Sciences,* **9**, pp. 891–900.

98. Mammen, M., Choi, S. K., and Whitesides, G. M. (1998). Polyvalent interactions in biological systems: Implications for design and use of multivalent ligands and inhibitors, *Angew. Chem. Int. Ed.,* **37**, pp. 2754–2794.

99. Rosa Borges, A. and Schengrund, C. L. (2005). Dendrimers and antivirals: A review, *Curr. Drug. Targets. Infect. Disord.,* **5**, pp. 247–254.

100. Thompson, J. P. and Schengrund, C. L. (1996). Oligo-dendrimer inhibition of cholera toxin binding to GM1, *FASEB J.,* **10**, pp. 1319–1319.

101. Schengrund, C. L., DasGupta, B. R., and Thompson, J. P. (1997). Inhibition of the adherence of botulinum toxin serotype A to immobilized GT1b by multivalent oligosaccharide GT1b-derivatized dendrimers, *J. Neurochem.*, **69**, pp. S17–S17.

102. Thompson, J. P. and Schengrund, C. L. (1997). Oligosaccharide-derivatized dendrimers: Defined multivalent inhibitors of the adherence of the cholera toxin B subunit and the heat labile enterotoxin of E-coli GM1, *Glycoconjugate J.*, **14**, pp. 837–845.

103. Thompson, J. P. and Schengrund, C. L. (1998). Inhibition of the adherence of cholera toxin and the heat-labile enterotoxin of *Escherichia coli* to cell-surface GM1 by oligosaccharide-derivatized dendrimers, *Biochem. Pharmacol.*, **56**, pp. 591–597.

104. Pike, L. J. (2009). The challenge of lipid rafts, *J. Lipid Res.*, **50**, pp. S323–S328.

105. Kensinger, R. D., Yowler, B. C., Benesi, A. J., and Schengrund, C.-L. (2004). Synthesis of novel, multivalent glycodendrimers as ligands for HIV-1 gp120, *Bioconjugate Chem.*, **15**, pp. 349–358.

106. Farzan, M., Mirzabekov, T., Kolchinsky, P., Wyatt, R., Cayabyab, M., Gerard, N. P., Gerard, C., Sodroski, J., and Choe, H. (1999). Tyrosine sulfation of the amino terminus of CCR5 facilitates HIV-1 entry, *Cell*, **96**, pp. 667–676.

107. Kensinger, R. D., Catalone, B. J., Krebs, F. C., Wigdahl, B., and Schengrund, C. L. (2004). Novel polysulfated galactose-derivatized dendrimers as binding antagonists of human immunodeficiency virus type 1 infection, *Antimicrob. Agents Chemother.*, **48**, pp. 1614–1623.

108. Bertozzi, C. R., Cook, D. G., Kobertz, W. R., Gonzalez-Scarano, F., and Bednarski, M. D. (1992). Carbon-linked galactosphingolipid analogs bind specifically to HIV-1 gp120, *J. Am. Chem. Soc.*, **114**, pp. 10639–10641.

109. Fantini, J., Hammache, D., Delézay, O., Yahi, N., André-Barrès, C., Rico-Lattes, I., and Lattes, A. (1997). Synthetic soluble analogs of galactosylceramide (GalCer) bind to the V3 domain of HIV-1 gp120 and inhibit HIV-1-induced fusion and entry, *J. Biol. Chem.*, **272**, pp. 7245–7252.

110. Blanzat, M., Perez, E., Rico-Lattes, I., Promé, D., Promé, J. C., and Lattes, A. (1999). New catanionic glycolipids. I. Synthesis, characterization, and biological activity of double-chain and gemini catanionic analogues of Galactosylceramide (GalCer), *Langmuir*, **15**, pp. 6163.

111. Jokela, P., Jönsson, B., and Khan, A. (1987). Phase equilibria of catanionic surfactant-water systems, *J. Phys. Chem.*, **91**, pp. 3291–3298.

112. Huang, J. B. and Zhao, G. X. (1995). Formation and coexistence of the micelles and vesicles in mixed solution of cationic and anionic surfactant, *Colloid Polym. Sci.*, **273**, pp. 156.

113. Kaler, E. W., Kamalakara Murthy, A., Rodriguez, B. E., and Zasadzinski, J. A. N. (1989). Spontaneous vesicles formation in aqueous mixtures of single-tailed surfactants, *Science*, **245**, pp. 1371.

114. Zemb, T., Dubois, M., Deme, B., and Gulik-Krzywicki, T. (1999). Self-assembly of flat nanodiscs in salt-free catanionic surfactant solutions, *Science*, **283**, pp. 816.

115. Kahn, A. and Marques, E. (1997). Catanionic surfactants. In: I. D. Robb (Ed.), *Specialist Surfactants* (pp. 37–80): Blackie Academic and Professional, an imprint of Chapman & Hall.

116. Dubois, M., Deme, B., Gulik-Krzywicki, T., Dedieu, J. C., Vautrin, C., Desert, S., Perez, E., and Zemb, T. (2001). Self-assembly of regular hollow icosahedra in salt-free catanionic solutions, *Nature*, **411**, pp. 672.

117. Blanzat, M., Perez, E., Rico-Lattes, I., and Lattes, A. (1999). Synthesis and anti-HIV activity of catanionic analogues of galactosylceramide, *New J. Chem.*, **23**, pp. 1063.

118. Angyal, S. J. (1989). *Adv. Carbohydate Chem. Biochem.*, **47**, pp. 1–43.

119. Soussan, E., Cassel, S., Blanzat, M., and Rico-Lattes, I. (2009). Drug delivery by soft matter: Matrix and vesicular carriers, *Angew. Chem. Int. Ed.*, **48**, pp. 274–288.

120. Blanzat, M., Massip, S., Spéziale, V., Perez, E., and Rico-Lattes, I. (2001). First example of helices and tubules in aqueous solution of new fluorescent catanionic sugar surfactant, *Langmuir*, **17**, pp. 3512–3514.

121. Boudier, A., Castagnos, P., Soussan, E., Beaune, G., Belkhelfa, H., Ménager, C., Cabuil, V., Haddioui, L., Roques, C., Rico-Lattes, I., and Blanzat, M. (2011). Polyvalent catanionic vesicles: Exploring the drug delivery mechanisms, *Int. J. Pharm.*, **403**, pp. 230–236.

122. Soussan, E., Mille, C., Blanzat, M., Bordat, P., and Rico-Lattes, I. (2008). Sugar-derived tricatenar catanionic surfactant: Synthesis, self-assembly properties, and hydrophilic probe encapsulation by vesicles, *Langmuir*, **24**, pp. 2326–2330.

123. Mauroy, C., Castagnos, P., Orio, J., Blache, M.-C., Rico-Lattes, I., Teissie, J., Rols, M.-P., and Blanzat, M. (2015). Versatile cellular uptake mediated

by catanionic vesicles: Simultaneous spontaneous membrane fusion and endocytosis, *Mol. Pharm.*, **12**, pp. 103–110.

124. Castagnos, P., Siqueira-Moura, M. P., Leme Goto, P., Perez, E., Franceschi, S., Rico-Lattes, I., Tedesco, A. C., and Blanzat, M. (2014). Catanionic vesicles charged with chloroaluminium phthalocyanine for topical photodynamic therapy. In vitro phototoxicity towards human carcinoma and melanoma cell lines, *RSC Advances*, **4**, pp. 39372–39377.

125. Bronshtein, T., Toledano, N., Danino, D., Pollack, S., and Machluf, M. (2011). Cell derived liposomes expressing CCR5 as a new targeted drug-delivery system for HIV infected cells, *J. Control. Release*, **151**, pp. 139–148.

126. Soussan, E., Blanzat, M., Rico-Lattes, I., Brun, A., Teixeira, C. V., Brezesinski, G., Al-Ali, F., Banu, A., and Tanaka, M. (2007). Physical study of the arrangement of pure catanionic glycolipids and interaction with phospholipids, in support of the optimisation of anti-HIV therapies, *Colloids Surf. A Physicochem. Eng. Asp.*, **303**, pp. 55–72.

127. Harris, A., Borgnia, M., Shi, D., Bartesaghi, A., He, H., Pejchal, R., Kang, Y., Depetris, R., Marozsan, A., Sanders, R., Klasse, P., Milne, J., Wilson, I., Olson, W., Moore, J., and Subramaniam, S. (2011). Trimeric HIV-1 glycoprotein gp140 immunogens and native HIV-1 envelope glycoproteins display the same closed and open quaternary molecular architectures, *Proc. Natl. Acad. Sci. USA*, **108**, pp. 11440–11445.

128. Clayton, R., Hardman, J., LaBranche, C. C., and McReynolds, K. D. (2011). Evaluation of the synthesis of sialic acid-PAMAM glycodendrimers without the use of sugar protecting groups, and the anti-HIV-1 properties of these compounds, *Bioconjugate Chem.*, **22**, pp. 2186–2197.

129. Kensinger, R. D., Catalone, B. J., Krebs, F. C., Wigdahl, B., and Schengrund, C. L. (2004). Novel polysulfated galactose-derivatized dendrimers as binding antagonists of human immunodeficiency virus type 1 infection, *Antimicrob. Agents Chemother.*, **48**, pp. 1614–1623.

130. Pedziwiatr-Werbickaa, E., Ferenca, M., Zaborskib, M., Gabarac, B., Klajnerta, B., and Bryszewska, M. (2011). Characterization of complexes formed by polypropylene imine dendrimers and anti-HIV oligonucleotides, *Colloids Surf. B Biointerfaces*, **83** pp. 360–366.

131. Mitsuya, H. and Broder, S. (1986). Inhibition of the *in vitro* infectivity and cytopathic effect of human T-lymphotrophic virus

type III/lymphadenopathy-associated virus (HTLV-III/LAV) by 2′,3′-dideoxynucleoside, *Proc. Natl. Acad. Sci. USA,* **83**, pp. 1911–1915.

132. Blanzat, M., Perez, E., Rico-Lattes, I., Lattes, A., and Gulik, A. (2003). Correlation between structure, aggregation behaviour and cellular toxicity of anti-HIV catanionic analogues of galactosylceramide, *Chem. Commun.,* pp. 244–245.

133. Teixeira, C. V., Blanzat, M., Koetz, J., Rico-Lattes, I., and Brezesinski, G. (2006). In-plane miscibility and mixed bilayer microstructure in mixtures of catanionic glycolipids and zwitterionic phospholipids, *Biochimica Et Biophysica Acta-Biomembranes,* **1758**, pp. 1797–1808.

134. Caminade, A.-M., Fruchon, S., Turrin, C.-O., Poupot, M., Ouali, A., Maraval, A., Garzoni, M., Maly, M., Furer, V., Kovalenko, V., Majoral, J.-P., Pavan, G. M., and Poupot, R. (2015). The key role of the scaffold on the efficiency of dendrimer nanodrugs, *Nat. Commun.,* **6**, 7722.

135. Doebner, O. (1902). Ueber die der Sorbinsäure homologen, ungesättigten Säuren mit zwei Doppelbindungen, *Ber. Dtsch. Chem. Ges.,* **35**, pp. 1136–1147.

136. Rico-Lattes, I., Garrigues, J. C., Perez, E., André-Barrès, C., Madelaine-Dupuich, C., Lattes, A., Linas, M. D., and Aubertin, A. M. (1995). *New J. Chem.,* **19**, pp. 341–344.

137. Mammen, M., Choi, S. K., and Whitesides, M. (1998). Polyvalent interactions in biological systems: Implications for design and use of multivalent ligands and inhibitors, *Angew. Chem. Int. Ed. Eng.,* **37**, pp. 2754.

138. Öztürk, K., Ertürk, A. S., Sarısözen, C., Tulu, M., and Çalış, S. (2014). Cytotoxicity and *in vitro* characterization studies of synthesized Jeffamine-cored PAMAM dendrimers, *J. Microencapsul.,* **31**, pp. 127–136.

139. Jevprasesphant, R., Penny, J., Attwood, D., McKeown, N. B., and D'Emanuele, A. (2003). Engineering of dendrimer surfaces to enhance transepithelial transport and reduce cytotoxicity, *Pharm. Res.,* **20**, pp. 1543–1550.

140. Kaminskas, L. M., Boyd, B. J., and Porter, C. J. H. (2012). Dendrimer pharmacokinetics: The effect of size, structure and surface characteristics on ADME properties (vol 6, pg 1063, 2011), *Nanomedicine,* **7**, pp. 167–168.

141. Pérez-Anes, A., Stefaniu-Bololoï, C., Moog, C., Majoral, J. P., Blanzat, M., Turrin, C. O., Caminade, A. M., and Rico-Lattes, I. (2009). Multivalent

catanionic GalCer analogs derived from first generation dendrimeric phosphonic acids, *Bioorg. Med. Chem.*, **18**, pp. 242–248.

142. Pérez-Anes, A., Spataro, G., Coppel, Y., Blanzat, M., Turrin, C.-O., Moog, C., Caminade, A.-M., Rico-Lattes, I., and Majoral, J.-P. (2009). Phosphonate terminated PPH dendrimers: Influence of pendant alkyl chains on the *in vitro* anti-HIV1 properties, *Org. Biomol. Chem.*, **7**, pp. 3491–3498.

143. McKenna, C. E., Higa, M. T., Cheung, N. H., and McKenna, M.-C. (1977). The facile dealkylation of phosphonic acid dialkyl esters by bromotrimethylsilane, *Tetrahedron Lett.*, **18**, pp. 155–158.

144. Caminade, A. M., Laurent, R., Turrin, C. O., Rebout, C., Delavaux-Nicot, B., Ouali, A., Zablocka, M., and Majoral, J. P. (2010). Phosphorus dendrimers as viewed by (31)P NMR spectroscopy: Synthesis and characterization, *C. R. Chimie*, **13**, pp. 1006–1027.

145. Fletcher, P. S., Wallace, G. S., Mesquita, P. M. M., and Shattock, R. J. (2006). Candidate polyanion microbicides inhibit HIV-1 infection abd dissemination pathways in human cervical explants, *Retrovirology*, **3**, pp. 46–56.

146. Macri, R. V., Karlovská, J., Doncel, G. F., Du, X., Maisuria, B. B., Williams, A. A., Sugandhi, E. W., III, J. O. F., Esker, A. R., and Gandour, R. D. (2009). Comparing anti-HIV, antibacterial, antifungal, micellar, and cytotoxic properties of tricarboxylato dendritic amphiphiles, *Bioorg. Med. Chem.*, **17**, pp. 3162–3168.

Chapter 7

Role of Dendrimers in the Development of New Dendritic Cells Immunotherapies against HIV-1 Infection

Rosa Reguera,[a] João Rodrigues,[b] Jose Correa,[c] M. Angeles Muñoz-Fernández[d]

[a]*Departamento de Ciencias Biomédicas, Universidad de León, Campus de Vegazana, León, Spain*
[b]*CQM-Centro de Química da Madeira (National Research Centre), Universidade da Madeira, Campus da Penteada, 9020-105 Funchal, Portugal*
[c]*Laboratorio de Modelado Molecular, Diseño de Fármacos y Bioinformática, Escuela Superior de Medicina-Instituto Politécnico Nacional, Mexico City 11340, Mexico*
[d]*Immunology Section, Spanish HIV HGM BioBank, Hospital General Universitario Gregorio Marañón, Instituto de Investigición Sanitaria Gregorio Marañón, C/Dr Esquerdo 4 28007 Madrid, Spain*
rmregt@unileon.es, joaor@uma.pt, jcorreab@ipn.mx, mmunoz.hgugum@gmail.com

7.1 Introduction

The United Nations Programme on Human Immunodeficiency Virus (HIV) and Acquired Immunodeficiency Syndrome (AIDS)

Phosphorus Dendrimers in Biology and Nanomedicine: Synthesis, Characterization, and Properties
Edited by Anne-Marie Caminade, Cédric-Olivier Turrin, and Jean-Pierre Majoral
Copyright © 2018 Pan Stanford Publishing Pte. Ltd.
ISBN 978-981-4774-33-8 (Hardcover), 978-1-315-11085-1 (eBook)
www.panstanford.com

estimates that in 2014 more than 36.9 million people lived with HIV-1. Although combined antiretroviral therapy (cART) has delayed disease progression and significantly decreased the morbidity and mortality rate in HIV-1 subjects [1], HIV-1 has not been eliminated. The number of people receiving cART continues to be increased, and clinical trials have confirmed the powerful impact that cART can have on the AIDS pandemic as part of an effective option for HIV-1 prevention [2, 3]. Moreover, still too many people are acquiring HIV-1 infection and only minorities of HIV-1 subjects globally have access to cART. Economic, social, cultural, and political issues impose major obstacles to the implementation of widespread cART in developing countries, and hence the infected population is likely to grow. In fact, only 41% of the individuals in need of treatment (15 millions) received standard cART. In consequence, HIV infection is not yet a curable disease. Efforts to prevent the transmission of HIV-1 are based on three approaches: behavioral change (safer sex), development of microbicides, and development of vaccines. There are two kinds of vaccination to fight against HIV-1: preventive and therapeutic vaccines. In this context, vaccination has been proposed as the best strategy to eradicate a long-term virus.

Preventive HIV vaccines are designed to protect non-HIV-1 subjects and to stop HIV-1 spreading by a gradual decrease in the number of new infections. Nevertheless, all attempts to develop an efficacious and effective HIV-1 preventive vaccine have failed [4–7]. Therapeutic HIV vaccines are designed to control HIV-1 infection in the individuals who have already been HIV-1 infected. Although cART has proved to be highly effective to prevent HIV clinical progression and death, by itself it is unable to eradicate the HIV-1 infection. Combined antiretroviral therapy needs to be taken along the whole life of an HIV-1 subject. In addition, development of resistance in virus, adverse effects in the medium and long term, and the significant cost of cART are important limitations for lifelong adherence to this therapy. Therapeutic vaccines have already shown efficacy against other virus such as herpes zoster using ZOSTAVAX® (Zoster Vaccine Live) [8].

7.2 Immune System Strategies: Antibodies and Vaccines

The immune system plays a crucial role in the control of HIV-1 infection, but in most HIV-1 subjects, immune escape precludes complete and lasting control. Although cART usually leads to a normalization of CD4+ T-cell numbers, it does not fully restore a normal immune status in HIV-1 subjects. More and more efforts have been devoted to influence the immune system in such a way that it can control the HIV-1 infection without the need for lifelong cART. Various classical strategies and other novel methodologies such as neutralizing antibodies or dendritic cell (DC)-based immunotherapies are being researched as therapeutic HIV vaccine candidates [4, 9–12]. In the case of broad-spectrum neutralizing antibodies, new screenings have promoted the discovery of novel candidates similar to those present in non-progressor HIV-1 subjects. These neutralizing antibodies could be used in passive vaccines or be employed as templates to create immunogenic epitopes, which are expressed in vectors, promoting specific antibodies production by adaptive immunity cells, such as B cells [13, 14].

DCs play a key role in linking innate and adaptive immunity. DCs capture antigens from pathogens and present them to T cells, stimulating CD4- and CD8-specific responses by MHC class-I and MHC class-II molecules [15]. DC-based immunotherapies have been applied successfully in cancer [16–18]. DCs loaded with tumor lysates, tumor antigen-derived peptides, or whole tumor proteins have all been shown to generate anti-cancer immune responses, including the capacity to induce complete regression of the tumor. In particular, a DC-based therapy, Sipuleucel-T, is the unique vaccine approved by the US Food and Drug Administration (FDA) for the treatment of advanced prostate cancer [19, 20]. Additional data in mice tumor models obtained by VUB (Vrije Universiteit Brussel) showed that intranodal immunization with a messenger RNA (mRNA)-based therapeutic vaccine (tumor-associated antigen-TriMix-mRNA) has the potential to efficiently increase the induction of tumor-specific immune responses compared to an mRNA-electroporated DC-based vaccine, suggesting that this strategy could provide the needed tool to be tested on humans [21].

In HIV-1 vaccination, various approaches such as HIV-derived peptides, viral proteins, DNA, RNA, or inactivate viral particles have been used to improve antigen loading in DCs and to enhance immune responses [22–27]. In this context, the most successful results in HIV DC-based clinical trials have been those using complete inactivated viruses. In a non-randomized study with non-treated HIV-1 infected individuals, Lu *et al.* showed that 8 out of 18 HIV-1 subjects treated with autologous AT-2 inactivated virus pulsed-DCs had a reduction of more than 90% in the viral load [28]. In addition, in randomized double-blind placebo-controlled trials carried out by García *et al.*, with cART treated and untreated HIV-1 subjects and involving heat-inactivated autologous virus pulsed-DCs, a modest significant control of plasma viral load was achieved in immunized recipients and was associated with a consistent increase in HIV-1-specific T-cell responses [21].

Although in all experimental immunotherapies against HIV-1 involving DCs, the security profile was excellent and specific responses against the virus were found. Only in four studies, an immunological response capable of controlling the viremia was observed. In none of these clinical trials, a real "functional cure" was accomplished. It has been shown that a DC-based vaccine (European patent application number EP12382078.9) suppressed, controlled significantly the viral load in vaccinated HIV-1 subjects with a mean peak reduction of viral load of 94%. However, a "functional cure" was not observed in any of the HIV-1 subjects, due to the induction of insufficiently strong antiviral immune responses [21].

Several key aspects of DC-based therapies should be meticulously analyzed in therapeutic vaccines development. It includes the election of target antigen, viral inactivation method, the DCs isolation procedure or the vaccination strategy, antigen doses, routes of administration, etc. [29].

7.3 Alternatives to Combined Antiretroviral Therapy for Life: The Role of Therapeutic Vaccines

Treatment resistance, adverse effects in the medium-long term, and the enormous costs of cART are important limitations for lifelong adherence to this therapy. Standard therapies do not fully restore health or a normal immune status in HIV-1 subjects, and patients still experience co-morbidities, such as increased cardiovascular disease, bone disorders, and cognitive impairment [30]. In addition, interruption of cART almost invariably leads to the re-emergence of detectable viral replication and the progression of AIDS [31]. Other features that impede the development of effective immunotherapeutic vaccines against HIV infection can be genetic diversity and mutations of HIV-1. The fact that immune cells are the main targets of HIV-1, HIV infection generates the hyper-activation of the immune system and that vaccines should induce specific new immune responses against subdominant HIV-1 epitopes; a suitable control of viral replication is crucial. New approaches should be explored, developed, and tested to fight against HIV-1 infection.

The feasibility of this approach is highlighted by the fact that exceptional individuals, the so-called "long-term elite controllers," a very small proportion of HIV-1 subjects, show a lack of clinical progression associated with strict control of viral replication in the absence of any cART. This so-called "functional cure" has been linked to potent HIV-specific immune responses observed in these HIV-1 subjects. The best-defined correlates of protection against disease progression seen in these HIV-1 subjects are low pro-viral load, low to absent levels of intracellular spliced and unspliced viral mRNA, and potent HIV-suppressive CD8+ T-cell responses [32, 33]. To achieve these characteristics in HIV-1 subjects unable to control viral replication on their own and, therefore, needs of sustained cART, therapeutic vaccinations have emerged as one of the most promising strategies that could restore HIV-specific T-cell responses in HIV-1 subjects and help them control viral replication without cART. The most promising approach so far has been the administration of *in vitro* modified autologous DCs. In fact, Van Gulck *et al.* showed these characteristics in HIV-1 "elite controller" subjects and after DCs vaccination in HIV-1-treated subjects [34].

García *et al.* have reported the most striking results in this field to date, demonstrating that a DC-based vaccine controlled significantly the viral load with a mean peak reduction of viral load of 94% in vaccinated HIV-1 subjects. However, a "functional cure" was not observed in any of the HIV-1 subjects due to the induction of insufficiently strong antiviral immune responses [21].

7.4 Route of Therapeutic Vaccine Administration

The route of administration is a crucial determinant for the quality of the immune response. Recent data obtained in a preclinical mouse model show that intranodal injection of mRNA results in a selective uptake by resident DCs and induces stronger immune responses and better survival of tumor-bearing mice than a DC-based vaccine [35]. However, intranodal immunization cannot be routinely applied in clinical settings. Thus, other routes of administration need to be explored. Given the natural sensitivity of mRNA to RNases, which are abundantly present in the environment, other administration routes such as intradermal or subcutaneous injection would require that the mRNA is stabilized and protected. This could be achieved by conjugating the different mRNA vaccine components with biodegradable nanoparticles in order to develop a novel "off-the-shelf" therapeutic vaccine against HIV-1 that can be easily formulated and stored, protect a wide range of subjects and commonly administration routes are used. The formulation of such mRNAs with chemical carriers should entail a greater specificity and internalization by DCs, contributing to the generation of increased immune responses and a reduced dose to be administered [36].

7.5 Nanotechnology and Nanomedicine in HIV-Vaccination Strategies

According to the European Science Foundation (ESF), nanomedicine is the process of diagnosing, treating, and preventing disease and traumatic injury of relieving pain, and preserving and improving human health, by using molecular tools and molecular knowledge of the human body [37]. The applications of nanomedicine involve delivery of pharmaceuticals, *in vitro* and *in vivo* diagnostics, including imaging, regenerative medicine, and implanted devices. Examples of nanomaterials with diagnostic applications in biology and medicine include liposomes, dendrimers, gold nanoparticles, polymeric micelles, quantum dots, fullerenes, or iron oxide crystals (Fig. 7.1) [38, 39]. In particular, dendrimers are promising candidates for application in medicine and deserve attention as they are used as solubility enhancers, anti-cancer, anti-inflammatory, and antiviral drugs, drug-delivery carriers, diagnosis and imaging agents, vaccines, adjuvants, and microbicides [40–42].

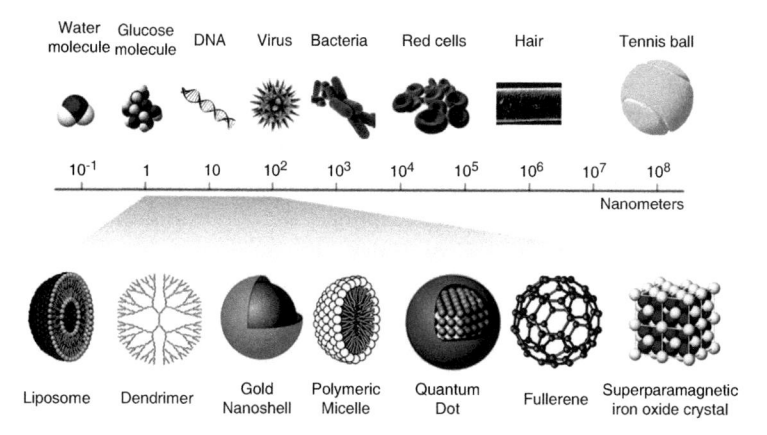

Figure 7.1 Nanomaterials commonly used in biomedicine compared with familiar items. Modified from (McNeil, 2005).

The application of nanotechnology for prevention and/or treatment of HIV-1 infection has already been a reality [43–50]. Applications of nanotechnology platforms enhance the current treatments and can be used as novel therapeutic agents in anti-HIV immunotherapy and gene therapy. Various nanosystems have been researched for *ex vivo* and *in vivo* targeting of DCs and for delivery of small molecules, proteins, and DNA showing potential for immunotherapy [47, 50–52]. These nanosystems release antigens in a controlled manner and effectively target DCs [44, 51, 52]. These nanosystems use different ways such as encapsulating antigens in their core or absorbing these small molecules on their functionalized surface with the purpose to deliver them. For instance, poly(ethylene glycol) (PEG), stabilized poly(propylene sulfide), polymer nanoparticles [53], cross-linked polymer nanoparticles with a pH-responsive core, and hydrophilic charged shell [54] or nanoparticles of the copolymer poly(D,L-lacticide-co-glycolide) (PLGA) [55] have been used to deliver antigens such as proteins to DCs. Other studies using HIV-1 gp160 or gp41 proteins encapsulated in liposomes [56, 57] or p24 protein adsorbed on the surface of anionic poly(D,L-lactide) (PLA) nanoparticles induced antigen-specific cellular immunity when targeted to DCs in a mice model [58, 59]. Nevertheless, nanoparticles have potential not only as carriers in immunotherapies but also as adjuvants in vaccine development [60]. One of the most advanced clinical applications of nanocompounds for HIV-1 immunotherapy is the DermaVir patch [61, 62]. This nanoparticle is based on poly(ethyleneimine) (PEI) mannose (PEIm), glucose and HIV-1 antigen coding DNA plasmid and delivered to epidermis. Antigens captured by Langerhans cells in the epidermis DCs mature and present the antigens to T cells, promoting an increased cellular immune response. DermaVir administered in skin path is in phase II clinical trial.

None of the tested immunotherapy vaccines using single antigens coupled to nanosystems have elicited a broadly neutralizing antibodies response to HIV-1 infection [47]. These nanosystems need to be improved to include and deliver a broad variety of HIV-1 epitopes that generate broader and stronger immune responses against the HIV-1 infection. Co-adsorption of gp120 and p24 proteins by PLA nanoparticles has elicited high antibodies titers in mice, showing the potential of multivalent immunotherapeutic vaccines [59]. Although the results are encouraging, some parameters should be optimized such as the size, targeting ligand, surface density, encapsulation efficiency, and route of administration to achieve better and more suitable vaccine delivery platforms.

7.6 Dendrimers in HIV-1 Immunotherapy Strategies

One crucial point in the development and potential use of dendrimers as non-viral vectors is a rational design of families of dendrimers to achieve targeted delivery of antigens. Various families of dendrimers can be potentially used as carriers in DC-based immunotherapies.

Recent progress in the design of biodegradable nanosystems, together with the regulation of dendrimer design and preparation, makes possible to precisely manipulate dendrimer architectures, molecular weight, and chemical composition, resulting in predictable tuning of their biocompatibility as well as their delivery ability.

Dendrimers are highly branched, star-shaped, and nano-sized molecules consisting of tree-like branches or arms constructed through the sequential addition of branching units from an initial core. Dendrimers are divided into three architectural components: nucleus, interior layers with repeating units or generations, and exterior with functional end groups [63, 64] (Fig. 7.2). Most dendrimers have diameters ranging from 1 to 20 nm [65]. The diameter of dendrimers increases linearly at the rate of around 1 nm/generation, whereas the surface groups raise exponentially at each generation [66]. The core and the number of the interior branching units affect the dendrimer morphology [67]. The core affects the three-dimensional shape of dendrimers, the interior affects the host–guest properties of dendrimers, and the charge of end groups determines a large number of potentially reactive sites [68]. The core and especially the generation number are relevant to the three-dimensional shape of dendrimers. Lower generations of dendrimers are more flexible and tend to be open and amorphous structures than dendrimers at higher generations, which can adopt spherical conformations [69].

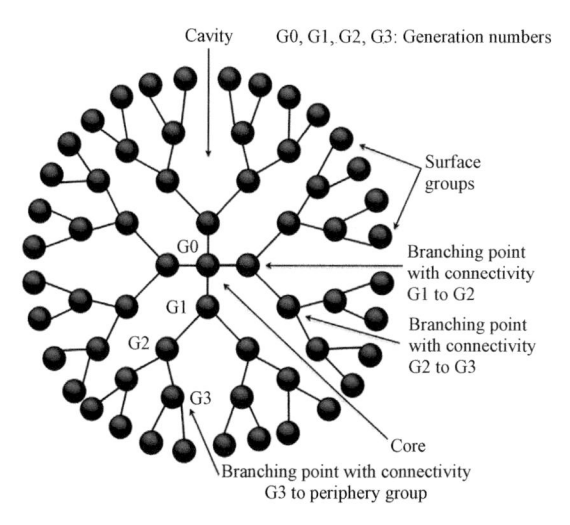

Figure 7.2 Schematic representation of dendrimer components. Dendrimers are formed by three components: an initiator core, scaffold layers or generations, and functional groups at the outer surface. The nucleus molecule is demonstrated by the generation 0 (G0), while successive addition of branching units leads to higher generations G1, G2, G3, …. Generations are defined as the number of repeating layers with branching units forming the dendrimer. End groups can possess positive, negative, or neutral charges, which will define their biological functionality.

Dendrimers can be engineered by manipulating the structure of the central core, the structure and number of branching units, or the composition and number of surface functional groups to obtain compounds with physicochemical, biological, and medical desired properties. One of the important characteristics of dendrimers is their multivalency due to the presence of numerous surface functional groups in the terminal branches. It enables multiple drugs or targeting ligands to be conjugated to a single dendrimer molecule. Dendrimers have the ability to encapsulate hydrophobic molecules in their core cavity.

Based on the chemical structure, dendrimers are classified by their size, generation, layers, and repetitive units. To date, dendrimers with diverse functionalities and architectures have been designed: PAMAM (polyamidoamine) dendrimers, PAMAMOS (polyamidoamine-organosilicon) dendrimers, phosphorus-based dendrimers, carbon/oxygen-based dendrimers (polyether, polyester, glycodendrimers), chiral dendrimers, metallodendrimers, peptide dendrimers, PLL (polylysine) dendrimers, hybrid dendrimers, porphyrin-based dendrimer, poly(propylenimine) (PPI) dendrimers, silicon-based dendrimers (silane, carbosilane, carbosiloxane, siloxane), and triazine dendrimers, [70–72] (Fig. 7.3). These dendrimers are very attractive in several biological and medical applications. They have been used in diagnosis and imaging [66, 73] as well as in various clinical strategies such as drug delivery, non-viral vectors in gene therapy, therapeutic agents as antimicrobial or microbicides, antitumors or anti-inflammatory drugs. Due to these applications of dendrimers, there is a critical need of their physicochemical characterization by employing a wide range of analytical techniques [74]. It is essential to clearly define the purpose and to know limitations of analytical tools, not only to determine chemical composition of dendrimers, but also their morphology, size/shape, purity, and their homogeneity, among other properties.

The surface charge of dendrimers plays a key role in interaction with cell membranes and plasma proteins. The cationic charges generate the most significant impact. Surface functionality has an important effect on absorption, distribution, metabolism, and elimination properties of dendrimers [65, 75]. Dendrimers with cationic surface groups tend to interact with negative lipid bilayer, enhancing the permeability and decreasing the integrity of membrane that finally causes its destabilization and cell lysis. A cationic functionalized dendrimer could be used as a carrier to target delivery of cationic biomolecules and as a drug such as nucleic acids or peptides forming dendriplexes. For example, PAMAM-based RNA vector down-regulated the expression of heat-shock protein 27 (Hsp27) in prostate cancer cells [76]. PPI dendrimers knocked down the expression of phosphoenolpyruvate carboxykinase (PEPCK) and of organic cationic transporter 1 (OCT 1) in a rat cell line [77].

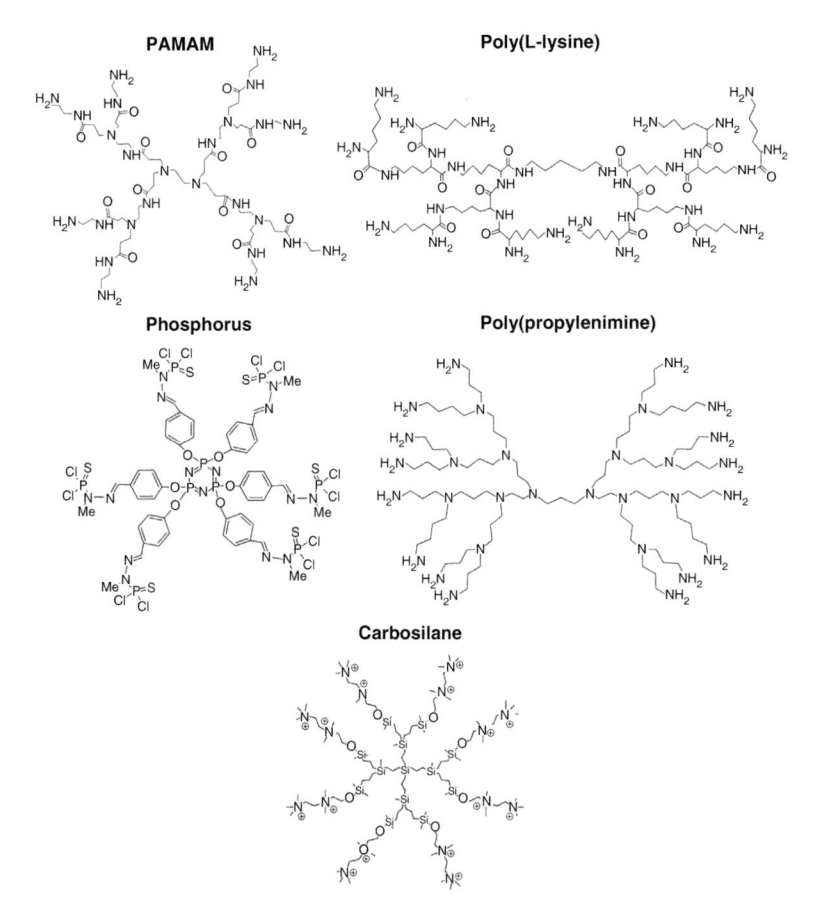

Figure 7.3 Chemical structures of commercially available dendrimers and commonly used as HIV-1 immunotherapies.

The primary limitation of gene therapy is the effective delivery of nucleic acids to the target cells. Dendrimers are nanoparticles that are used as nucleic acid vehicles. "Si–C" amino-terminated carbosilane dendrimers [GnO3(NMe3)m](m+) functionalized with quaternary ammonium [NMe3(+)] terminal groups via hydrosilylation of allyl dimethylamine with the corresponding GnO3(SiH) m dendrimers and further addition of MeI are soluble in water. The charge and size of the dendriplexes (complexes of "Si–C" dendrimers with ANTITAR and GEM91, siRNA siP24 nucleic acids) possessed charges of +5 to +40 mV and sizes of 60–600 nm (zetasizer) or 50–100 nm (atomic force microscopy) suitable for cell transfection. The effects of dendriplexes on PBMCs are 10 times less cytotoxic than the pure dendrimers. The ability of carbosilane dendrimer 2G-[Si{O(CH(2))(2)N(Me)(2) (+)(CH(2))(2)NMe(3) (+) (I(–))(2)}](8) (NN16) to transfect a wide range of cell types, PBMCs and immortalized suspension cells (lymphocytes), primary macrophages and DCs, and immortalized adherent cells (astrocytes and trophoblasts), as well as the possible biomedical application in direct or indirect inhibition of HIV-1 replication was demonstrated. Transfection efficiency and gene knockdown were performed using dendrimer-delivered antisense oligonucleotides and small interfering RNA (siRNA). Dendrimer-bound siRNAs are resistant to degradation by RNase. Next, using flow cytometry and confocal microscopy, lymphocytes were seen to be successfully transfected by fluorochrome-labeled siRNA either naked or complexed with carbosilane dendrimers. Finally, dendriplexes were shown to silence GAPDH expression and reduce HIV-1 replication in SupT1 and PBMCs. Dendrimers demonstrated the ability to transfect genetic material into a vast array of cells relevant to HIV-1 pathology, combining high efficacy with low toxicity. Dendrimers can be used to deliver and transfect siRNA into lymphocytes, thus allowing the use of RNA interference as a potential alternative therapy for HIV-1 infection [77–85].

The rich diversity of the chemistry of phosphorus, even when applied to nano-objects such as dendrimers, has been demonstrated. Phosphorus-derived dendrimers can be potentially used as nanocarriers in biological systems [81, 86, 87]. The presence of phosphorus at branching points of the dendrimeric structure plays an important role and is directly associated with the properties of these nanosystems [88]. The versatility of phosphorus chemistry enables diversified organic chemistry to synthesize dendrimers. These phosphorus-based dendrimers, using a tetravalent thiophosphoryl trichloride as branching points and aromatic rings as repeating units, present unique features such as globular shape, rigid scaffold due to the multiple double bond and the aromatic rings forming the backbone, an hydrophobic interior with well-defined cavity, high thermal stability, and highly versatile surface functions [89, 90].

A large panel of organophosphorus reactions has been used for the synthesis of phosphorus-containing dendrimers. Besides the efficiency of these reactions, the simplicity of characterization of these large compounds by ^{31}P-NMR must be emphasized. In fact, even highly sophisticated structures can be totally analyzed by ^{31}P-NMR. The presence of phosphorus leads to unprecedented properties, particularly in the fields of catalysis, materials, and biology. In most cases, the water solubility of phosphorus-containing dendrimers is mainly due to the presence of hydrophilic end groups, which bear either positive or negative charges. Some of these dendrimers also possess interesting biological properties and can be used as *in vitro* DNA transfecting agents or *in vivo* anti-prion agents. Phosphorus-containing dendrimers G4(NH+Et2Cl–)96 are delivery agent of ODNs and siRNAs. G4(NH+Et2Cl–)96 formed stable complexes with ODNs or siRNAs and exhibited very low cytotoxicity in Sup T1 cells or PBMCs. Functional validation was performed by using specific siRNA against HIV-1 Nef, siNEF to interfere in HIV-1 replication. G4(NH+Et2Cl–)96/siNEF dendriplex showed a high efficiency in Nef silencing. Furthermore, *in vitro* treatment of HIV-infected PBMCs with G4(NH+Et2Cl–)96/siNEF dendriplex significantly reduced the viral replication. These results prove the usefulness of phosphorus-containing dendrimers to deliver and transfect siRNA into CD4 T cells as a potential alternative therapy in the HIV-1 infection [81].

Carbosilane and phosphorus dendrimers/siRNA complexes have shown high efficiency in HIV-Nef silencing, decreasing HIV replication in SupT1 T-cell line and in human PBMCs, and becoming an alternative strategy to fight against HIV-1 infection [78–82]. Both have shown great properties as non-viral vectors [91–99]. These dendrimers have been described as carriers of siRNA and oligonucleotides in gene therapy against HIV infection, cancer, prion diseases, or Alzheimer [80, 100]. Furthermore, carbosilane dendrimers have shown antiviral and antimicrobial activity and potential as microbicide compounds [101–103].

The fourth-generation maltose-decorated glycodendrimers with PPI-derived structure [84] present cationic groups around their surface that can be localized at the same level of maltose units or that can be placed outside the dendrimer core using spacer arms, facilitating the interaction of functionalized dendrimer's groups with anionic antigens. A dense shell architecture in DS-PPIg4 is suited to undergo H-bonds driven interactions. In the dense shell DS-PPIg4-3(NH2), DS-PPIg4-6(NH2), and the open shell OS-PPig4 glycodendrimers, there is a specific shell composition where both glycodendrimers possess an ambipolar shell with excess of neutral maltose units and randomly distributed cationic alkyl-spacered peripheral amino groups. In these cases, H-bonds and electrostatic interactions can simultaneously occur in the outer shell. These sugar-decorated dendrimers present some advantages in comparison with other groups, since sugar moieties increase dendrimer biocompatibility and also permit dendrimers interaction with lectins and other molecules in immune cells' surface that can be involved in immune response modulation [104–107]. Maltose sugar moiety is not considered a common immune enhancer. However, some studies have shown that the presence of aggregates of maltose or maltosylated compounds can stimulate the immune system in comparison to maltose alone [108, 109]. Some *in vivo* studies using maltosylated PEI nanoparticles have demonstrated that toxicity and transfection capacity were modified regarding the number of maltose-coupled residues to these nanoparticles [110]. It has recently been described that DCs stimulation by sugar moieties-functionalized nanoparticles could be associated to DCs sensibilization, leading to an enhanced antigen presentation, DCs activation, and thus, influencing the potency of the immune response [111].

PAMAM, polyglycerols, and peptide-derived dendrimers have also shown ability as nanocarriers. PAMAM dendrimers are characterized by an easy synthesis with controlled structure and size, minimal cytotoxicity, biodegradability, and high transfection efficiencies [112]. Dendritic polyglycerols exhibit good chemical stability and inertness under biological conditions and are highly biocompatible. They have shown several applications in nanomedicine as gene delivery systems, as well as in regenerative medicine in the form of non-fouling surfaces and matrix materials [113]. In the case of peptide dendrimers, they are branched macromolecules consisting of a peptide branching core and/or covalently attached surface functional units [114].

PPI-derived glycodendrimers, carbosilane dendrimers, and phosphorus dendrimers have been used as vectors to deliver well-defined antigenic motifs to DCs in HIV-1 immunotherapeutic vaccine strategies. Different HIV-1-derived peptides from gp160, p24, and Nef proteins have been used as viral antigens [83–87]. Immunostimulatory properties of maltose-decorated neutrally and positively charged G4 glycodendrimers on human DCs were evaluated in the context of HIV-1 infection. DCs treated with glycodendrimers were fully functional with respect to viability, maturation, and HIV-derived antigens uptake. iDC and mDC phenotypes as well as mDC functions such as migration ability and cytokines profile production were changed. The potential carrier property of glycodendrimers to activate the immune system by the way of DC stimulation was demonstrated. The use of maltose-functionalized dendrimers-peptides complexes could be a potential DC-based vaccine candidate.

On the other hand, iDCs and mDCs captured efficiently water-soluble carbosilane dendrimer (2G-NN16) and did not induce changes in maturation markers levels at the DCs surface. Carbosilane dendrimer-loaded mDCs migrated as efficiently as unloaded DCs toward CCL19 or CCL21. Furthermore, DCs viability, activation of allogenic naïve CD4+ T cells by mDCs, and secretion of cytokines were not significantly changed by 2G-NN16 dendrimer loading. Carbosilane dendrimer 2G-NN16 has no negative effects on the pivotal properties of DCs *in vitro*. It should, therefore, be feasible to further develop this antigen-loading strategy for clinical use in immunotherapy against viral infections.

However, phosphorus dendrimers from second and third generations induced important changes in the DCs phenotype. The treatment of mDCs with the second-generation dendrimer and derivated dendriplexes modified cellular migratory properties, altered their capacity to stimulate allogenic naïve T cells *in vitro* and impeded the production of pro-inflammatory cytokines. The phosphorus dendrimers cannot be used as DCs vaccines because they would not have the ability to induce an immune response. The cationic phosphorus dendrimers associated with HIV-derived peptides have the ability to deliver peptides as non-viral vectors.

However, there are other potential therapeutic applications of these compounds, for instance as topical anti-inflammatory agents, as compounds for allograft rejection or autoimmune diseases, and as agents inducing specific tolerance with antigen-loaded DCs against allergy reaction.

7.7 Dendritic Cells Approved by the US FDA for Vaccination Clinical Trial

The FDA has approved DCs generated *in vitro* for cancer and vaccination clinical trials [115–117]. The isolation and generation of DCs are key points in DC-based immunotherapies. These processes must be performed in optimal, secure, and sterilized conditions to assure the correct differentiation of the DCs and the safety of the HIV-1 subjects. The most accepted and used method to generate *ex vivo* DCs is from peripheral blood CD14+ monocytes isolated from PBMCs [118]. This chosen method has an impact on the subsequent function of DCs by affecting their ability to express co-stimulatory molecules, maturation marker, and to secrete immunomodulatory cytokines [119, 120]. To mature DCs, LPS is commonly used. DCs can also be matured by polyinosinic polycytidylic acid (poly (I: C)) or by a mix of cytokines [121]. Because of the wide diversity of DCs in humans and their roles driving various types of immune responses, it is very crucial to analyze the phenotype of the obtained monocyte-derived DCs.

7.8 *Ex Vivo* and *In Vivo* Assays

Ex vivo loaded DC-based immunotherapies have been extensively studied in a variety of experimental models and clinical trials in the case of cancer [10, 20, 122]. Thus, poly(γ-glutamin acid) and poly(D,L-lactic-co-glycolic acid) nanoparticles have shown efficacy as antigen-delivery carriers in DC-based cancer vaccines [52–54]. These studies have demonstrated that this approach is safe, well tolerated, and capable of inducing cellular immune responses. However, the overall rate of clinical response in patients is still very low, mainly because the migration of *ex vivo* generated DCs to the lymph nodes is very inefficient.

Nevertheless, *ex vivo* loaded DCs present other constraints that make their real development for human use difficult. The most important one is that *ex vivo* loaded DCs have to be tailor made for each individual. Thus, the process of vaccine development is time consuming, requires extensive laboratory work, and standard culture/activation protocols for the generation of clinical grade DCs, and, therefore, is extremely expensive. Finally, existence of several variable parameters in the process (*e.g.*, dose of DCs, route and frequency of administration) makes the process hardly reproducible.

Several nanoparticles such as chitosan, PLGA, PLA-derived platform carrying various HIV-1 antigens have been tested in animal models as HIV-1 immunotherapies [47, 48, 51, 52]. Since HIV-1 causes disease only in humans, sensitive models to HIV-1 infection should be used or engineered, such as macaques or humanized mice. Thereby, p24-loaded PLA nanoparticles subcutaneously injected to mice, rabbits, and macaques elicited significantly higher antibodies titers, including strong cytotoxic T-lymphocyte (CTL) responses *in vivo* [59]. Moreover, in DC-based assays, DCs treated with p24-PLA nanoparticles induced high antibody titers in mice [123]. Poly-amino acids such as poly-g-glutamic acid (PGA) nanoparticles [60], surface-modified polystyrene nanoparticles (PS-NP) [124], or polymethylmethacrylate (PMMA) [125, 126] based nanocarriers for delivering HIV-1 antigens have also been evaluated as vaccine candidates in mice.

An alternative to these *ex vivo* DC-based strategies is to load DCs *in vivo* with HIV-1 antigens using targeted nanoparticle-based delivery systems [10, 122]. It permits antigens to be targeted to multiple DC subjects by targeting multiple receptors, and DCs are reached and activated within their natural environment and at multiple sites. In addition, a major advantage of vaccines based on strategies targeting antigens to DCs *in vivo* is that they can be produced on large scale with lower costs, equal product quality among different locations and accessibility to a large number of patients. However, this approach presents some limitations: Most of the receptors used for *in vivo* DCs targeting strategies are expressed by other cells, limiting the specificity, and *in vivo* targeting of DCs is linked with a poor control of their maturation and activation.

Different cell-surface molecules expressed by DCs are being explored as targets to deliver antigens *in vivo*, such as the C-type lectin mannose receptor, CD205, and DC-specific intercellular adhesion molecule 3 (ICAM3)-grabbing non-integrin (DC-SIGN) [127–132]. The outcome of the *in vivo* DC-based therapy will be influenced by intracellular routing of the targeted receptor. Specific cell-surface receptors trigger distinct intracellular signaling pathways on ligand binding, thereby modulating immune responses. Moreover, what density of ligand should be arrayed on the nanoparticles surface to interact most efficiently with DC is an open question that must be evaluated.

The use of different tailor-engineered dendrimers targeting DC receptors is a promising approach in targeted delivery vaccination strategies. Mannose surface-modified PAMAM dendrimers have been proposed as carriers to facilitate the delivery via C-type mannose receptors of antigens into DCs *in vivo* [133]. Covalently attached CMV pp65-derived peptides to polyamidoamine (PAMAM) dendrimers and coupled to an anti-biotin antibody targeted specifically large amounts of peptides via CD36 biotin antibody to blood DCs for effective stimulation of autologous CMV specific T cells. Furthermore, PLGA polymeric nanoparticles surface-modified with anti-DEC 205 targeted DCs *in vivo* and induced efficient humoral and cellular responses in mice [51, 134].

Nevertheless, to be suitable for this *in vivo* application, first it is essential to perform different studies to evaluate dendrimers toxicity, immunogenicity, or body distribution.

Next improvements in rational synthesis and engineering of dendrimers as well as new strategies in HIV-1 epitopes selection and antigen design (overlapping peptides, bioinformatic-designed mosaic antigens, or immunogenic broadly neutralizing antibodies-derived peptides) will permit the design of novel, safe, and immunogenic nano-vaccines that effectively target antigen delivery *in vivo*, replacing the expensive and unbeatable *ex vivo* culturing techniques and facilitating large-scale application of DC-based vaccination therapies.

Acknowledgments

This work has been (partially) funded by the CYTED 214RT0482; CIBER-BBN is an initiative funded by the VI National R&D&i Plan 2008–2011, IniciativaIngenio 2010, the Consolider Program, and

CIBER Actions and financed by the Instituto de Salud Carlos III with assistance from the European Regional Development Fund. The partial support of FCT-Fundação para a Ciência e a Tecnologia (Project PEst-OE/QUI/UI0674/2013, CQM, Portuguese Government funds) and by ARDITI-Agência Regional para o Desenvolvimento da Investigação Tecnologia e Inovação through the project M1420-01-0145-FEDER-000005 - Centro de Química da Madeira - CQM+ (Madeira 14-20) is also acknowledged.

References

1. Perelson, A. S., Essunger, P., Cao, Y., Vesanen, M., Hurley, A., Saksela, K., Markowitz, M., and Ho, D. D. (1997). Decay characteristics of HIV-1-infected compartments during combination therapy, *Nature*, **387**(6629), pp. 188–191.

2. Lima, V. D., Lourenco, L., Yip, B., Hogg, R. S., Phillips, P., and Montaner, J. S. G. (2015). AIDS incidence and AIDS-related mortality in British Columbia, Canada, between 1981 and 2013: A retrospective study, *Lancet HIV*, **2**, pp. e92–e97.

3. Marrazzo, J. M., del Rio, C., Holtgrave, J. R., Cohen, M. S., Kalichman, S. C., Mayer, K. H., Montaner, J. S. G., Wheeler, D. P., Grant, R. M., Grinsztejn, B., Kumarasamy, N., Shoptaw, S., Walensky, R. P., Dabis, F., Sugarman, J., and Benson, C. A. (2014). HIV prevention in clinical care settings: 2014 recommendations of the International Antiviral Society-USA Panel, *JAMA*, **312**, pp. 390–409.

4. Scherer, E., Douek, D., and Mcmichael, A. (2008). 25 years of HIV research on virology, virus restriction, immunopathogenesis, genes and vaccines, *Clin. Exp. Immunol.*, **154**, pp. 6–14.

5. Munier, C. M., Andersen, C. R., and Kelleher, A. D. (2011). HIV vaccines: Progress to date, *Drugs*, **71**, pp. 387–414.

6. Rerks-Ngarm, S., Pitisuttithum, P., Nitayaphan, S., Kaewkungwal, J., Chiu, J., Paris, R., Premsri, N., Namwat, C., de Souza, M., Adams, E., Benenson, M., Gurunathan, S., Tartaglia, J., McNeil, J. G., Francis, D. P., Stablein, D., Birx, D. L., Chunsuttiwat, S., Khamboonruang, C., Thongcharoen, P., Robb, M. L., Michael, N. L., Kunasol, P., Kim, J. H., and MOPH-TAVEG Investigators. (2009). Vaccination with ALVAC and AIDSVAX to prevent HIV-1 infection in Thailand, *N. Engl. J. Med.*, **361**, pp. 2209–2220.

7. Pitisuttithum, P., Rerks-Ngarm, S., Bussaratid, V., Dhitavat, J., Maekanantawat, W., Pungpak, S., Suntharasamai, P., Vanijanonta, S., Nitayapan, S., Kaewkungwal, J., Benenson, M., Morgan, P., O'Connell, R.

J., Berenberg, J., Gurunathan, S., Francis, D. P., Paris, R., Chiu, J., Stablein, D., Michael, N. L., Excler, J. L., Robb, M. L., and Kim, J. H. (2011). Safety and reactogenicity of canarypox ALVAC-HIV (vCP1521) and HIV-1 gp120 AIDSVAX B/E vaccination in an efficacy trial in Thailand, *PLoS One*, **6**, pp. e27837.

8. Mills, R., Tyring, S. K., Levin, M. J., Parrino, J., Li, X., Coll, K. E., Stek, J. E., Schlienger, K., Chan, I. S., and Silber, J. L. (2010). Safety, tolerability, and immunogenicity of zoster vaccine in subjects with a history of herpes zoster, *Vaccine*, **28**, pp. 4204–4209.

9. Angel, J. B., Routy, J. P., Tremblay, C., Ayers, D., Woods, R., Singer, J., Bernard, N., Kovacs, C., Smaill, F., Gurunathan, S., and Sekaly, R. P. (2011). A randomized controlled trial of HIV therapeutic vaccination using ALVAC with or without Remune, *AIDS*, **25**, pp. 731–739.

10. Shimada, M., Wang, H. B., Kondo, A., Xu, X. P., Yoshida, A., Shinoda, K., Ura, T., Mizuguchi, H., Klinman, D., Luo, J. L., Bai, H., and Okuda, K. (2009). Effect of therapeutic immunization using Ad5/35 and MVA vectors on SIV infection of rhesus monkeys undergoing antiretroviral therapy, *Gene Ther.*, **16**, pp. 218–228.

11. Tacken, P. J., De Vries, I. J., Torensma, R., and Figdor, C. G. (2007). Dendritic-cell immunotherapy: From *ex vivo* loading to *in vivo* targeting, *Nat. Rev. Immunol.*, **7**, pp. 790–802.

12. Vanham, G. and Van Gulck, E. (2012). Can immunotherapy be useful as a "functional cure" for infection with Human Immunodeficiency Virus-1? *Retrovirology*, **9**, pp. 72.

13. Van Gils, M. J. and Sanders, R. W. (2013). Broadly neutralizing antibodies against HIV-1: Templates for a vaccine, *Virology*, **435**, pp. 46–56.

14. Walker, L. M., Huber, M., Doores, K. J., Falkowska, E., Pejchal, R., Julien, J. P., Wang, S. K., Ramos, A., Chan-Hui, P. Y., Moyle, M., Mitcham, J. L., Hammond, P. W., Olsen, O. A., Phung, P., Fling, S., Wong, C. H., Phogat, S., Wrin, T., Simek, M. D., Protocol G Principal Investigators, Koff, W. C., Wilson, I. A., Burton, D. R., and Poignard, P. (2011). Broad neutralization coverage of HIV by multiple highly potent antibodies, *Nature*, **477**(7365), pp. 466–470.

15. Steinman, R. M. (2012). Decisions about dendritic cells: Past, present, and future, *Annu. Rev. Immunol.*, **30**, pp. 1–22.

16. Palucka, K. and Banchereau, J. (2013). Dendritic-cell-based therapeutic cancer vaccines, *Immunity*, **39**, pp. 38–48.

17. Thara, E., Dorff, T. B., Pinski, J. K., and Quinn, D. I. (2013). Vaccine therapy with sipuleucel-T (Provenge) for prostate cancer, *Maturitas*, **69**, pp. 296–303.

18. Trepiakas, R., Berntsen, A., Hadrup, S. R., Bjørn, J., Geertsen, P. F., Straten, P. T., Andersen, M. H., Pedersen, A. E., Soleimani, A., Lorentzen, T., Johansen, J. S., and Svane, I. M. (2010). Vaccination with autologous dendritic cells pulsed with multiple tumor antigens for treatment of patients with malignant melanoma: Results from a phase I/II trial, *Cytotherapy*, **12**, pp. 721–734.

19. Vacchelli, E., Vitale, I., Eggermont, A., Fridman, W. H., Fučíková, J., Cremer, I., Galon, J., Tartour, E., Zitvogel, L., Kroemer, G., and Galluzzi, L. (2013). Trial watch: Dendritic cell-based interventions for cancer therapy, *Oncoimmunology*, 2(10), pp. e25771.

20. Cheever, M. A. and Higano, C. S. (2011). PROVENGE (Sipuleucel-T) in prostate cancer: The first FDA-approved therapeutic cancer vaccine, *Clin. Cancer Res.*, **17**, pp. 3520–3526.

21. Garcia, F., Climent, N., Guardo, A. C., Gil, C., León, A., Autran, B., Lifson, J. D., Martínez-Picado, J., Dalmau, J., Clotet, B., Gatell, J. M., Plana, M., and Gallart, T. (2013). A dendritic cell-based vaccine elicits T-cell responses associated with control of HIV-1 replication, *Sci. Transl. Med.*, **5**(166), pp. 166ra2.

22. Rinaldo, C. R. (2009). Dendritic cell-based human immunodeficiency virus vaccine, *J. Intern. Med.*, **265**, pp. 138–158.

23. Yoshida, A., Tanaka, R., Murakami, T., Takahashi, Y., Koyanagi, Y., Nakamura, M., Ito, M., Yamamoto, N., and Tanaka, Y. (2003). Induction of protective immune responses against R5 human immunodeficiency virus type 1 (HIV-1) infection in hu-PBL-SCID mice by intrasplenic immunization with HIV-1-pulsed dendritic cells: Possible involvement of a novel factor of human CD4(+) T-cell origin, *J. Virol.*, **77**, pp. 8719–8728.

24. Van Tendeloo, V. F., Ponsaerts, P., Lardon, F., Nijs, G., Lenjou, M., Van Broeckhoven, C., Van Bockstaele, D. R., and Berneman, Z. N. (2001). Highly efficient gene delivery by mRNA electroporation in human hematopoietic cells: Superiority to lipofection and passive pulsing of mRNA and to electroporation of plasmid cDNA for tumor antigen loading of dendritic cells, *Blood*, **98**, pp. 49–56.

25. Ahlers, J. D. and Belyakov, I. M. (2009). Strategies for recruiting and targeting dendritic cells for optimizing HIV vaccines, *Trends Mol. Med.*, **15**, pp. 263–274.

26. Trumpfheller, C., Longhi, M. P., Caskey, M., Idoyaga, J., Bozzacco, L., Keler, T., Schlesinger, S. J., and Steinman, R. M. (2012). Dendritic cell-targeted protein vaccines: A novel approach to induce T-cell immunity, *J. Intern. Med.*, **271**, pp. 183–192.

27. Pavot. V., Climent, N., Rochereau, N., Garcia, F., Genin, C., Tiraby, G., Vernejoul, F., Perouzel, E., Lioux, T., Verrier, B., and Paul, S. (2016). Directing vaccine immune responses to mucosa by nanosized particulate carriers encapsulating NOD ligands, *Biomaterials*, **75**, pp. 327–339.

28. Lu, W., Arraes, L. C., Ferreira, W. T., and Andrieu, J. M. (2004). Therapeutic dendritic-cell vaccine for chronic HIV-1 infection, *Nat. Med.*, **10**, pp. 1359–1365.

29. Steinman, R. M. and Nussenzweig, M. C. (2002). Avoiding horror autotoxicus: The importance of dendritic cells in peripheral T-cell tolerance, *Proc. Natl. Acad. Sci. USA*, **99**, pp. 351–358.

30. Martinez, E., Milinkovic, A., Buira, E., de Lazzari, E., León, A., Larrousse, M., Loncá, M., Laguno, M., Blanco, J. L., Mallolas, J., García, F., Miró, J. M., and Gatell, J. M. (2007). Incidence and causes of death in HIV-infected persons receiving highly active antiretroviral therapy compared with estimates for the general population of similar age and from the same geographical area, *HIV Med.*, **8**, pp. 251–258.

31. El-Sadr, W. M., Lundgren, J., Neaton, J. D., Gordin, F., Abrams, D., Arduino, R. C., Babiker, A., Burman, W., Clumeck, N., Cohen, C. J., Cohn, D., Cooper, D., Darbyshire, J., Emery, S., Fätkenheuer, G., Gazzard, B., Grund, B., Hoy, J., Klingman, K., Losso, M., Markowitz, N., Neuhaus, J., Phillips, A., and Rappoport, C. (2006). CD4+ count-guided interruption of antiretroviral treatment, *N. Engl. J. Med.*, **355**, pp. 2283–2296.

32. Deeks, S. G., Autran, B., Berkhout, B., Benkirane, M., Cairns, S., Chomont, N., Chun, T. W., Churchill, M., Di Mascio, M., Katlama, C., Lafeuillade, A., Landay, A., Lederman, M., Lewin, S. R., Maldarelli, F., Margolis, D., Markowitz, M., Martinez-Picado, J., Mullins, J. I., Mellors, J., Moreno, S., O'Doherty, U., Palmer, S., Penicaud, M. C., Peterlin, M., Poli, G., Routy, J. P., Rouzioux, C., Silvestri, G., Stevenson, M., Telenti, A., Van Lint, C., Verdin, E., Woolfrey, A., Zaia, J., and Barré-Sinoussi, F. (2012). Towards an HIV cure: A global scientific strategy, *Nat. Rev. Immunol.*, **12**, pp. 607–614.

33. Garcia, F., Plana, M., Climent, N., León, A., Gatell, J. M., and Gallart, T. (2013). Dendritic cell based vaccines for HIV infection: The way ahead, *Hum. Vaccine Immunother.*, **9**, pp. 2445–2452.

34. Van Gulck, E., Bracke, L., Heyndrickx, L., Coppens, S., Atkinson, D., Merlin, C., Pasternak, A., Florence, E., and Vanham, G. (2012). Immune and viral correlates of "secondary viral control" after treatment interruption in chronically HIV-1 infected patients, *PLoS One*, **7**, pp. e37792.

35. Van Lint, S., Goyvaerts, C., Maenhout, S., Goethals, L., Disy, A., Benteyn, D., Pen, J., Bonehill, A., Heirman, C., Breckpot, K., and Thielemans, K. (2012). Preclinical evaluation of TriMix and antigen mRNA-based antitumor therapy, *Cancer Res.*, **72**, pp. 1661–1671.

36. Pollard, C., De Doker, S., Saelens, X., Vanham, G., and Grooten, J. (2013). Challenges and advances towards the rational design of mRNA vaccines, *Trends Mol. Med.*, **19**, pp. 705–713.

37. http://archives.esf.org/fileadmin/Public_documents/Publications/Nanomedicine.pdf

38. Kim, B. Y, Rutka, J. T, and Chan, W. C. (2010). Nanomedicine, *N. Engl. J. Med.*, **363**, pp. 2434–2443.

39. Moghimi, S. M., Hunter, A. C., and Murray, J. C. (2005). Nanomedicine: Current status and future prospects, *FASEB J.*, **19**, pp. 311–330.

40. Kannan, R. M., Nance, E., Kannan, S., and Tomalia, D. A. (2014). Emerging concepts in dendrimer-based nanomedicine: From design principles to clinical applications, *J. Intern. Med.*, **276**, pp. 579–617.

41. Madaan, K., Kumar, S., Poonia, N., Lather, V., and Pandita, D. (2014). Dendrimers in drug delivery and targeting: Drug-dendrimer interactions and toxicity issues, *J. Pharm. Bioallied Sci.*, **6**, pp. 139–150.

42. Svenson, S. (2015). The dendrimer paradox-high medical expectations but poor clinical translation, *Chem. Soc. Rev.*, **44**, pp. 4131–4144.

43. Mallipeddi, R. and Rohan, L. C. (2010). Progress in antiretroviral drug delivery using nanotechnology, *Int. J. Nanomedicine*, **5**, pp. 533–547.

44. Mahajan, S. D., Aalinkeel, R., Law, W. C., Reynolds, J. L., Nair, B. B., Sykes, D. E., Yong, K. T., Roy, I., Prasad, P. N., and Schwartz, S. A. (2012). Anti-HIV-1 nanotherapeutics: Promises and challenges for the future, *Int. J. Nanomedicine*, **7**, pp. 5301–5314.

45. Siccardi, M., Martin, P., Mcdonald, T. O., Liptrott, N. J., Giardiello, M., Rannard, S., and Owen, A. (2013). Nanomedicines for HIV therapy, *Ther. Deliv.*, **4**, pp. 153–156.

46. Zhang, J., Mulvenon, A., Makarov, E., Wagoner, J., Knibbe, J., Kim, J. O., Osna, N., Bronich, T. K., and Poluektova, L. Y. (2013). Antiviral peptide nanocomplexes as a potential therapeutic modality for HIV/HCV co-infection, *Biomaterials*, **34**, pp. 3846–3857.

47. Date, A. A. and Destache, C. J. (2013). A review of nanotechnological approaches for the prophylaxis of HIV/AIDS, *Biomaterials*, **34**, pp. 6202–6228.

48. Kim, P. S. and Read, S. W. (2010). Nanotechnology and HIV: Potential applications for treatment and prevention, *Wiley Interdiscip. Rev. Nanomed. Nanobiotechnol.*, **2**, pp. 693–702.

49. Mamo, T., Moseman, E. A., Kolishetti, N., Salvador-Morales, C., Shi, J., Kuritzkes, D. R., Langer, R., von Andrian, U., and Farokhzad, O. C. (2010). Emerging nanotechnology approaches for HIV/AIDS treatment and prevention, *Nanomedicine (Lond.)*, **5**, pp. 269–285.

50. Boyapalle, S. and Mohapatra, S. (2012). Nanotechnology applications to HIV vaccines and microbicides, *J. Glob. Infect. Dis.*, **4**, pp. 62–68.

51. Fahmy, T. M., Demento, S. L., Caplan, M. J., Mellman, I., and Saltzman, W. M. (2008). Design opportunities for actively targeted nanoparticle vaccines, *Nanomedicine (Lond.)*, **3**, pp. 343–355.

52. Hamdy, S., Haddadi, A., Hung, R. W., and Lavasanifar, A. (2011). Targeting dendritic cells with nano-particulate PLGA cancer vaccine formulations, *Adv. Drug Deliv. Rev.*, **63**, pp. 943–955.

53. Reddy, S. T., Rehor, A., Schmoekel, H. G., Hubbell, J. A., and Swartz, M. A. (2006). In vivo targeting of dendritic cells in lymph nodes with poly(propylene sulfide) nanoparticles, *J. Control. Release*, **112**, pp. 26–34.

54. Hori, Y., Winans, A. M., Huang, C. C., Horrigan, E. M., and Irvine, D. J. (2008). Injectable dendritic cell-carrying alginate gels for immunization and immunotherapy, *Biomaterials*, **29**, pp. 3671–3682.

55. Elamanchili, P., Diwan, M., Cao, M., and Samuel, J. (2004). Characterization of poly(D,L-lactic-co-glycolic acid) based nanoparticulate system for enhanced delivery of antigens to dendritic cells, *Vaccine*, **22**, pp. 2406–2412.

56. Singh, S. K. and Bisen, P. S. (2006). Adjuvanticity of stealth liposomes on the immunogenicity of synthetic gp41 epitope of HIV-1, *Vaccine*, **24**, pp. 4161–4166.

57. Wagner, A., Stiegler, G., Vorauer-Uhl, K., Katinger, H., Quendler, H., Hinz, A., and Weissenhorn, W. (2007). One step membrane incorporation of viral antigens as a vaccine candidate against HIV, *J. Liposome Res.*, **17**, pp. 139–154.

58. Aline, F., Brand, D., Pierre, J., Roingeard, P., Séverine, M., Verrier, B., and Dimier-Poisson, I. (2009). Dendritic cells loaded with HIV-1 p24 proteins adsorbed on surfactant-free anionic PLA nanoparticles induce enhanced cellular immune responses against HIV-1 after vaccination, *Vaccine*, **27**, pp. 5284–5291.

59. Lamalle-Bernard, D., Munier, S., Compagnon, C., Charles, M. H., Kalyanaraman, V. S., Delair, T., Verrier, B., and Ataman-Onal, Y. (2006). Coadsorption of HIV-1 p24 and gp120 proteins to surfactant-free anionic PLA nanoparticles preserves antigenicity and immunogenicity, *J. Control. Release*, **115**, pp. 57–67.

60. Wang, X., Uto, T., Akagi, T., Akashi, M., and Baba, M. (2008). Poly(gamma-glutamic acid) nanoparticles as an efficient antigen delivery and adjuvant system: Potential for an AIDS vaccine, *J. Med. Virol.*, **80**, pp. 11–19.

61. Lisziewicz, J., Bakare, N., Calarota, S. A., Bánhegyi, D., Szlávik, J., Ujhelyi, E., Tőke, E. R., Molnár, L., Lisziewicz, Z., Autran, B., and Lori, F. (2012). Single DermaVir immunization: Dose-dependent expansion of precursor/memory T cells against all HIV antigens in HIV-1 infected individuals, *PLoS One*, **7**, pp. e35416.

62. Lori, F. (2011). DermaVir: A plasmid DNA-based nanomedicine therapeutic vaccine for the treatment of HIV/AIDS, *Expert Rev. Vaccines*, **10**, pp. 1371–1384.

63. Tomalia, D. A. (1996). Dendrimer molecules, *Sci. Am.*, **272**, pp. 62–66.

64. Tomalia, D. A. (1996). Starburst dendrimers-nanoscopic supermolecules according to dendritic rules and principles, *Macromol. Symp.*, **101**, pp. 243–255.

65. Kaminskas, L. M., Boyd, B. J., and Porter, C. J. (2011). Dendrimer pharmacokinetics: The effect of size, structure and surface characteristics on ADME properties, *Nanomedicine (Lond.)*, **6**, pp. 1063–1084.

66. Svenson, S. and Tomalia, D. A. (2005). Dendrimers in biomedical applications-reflections on the field, *Adv. Drug Deliv. Rev.*, **57**, pp. 2106–2129.

67. Mintzer, M. A. and Grinstaff, W. W. (2011). Biomedical applications of dendrimers: A tutorial, *Sev. Soc. Rev.*, **40**, pp. 173–190.

68. Kannan, R. M., Nance, E., Kannan, S., and Tomalia, D. A. (2014). Emerging concepts in dendrimer-based nanomedicine: From design principles to clinical applications, *J. Intern. Med.*, **276**, pp. 579–617.

69. Jain, K., Kesharwani, P., Gupta, U., and Jain, N. K. (2012). A review of glycosilated carriers for drug delivery, *Biomaterials*, **33**, pp. 4166–4186.

70. Kesharwani, P., Jain, K., and Jain, N. K. (2014). Dendrimer as nanocarrier for drug delivery, *Prog. Polym. Sci.*, **39**, pp. 268–307.

71. Nanjwade, B. K., Bechra, H. M., Derkar, G. K., Manvi, F. V., and Nanjwade, V. K. (2009). Dendrimers: Emerging polymers for drug-delivery systems, *Eur. J. Pharm. Sci.*, **38**, pp. 185–196.

72. Vögtle, F., Richardt, G., and Werner, N. (2009). Types of dendrimers and their syntheses. In *Dendrimer Chemistry: Concepts, Syntheses, Properties, Applications*, W. Wiley-VCH Verlag GmbH & Co. KGaA, Germany, pp. 81–167.

73. Gunay, M. S., Ozer, A. Y., and Chalon, S. (2016). Drug delivery systems for imaging and therapy of Parkinson's disease, *Curr. Neuropharmacol.*, **14**, pp. 376–391.

74. Caminade, A. M., Laurent, R., and Majoral, J. P. (2005). Characterization of dendrimers, *Adv. Drug Deliv. Rev.*, **57**, pp. 2130–2146.

75. Miyake, Y., Ishikawa, S., and Kimura, Y. (2015). Pharmacokinetics of chiral dendrimer-triamine-coordinated gd-mri contrast agents evaluated by *in vivo* MRI and estimated by *in vitro* QCM, *Sensors (Basel)*, **5**, pp. 31973–31986.

76. Liu, X. X., Rocchi, P., Qu, F. Q., Zheng, S. Q., Liang, Z. C., Gleave, M., Iovanna, J., and Peng, L. (2009). PAMAM dendrimers mediate siRNA delivery to target Hsp27 and produce potent antiproliferative effects on prostate cancer cells, *ChemMedChem*, **4**, pp. 1302–1310.

77. Shcharbin, D. G., Klajnert, B., and Bryszewska, M. (2009). Dendrimers in gene transfection, *Biochemistry (Mosc)*, **74**, pp. 1070–1079.

78. Pedziwiatr-Werbicka, E., Fuentes, E., Dzmitruk, V., Sanchez-Nieves, J., Sudas, M., Drozd, E., Shakhbazau, A., Shcharbin, D., de la Mata, F. J., Gomez-Ramirez, R., Munoz-Fernandez, M. A., and Bryszewska, M. (2013). Novel 'SiC' carbosilane dendrimers as carriers for anti-HIV nucleic acids: Studies on complexation and interaction with blood cells, *Colloids Surf. B Biointerfaces*, **109**, pp. 183–189.

79. Weber, N., Ortega, P., Clemente, M. I., Shcharbin, D., Bryszewska, M., de la Mata, F. J., Gomez, R., and Munoz-Fernandez, M. A. (2008). Characterization of carbosilane dendrimers as effective carriers of siRNA to HIV-infected lymphocytes, *J. Control. Release*, **132**, pp. 55–64.

80. Jimenez, J. L., Clemente, M. I., Weber, N. D., Sanchez, J., Ortega, P., de la Mata, F. J., Gomez, R., Garcia, D., Lopez-Fernandez, L. A., and Munoz-Fernandez, M. A. (2010). Carbosilane dendrimers to transfect human astrocytes with small interfering RNA targeting human immunodeficiency virus, *BioDrugs*, **24**, pp. 331–343.

81. Briz, V., Serramia, M. J., Madrid, R., Hameau, A., Caminade, A. M., Majoral, J. P., and Munoz-Fernandez, M. A. (2012). Validation of a generation

4 phosphorus-containing polycationic dendrimer for gene delivery against HIV-1, *Curr. Med. Chem.*, **19**, pp. 5044–5051.

82. Gonzalo, T., Clemente, M. I., Chonco, L. Weber, N. D., Diaz, L., Serramia, M. J., Gras, R., Ortega, P., de la Mata, F. J., Gomez, R., Lopez-Fernandez, L. A., Munoz-Fernandez, M. A., and Jimenez, J. L. (2010). Gene therapy in HIV-infected cells to decrease viral impact by using an alternative delivery method, *ChemMedChem*, **5**, pp. 921–929.

83. Pion, M., Serramia, M. J., Diaz, L., Bryszewska, M., Gallart, T., Garcia, F., Gomez, R., de la Mata, F. J., and Munoz-Fernandez, M. A. (2010). Phenotype and functional analysis of human monocytes-derived dendritic cells loaded with a carbosilane dendrimer, *Biomaterials*, **31**, pp. 8749–8758.

84. Cordoba, E. V., Pion, M., Rasines, B., Filippini, D., Komber, H., Ionov, M., Bryszewska, M., Appelhans, D., and Munoz-Fernandez, M. A. (2013). Glycodendrimers as new tools in the search for effective anti-HIV DC-based immunotherapies, *Nanomedicine*, **9**, pp. 972–984.

85. Vacas-Cordoba, E. V., Bastida, H., Pion, M., Hameau, A., Ionov, M., Bryszewska, M., Caminade, A. M., Majoral, J. P., and Muñoz-Fernández, M. A. (2014). HIV-antigens charged on phosphorus dendrimers as tools for tolerogenic dendritic cells-based immunotherapy, *Curr. Med. Chem.*, **21**, pp. 1898–1909.

86. Caminade, A. M. and Majoral, J. P. (2005). Water-soluble phosphorus-containing dendrimers, *Prog. Polym. Sci.*, **30**, pp. 491–505.

87. Caminade, A. M., Turrin, C. O., and Majoral, J. P. (2010). Biological properties of phosphorus dendrimers, *New J. Chem.*, **34**, pp. 1512–1524.

88. Caminade, A. M., Laurent, R., Zablocka, M., and Majoral, J. P. (2012). Organophosphorus chemistry for the synthesis of dendrimers, *Molecules*, **17**, pp. 13605–13621.

89. Caminade, A. M. and Majoral, J. P. (2016). Bifunctional phosphorous dendrimers and their properties, *Molecules*, **21**, pp. 538

90. Caminade, A. M., Ouali, A., Laurent, R., Turrin, C. O., and Majoral, J. P. (2015). The dendritic effect illustrated with phosphorous dendrimers, *Chem. Soc. Rev.*, **44**, pp. 3890–3899.

91. Pedziwiatr, E., Shcharbin, D., Chonco, L., Ortega, P., de la Mata, F., Gomez, R., Klajnert, B., Bryszewska, M., and Munoz-Fernandez, M. A. (2009). Binding properties of water-soluble carbosilane dendrimers, *J. Fluoresc.*, **19**, pp. 267–275.

92. Bermejo, J. F., Ortega, P., Chonco, L., Eritja, R., Samaniego, R., Mullner, M., de Jesus, E., de la Mata, F. J., Flores, J. C., Gomez, R., and Munoz-Fernandez, A. (2007). Water-soluble carbosilane dendrimers: Synthesis biocompatibility and complexation with oligonucleotides; evaluation for medical applications, *Chem. Eur. J.*, **13**, pp. 483–495.

93. Vacas Córdoba, E. V., Arnaiz, E., Relloso, M., Sánchez-Torres, C., García, F., Pérez-Álvarez, L., Gómez, R., de la Mata, F. J., Pion, M., and Muñoz-Fernández, M. A. (2013). Development of sulphated and naphthylsulfonated carbosilane dendrimers as topical microbicides to prevent HIV-1 sexual transmission, *AIDS*, **27**, pp. 1219–1229.

94. Rasines, B., Sanchez-Nieves, J., Molina, I. T., Guzman, M., Munoz-Fernandez, M. A., Gomez, R., and de la Mata F. J. (2012). Synthesis and fluorescent properties of cationic carbosilane dendrimers containing eugenol linkers for their use in biomedical applications, *New J. Chem.*, **36**, pp. 360–370.

95. Rasines, B., Hernandez-Ros, J. M., De Las Cuevas, N., Copa-Patino, J. L., Soliveri, J., Munoz-Fernandez, M. A., Gomeza, R., and de la Mata, F. J. (2009). Water-stable ammonium-terminated carbosilane dendrimers as efficient antibacterial agents, *Dalton Trans.*, **40**, pp. 8704–8713.

96. Rasines, B., Sanchez-Nieves, J., Maiolo, M., Maly, M., Chonco, L., Jimenez, J. L., Munoz-Fernandez, M. A., de la Mata, F. J., and Gomez, R. (2012). Synthesis, structure and molecular modelling of anionic carbosilane dendrimers, *Dalton Trans.*, **41**, pp. 12733–12748.

97. Sanchez-Nieves, J., Fransen, P., Pulido, D., Lorente, R., Munoz-Fernandez, M. A., Albericio, F., Royo, M., Gomez, R., and de la Mata, F. J. (2014). Amphiphilic cationic carbosilane-PEG dendrimers: Synthesis and applications in gene therapy, *Eur. J. Med. Chem.*, **76**, pp. 43–52.

98. De Las Cuevas, N., Garcia-Gallego, S., Rasines, B., de la Mata, F. J., Guijarro, L. G., Munoz-Fernandez, M. A., and Gomez, R. (2012). In vitro studies of water-stable cationic carbosilane dendrimers as delivery vehicles for gene therapy against HIV and hepatocarcinoma, *Curr. Med. Chem.*, **19**, pp. 5052–5061.

99. Posadas, I., Lopez-Hernandez, B., Clemente, M. I., Jimenez, J. L., Ortega, P., de la Mata, J., Gomez, R., Munoz-Fernandez, M. A., and Cena, V. (2009). Highly efficient transfection of rat cortical neurons using carbosilane dendrimers unveils a neuroprotective role for HIF-1alpha in early chemical hypoxia-mediated neurotoxicity, *Pharm. Res.*, **26**, pp. 1181–1191.

100. Ionov, M., Ciepluch, K., Klajnert, B., Glinska, S., Gomez-Ramirez, R., de la Mata, F. J., Munoz-Fernandez, M. A., and Bryszewska, M. (2013).

Complexation of HIV derived peptides with carbosilane dendrimers, *Colloids Surf. B Biointerfaces*, **101**, pp. 236–242.

101. Chonco, L., Pion, M., Vacas, E., Rasines, B., Maly, M., Serramia M. J., Lopez-Fernandez, L., De la Mata, J., Alvarez, S., Gomez, R., and Munoz-Fernandez, M. A. (2012). Carbosilane dendrimer nanotechnology outlines of the broad HIV blocker profile, *J. Control. Release*, **161**, pp. 949–958.

102. Sepulveda-Crespo, D., Lorente, R., Leal, M., Gomez, R., De la Mata, F. J., Jimenez, J. L., and Munoz-Fernandez, M. A. (2014). Synergistic activity profile of carbosilane dendrimer G2-STE16 in combination with other dendrimers and antiretrovirals as topical anti-HIV-1 microbicide, *Nanomedicine*, **10**, pp. 609–618.

103. Cordoba, E. V., Arnaiz, E., De La Mata, F. J., Gomez, R., Leal, M., Pion, M., and Munoz-Fernandez, M. A. (2013). Synergistic activity of carbosilane dendrimers in combination with maraviroc against HIV *in vitro*, *AIDS*, **27**, pp. 2053–2058.

104. Garcia-Vallejo, J. J., Koning, N., Ambrosini, M., Kalay, H., Vuist, I., Sarrami-Forooshani, R., Geijtenbeek, T. B. H., and van Kooyk, Y. (2013). Glycodendrimers prevent HIV transmission via DC-SIGN on dendritic cells, *Int. Immunol.*, **25**, pp. 221–233.

105. Klajnert, B., Appelhans, D., Komber, H., Morgner, N., Schwarz, S., Richter, S., Brutschy, B., Ionov, M., Tonkikh, A. K., Bryszewska, M., and Voit, B. (2008). The influence of densely organized maltose shells on the biological properties of poly(propylene imine) dendrimers: New effects dependent on hydrogen bonding, *Chem. Eur. J.*, **14**, pp. 7030–7041.

106. Klementieva, O., Benseny-Cases, N., Gella, A., Appelhans, D., Voit, B., and Cladera, J. (2011). Dense shell glycodendrimers as potential nontoxic anti-amyloidogenic agents in Alzheimer's disease. Amyloid--dendrimer aggregates morphology and cell toxicity, *Biomacromolecules*, **12**, pp. 3903–3909.

107. Ionov, M., Ciepluch, K., Moreno, B. R., Appelhans, D., Sanchez-Nieves, J., Gomez, R., de la Mata, F. J., Munoz-Fernandez, M. A., and Bryszewska, M. (2013). Biophysical characterization of glycodendrimers as nano-carriers for HIV peptides, *Curr. Med. Chem.*, **20**, pp. 3935–3943.

108. Cho, H. J., Han, S. E., Im, S., Lee, Y., Kim, Y. B., Chun, T., and Oh, Y. K. (2011). Maltosylated polyethylenimine-based triple nanocomplexes of human papillomavirus 16L1 protein and DNA as a vaccine co-delivery system, *Biomaterials*, **32**, pp. 4621–4629.

109. Irache, J. M., Salman, H. H., Gamazo, C., and Espuelas, S. (2008). Mannose-targeted systems for the delivery of therapeutics, *Expert Opin. Drug Deliv.*, **5**, pp. 703–724.

110. Hobel, S., Loos, A., Appelhans, D., Schwarz. S., Seidel, J., Voit, B., and Aigner, A. (2011). Maltose- and maltotriose-modified, hyperbranched poly(ethylene imine)s (OM-PEIs): Physicochemical and biological properties of DNA and siRNA complexes, *J. Control. Release*, **149**, pp. 146–158.

111. Carrillo-Conde, B., Song, E. H., Chavez-Santoscoy, A., Phanse, Y., Ramer-Tait, A. E., Pohl, N. L., Wannemuehler, M. J., Bellaire, B. H., and Narasimhan, B. (2011). Mannose-functionalized "pathogen-like" polyanhydride nanoparticles target C-type lectin receptors on dendritic cells, *Mol. Pharm.*, **8**, pp. 1877–1886.

112. Braun, C. S., Vetro, J. A., Tomalia, D. A., Koe, G. S., Koe, J. G., and Middaugh, C. R. (2005) Structure/function relationships of polyamidoamine/DNA dendrimers as gene delivery vehicles, *J. Pharm. Sci.*, **94**, pp. 423–436.

113. Khandare, J., Calderon, M., Dagia, N. M., and Haag, R. (2012). Multifunctional dendritic polymers in nanomedicine: Opportunities and challenges, *Chem. Soc. Rev.*, **41**, pp. 2824–2848.

114. Sadler, K. and Tam, J. P. (2002). Peptide dendrimers: Applications and synthesis, *Rev. Mol. Biotechnol.*, **90**, pp. 195–229.

115. Kantoff, P. W., Higano, C. S., Shore, N. D., Berger, E. R., Small, E. J., Penson, D. F., Redfern, C. H., Ferrari, A. C., Dreicer, R., Sims, R. B., Xu, Y., Frohlich, M. W., Schellhammer, P. F., and IMPACT Study Investigators. (2010). Sipuleucel-T immunotherapy for castration-resistant prostate cancer, *N. Engl. J. Med.*, **363**, pp. 411–422.

116. Liu, Y. J. (2005). IPC: Professional type 1 interferon-producing cells and plasmacytoid dendritic cell precursors, *Annu. Rev. Immunol.*, **23**, pp. 275–306.

117. Tel, J., Aarntzen, E. H., Baba, T., Schreibelt, G., Schulte, B. M., Benitez-Ribas, D., Boerman, O. C., Croockewit, S., Oyen, W. J., van Rossum, M., Winkels, G., Coulie, P. G., Punt, C. J., Figdor, C. G., and de Vries, I. J. (2013). Natural human plasmacytoid dendritic cells induce antigen-specific T-cell responses in melanoma patients, *Cancer Res.*, **73**, pp. 1063–1075.

118. Romani, N., Gruner, S., Brang, D., Kämpgen, E., Lenz, A., Trockenbacher, B., Konwalinka, G., Fritsch, P. O., Steinman, R. M., and Schuler, G. (1994). Proliferating dendritic cell progenitors in human blood, *J. Exp. Med.*, **180**, pp. 83–93.

119. Elkord, E., Williams, P. E., Kynaston, H., and Rowbottom, A. W. (2005). Human monocyte isolation methods influence cytokine production from *in vitro* generated dendritic cells, *Immunology*, **114**, pp. 204–212.

120. Hiasa, M., Abe, M., Nakano, A., Oda, A., Amou, H., Kido, S., Takeuchi, K., Kagawa, K., Yata, K., Hashimoto, T., Ozaki, S., Asaoka, K., Tanaka, E., Moriyama, K., and Matsumoto, T. (2009). GM-CSF and IL-4 induce dendritic cell differentiation and disrupt osteoclastogenesis through M-CSF receptor shedding by up-regulation of TNF-alpha converting enzyme (TACE), *Blood*, **114**, pp. 4517–4526.

121. Matera, L. and Galetto, A. (2003). In vitro maturation of dendritic cells from blood progenitors, *Methods Mol. Biol.*, **215**, pp. 417–426.

122. Tacken, P. J. and Figdor, C. G. (2011). Targeted antigen delivery and activation of dendritic cells *in vivo*: Steps towards cost effective vaccines, *Semin. Immunol.*, **23**, pp. 12–20.

123. Liard, C., Munier, S., Arias, M., Joulin-Giet, A., Bonduelle, O., Duffy, D., Shattock, R. J., Verrier, B., and Combadière, B. (2011) Targeting of HIV-p24 particle-based vaccine into differential skin layers induces distinct arms of the immune responses, *Vaccine*, **29**, pp. 6379–6391.

124. Kawamura, M., Naito, T., Ueno, M., Akagi, T., Hiraishi, K., Takai, I., Makino, M., Serizawa, T., Sugimura, K., Akashi, M., and Baba, M. (2002). Induction of mucosal IgA following intravaginal administration of inactivated HIV-1-capturing nanospheres in mice, *J. Med. Virol.*, **66**, pp. 291–298.

125. Castaldello, A., Brocca-Cofano, E., Voltan, R., Triulzi, C., Altavilla, G., Laus, M., Sparnacci, K., Ballestri, M., Tondelli, L., Fortini, C., Gavioli, R., Ensoli, B., and Caputo, A. (2006). DNA prime and protein boost immunization with innovative polymeric cationic core-shell nanoparticles elicits broad immune responses and strongly enhance cellular responses of HIV-1 Tat DNA vaccination, *Vaccine*, **24**, pp. 5655–5669.

126. Bettencour, A. and Almeida, A. (2012). Poly(methyl methacrylate) particulate carriers in drug delivery, *J. Microencapsul.*, **29**, pp. 353–367.

127. Figdor, C. G, Van Kooyk, Y., and Adema, G. J. (2002). C-type lectin receptors on dendritic cells and Langerhans cells, *Nat. Rev. Immunol.*, **2**, pp. 77–84.

128. Keler, T., Ramakrishna, V., and Fanger, M. W. (2004). Mannose receptor-targeted vaccines, *Expert Opin. Biol. Ther.*, **4**, pp. 1953–1962.

129. Ramakrishna, V., Treml, J. F., Vitale, L., Connolly, J. E., O'Neill, T., Smith, P. A., Jones, C. L., He, L. Z., Goldstein, J., Wallace, P. K., Keler, T., and Endres, M. J. (2004). Mannose receptor targeting of tumor antigen pmel17

to human dendritic cells directs anti-melanoma T-cell responses via multiple HLA molecules, *J. Immunol.*, **172**, pp. 2845–2852.

130. Mahnke, K., Guo, M., Lee, S., Sepulveda, H., Swain, S. L., Nussenzweig, M., and Steinman, R. M. (2000). The dendritic cell receptor for endocytosis, DEC-205, can recycle and enhance antigen presentation via major histocompatibility complex class II-positive lysosomal compartments, *J. Cell. Biol.*, **151**, pp. 673–684.

131. Bonifaz, L., Bonnyay, D., Mahnke, K., Rivera, M., Nussenzweig, M. C., and Steinman, R. M. (2002). Efficient targeting of protein antigen to the dendritic cell receptor DEC-205 in the steady state leads to antigen presentation on major histocompatibility complex class I products and peripheral CD8+ T-cell tolerance, *J. Exp. Med.*, **196**, pp. 1627–1638.

132. Bonifaz, L. C., Bonnyay, D. P., Charalambous, A., Darguste, D. I., Fujii, S., Soares, H., Brimnes, M. K., Moltedo, B., Moran, T. M., and Steinman, R. M. (2004). In vivo targeting of antigens to maturing dendritic cells via the DEC-205 receptor improves T-cell vaccination, *J. Exp. Med.*, **199**, pp. 815–824.

133. Lewis, J. S., Zaveri, T. D., Crooks, C. P., and Keselowsky, B. G. (2012). Microparticle surface modifications targeting dendritic cells for non-activating applications, *Biomaterials*, **33**, pp. 7221–7232.

134. Sheng, K. C., Kalkanidis, M., Pouniotis, D. S., Esparon, S., Tang, C. K., Apostolopoulos, V., and Pietersz, G. A. (2008). Delivery of antigen using a novel mannosylated dendrimer potentiates immunogenicity *in vitro* and *in vivo*, *Eur. J. Immunol.*, **38**, pp. 424–436.

Chapter 8

Phosphorus Dendrimers as Vectors for Gene Therapy in Cancer

Dzmitry Shcharbin,[a] Natallia Shcharbina,[b]
Elzbieta Pedziwiatr-Werbicka,[c] Javier de la Mata,[d]
Rafael Gomez-Ramirez,[d] Serge Mignani,[e]
Vladimir A. Kulchitsky,[f] Maria-Angeles Muñoz-Fernández,[g]
Anne-Marie Caminade,[h] Jean-Pierre Majoral,[h] and
Maria Bryszewska[c]

[a]*Institute of Biophysics and Cell Engineering of NASB, Minsk, Belarus*
[b]*Republican Research and Practical Center of Neurology and Neurosurgery, Minsk, Belarus*
[c]*Department of General Biophysics, Faculty of Biology and Environmental Protection, University of Lodz, Lodz, Poland*
[d]*Departamento Química Orgánica y Química Inorgánica, Universidad de Alcalá, Alcalá de Henares, Spain*
[e]*Université Paris Descartes, PRES Sorbonne Paris Cité, Paris, France*
[f]*Institute of Physiology of NASB, Minsk, Republic of Belarus*
[g]*Laboratorio de Inmunobiología Molecular, Hospital General Universitario Gregorio Marañón, Madrid, Spain*
[h]*Laboratoire de Chimie de Coordination, CNRS, Toulouse, France*
marbrys@biol.uni.lodz.pl

Phosphorus dendrimers are promising new tools for the delivery of drugs and genes to targets such as tumors. This review discusses

Phosphorus Dendrimers in Biology and Nanomedicine: Synthesis, Characterization, and Properties
Edited by Anne-Marie Caminade, Cédric-Olivier Turrin, and Jean-Pierre Majoral
Copyright © 2018 Pan Stanford Publishing Pte. Ltd.
ISBN 978-981-4774-33-8 (Hardcover), 978-1-315-11085-1 (eBook)
www.panstanford.com

and summarizes advances in the ability of phosphorus dendrimers to deliver genes into nuclei of cells and small interfering RNAs into the cytoplasm as a molecular basis for gene therapy in cancer. Their cytotoxicity *in vitro* and toxicity *in vivo* will also be discussed. Several low toxicity and efficient phosphorus dendrimers will be described as promising candidates for gene delivery; however, there is much needed to be done before they can be effectively applied in human gene therapy.

8.1 Gene Therapy and Systems for Gene Delivery: The Present Situation

The 2015 revolution in gene therapy based on genetic modification of human embryos by Chinese scientists [1] opened the door to the completely new world; it will allow us to create the new kinds of human beings and their chimeras depending on which genes are added or deleted. However, even if CRISPR/Cas9 applied to human pre-implantation embryos become widely used, "new" human beings will continue to experience the common age and immune system related diseases (infections, cancer, neurodegenerative diseases, stroke, etc.) that cannot as yet be eliminated at the genomic level. Thus, we still need the classic drugs and gene-based drugs to treat the diseases. In this regard, gene therapy is a completely new way to treat major infectious diseases, cancer, and genetic disorders [2]. There are three different directions in gene therapy: (a) the construction of human genome to create meta-homo sapiens [1], (b) the delivery of therapeutic genes into cell nuclei to have these genes permanently expressing themselves [2], and (c) the (temporary) silencing of unwanted genes [3] (Fig. 8.1).

Each of the three directions has advantages and drawbacks. The first is completely new and nothing as yet is known about it. The second requires efficient delivery of genes to nuclear DNA, with viral vectors being most efficient [2]. Because of their low pathogenicity, infectious properties, wide tropism, high level of expression of viral proteins during replication, and the natural delivery of the viral genome into the nucleus, viruses have been considered the best candidates for gene therapy since its inception [2–4]. However, some have drawbacks, including high immunogenicity and levels of pre-existing immunity, risk of insertional mutagenesis [2–5], transient expression of transgenes, and low capacity in accommodating some genes required for clinical applications [3, 4].

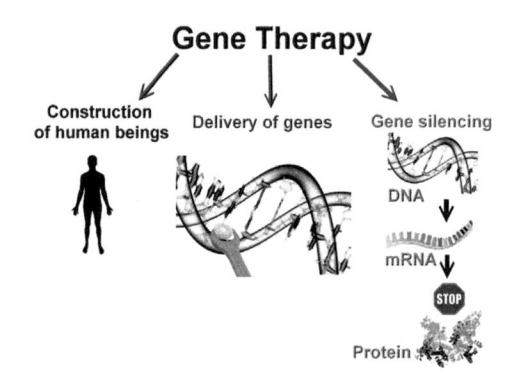

Figure 8.1 Construction of human genome to create meta-homo sapiens (a), delivery of therapeutic genes into a cell nucleus (b), and silencing of unwanted genes with disruption of protein expression (c).

The fear of insertional mutagenesis (and oncogenesis) is one of the major hurdles in integrating vectors, bringing implications on their use as gene-delivery vehicles in the clinic [2–6]. The third is the delivery of small RNAs (siRNA, microRNA, etc.) [3, 7] into the cytoplasm to silence unwanted genes at the mRNA level and prevent the expression of their proteins [3, 7, 8]. In this regard, non-viral systems (first of all, nanomaterials) are more effective in delivering small RNAs into cytoplasm [9, 10]. Both of these research fields are rapidly developing (Fig. 8.2) and might have promising futures.

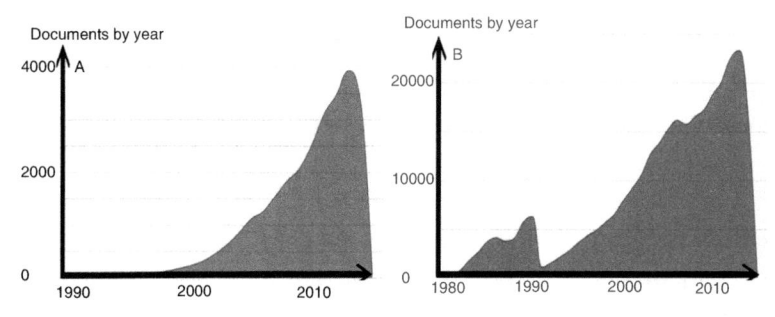

Figure 8.2 Publications on nanomaterials (A) and gene therapy (B). Analysis was made by database Scopus TM by keywords "nanomaterials" and "gene therapy."

8.2 Nanomaterials for Biology and Medicine: Advantages and Drawbacks

Nanotechnology development has offered biologists and physicians a wide new prospective of engineered nanomaterials, including nanoparticles of metals, quantum dots, fullerenes, carbon nanotubes (CNTs), and dendrimers [11]. Nanoparticles of metals can be used for magnetic resonance imaging applications, their optical properties being determined by changing size, shape, and surface properties [12]. Quantum dots were introduced as a new kind of fluorescent reporter in immunoassays, microarrays, and other fluorescent imaging applications [13]. Fullerenes and CNTs have high surface areas and internal volumes for loading drugs and imaging agents, but they are insoluble in most organic or aqueous solutions, rendering them generally toxic [14]. Dendrimers are branching polymer structures formed by monomeric subunit branches diverging on all sides from a central nucleus [15]. Dendrimers can be used as contrast agents for magnetic resonance imaging, synthetic vectors for gene therapy, drug-delivery carriers, drugs for treatment of prion diseases and neurodegenerative disorders, and antibacterial and antiviral agents, detoxification agents, antioxidants, and immuno-stimulatory components (adjuvants) [16]. Comparative analysis of their application in biology and medicine showed interestingly that, although there are more publications on fullerenes, graphene, CNTs, metal nanoparticles, and quantum dots than on dendrimers, publications concerning the application of dendrimers in biology and medicine outnumber other nanomaterials: dendrimers in biology and medicine—39%, metal nanoparticles—29%, fullerenes—13%, quantum dots—11%, CNTs—9%, graphene—>1% (Fig. 8.3); for a detailed analysis, see Ref. [17].

The data suggest that there is a significantly higher biocompatibility of dendrimers than other kinds of nanomaterials [17–20]. In this review, we present the phosphorus dendrimers as gene carriers for gene therapy of cancer.

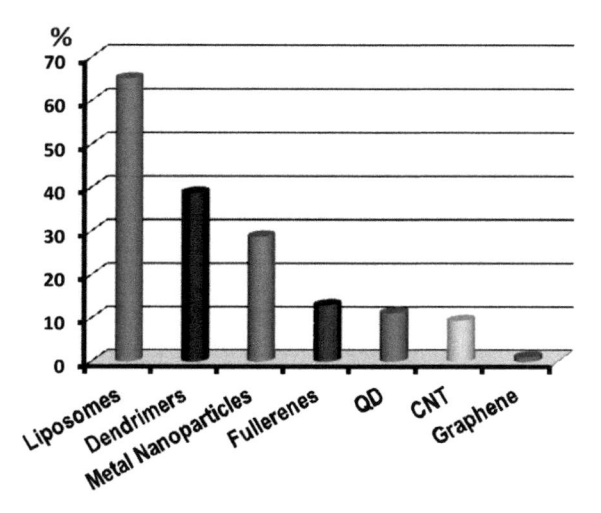

Figure 8.3 Percentage of publications on nanomaterials in biology and medicine [17]. QD: quantum dots, CNT: carbon nanotubes

8.3 Phosphorus Dendrimers *In Vivo*: Questions on Toxicity

Phosphorus (or phosphorus-containing) dendrimers were developed by Majoral and Caminade [21–23]. Briefly, classic phosphorus dendrimers are monodisperse branching polymers in a form of monomeric branches diverging on all sides from a central nucleus [21–23]. Lower generations have an open, flattened, and asymmetric shape, but as the generation increases, the structure becomes globular and densely packed at the periphery. Dendrimers are empty inside. Finally, phosphorus dendrimers possess many functional end groups responsible for their high solubility and reactivity [21–23]. Detailed analysis of them can be found in other chapters of this book, so here we will briefly mention their bioavailability *in vivo*. Solassol *et al.* [24] were the first to report the successful *in vivo* application of phosphorus dendrimers; 50 and 100 mg phosphorus dendrimers of fourth generation significantly inhibited PrP^{Sc} accumulation in mouse spleens at non-cytotoxic doses, proving that they were effective anti-prion agents of high bioavailability [24]. Phosphorus-containing dendrimers with one quaternary ammonium salt as the core and carboxylic acid terminal groups were used as a vehicle for ocular delivery of carteolol to rabbits [24], with no irritation noted after several hours [24]. A series of phosphorus dendrimers having the chromophore for two-photon excited fluorescence at the core and several ammonium groups as terminal functions were injected intravenously to rats, allowing two-photon absorption and imaging of the vascular network in the dorsal region of the olfactory bulb at a depth of 200 mm [25]. No marked adverse effects occurred [25]. Intravenous injections of azabisphosphonate-capped dendrimers inhibited the development of inflammatory arthritis in IL-1ra(−/−) mice and mice undergoing K/BxN serum transfer, with no adverse effects as followed up from normalization of synovial membranes, reduction of the levels of inflammatory cytokines, and absence of cartilage destruction and bone erosion. These dendrimers also had anti-osteoclastic activity on mouse and human cells [27]. Nontoxic fluorescent phosphorus dendrimers have a robust spectral shift in their emission in response to polarization conditions inside macrophages of mice cells *in vivo*. Their fluorescence properties also assisted the identification of macrophages and their phenotype status at different time-points after spinal cord injury in mice [28].

Summarizing, several effective and nontoxic phosphorus dendrimers have been synthesized and evaluated *in vitro* and *in vivo* as anti-prion agents, ocular drug carriers, and fluorescence imaging markers. The data open up the perspective of using phosphorus dendrimers as gene carriers.

8.4 Phosphorus Dendrimers versus Nucleic Acids: Mechanisms of Interaction and Paradigms of Transfection

The mechanisms of interaction between phosphorus dendrimers and nucleic acids, and the gene transfer mediated by these dendrimers, are practically the same as for poly(amidoamine) dendrimers [10, 29]. Briefly, (1) the complexing is based mainly on the interaction between the anionic phosphate groups of the nucleic acid and cationic groups on the dendrimers; (2) when charged, these complexes are colloidally stable, *i.e.*, an excess of the cationic dendrimer has to be present; (3) nucleic acid–dendrimer complexes are internalized by endocytosis; (4) decomplexing of nucleic acid from dendrimers inside cells occurs in endosomes or lysosomes due to a "proton-sponge" effect; (5) optimally flexible middle generations of cationic dendrimers are the most effective for gene delivery; (6) complete condensation of nucleic acid is not necessary for efficient gene transfer; (7) growth in dendrimer generations leads to greater cytotoxicity; (8) the efficiency of transfection by a dendrimer can be significantly enhanced by partial removal of its branches; (9) transfection efficiency of dendrimers and their cytotoxicity are tightly related to their internal hydrophobicity; and (10) the structure of the dendrimer nucleus is important for its transfection efficiency [10]. The recent findings showed also (11) the importance of the length of corresponding DNA for DNA–dendrimer complexes [30] (Fig. 8.4). Binding of dendrimer to ssDNA strongly depends on the charge of the dendrimer and the length of the ssDNA. Complex with a non-protonated dendrimer can maintain a DNA length-dependent inter-dendrimer distance. In contrast, the inter-dendrimer distance is independent of the DNA length in complexes with a protonated dendrimer. This phenomenon was explained by the electrostatic complexation of a negatively charged DNA strand with the positively charged protonated dendrimer [30].

The strength of binding between dendrimers and nucleic acids is also very important for successful transfection (12). If the interaction is too strong, nucleic acid cannot be released from dendrimer in the endosomes. If the interaction is too weak, the complex can be dissociated by protein, heparin, etc. Shcharbin *et al.* [31] proposed the use of the anionic hydrophobic fluorescent probe, 8-anilinonaphthalene-1-sulfonic acid (ANS), for estimating a dendrimer's binding constant and the binding capacity of cationic phosphorus dendrimers [31]. The pure ANS probe in aqueous solution has a weak fluorescence at 400–600 nm with a maximum at 520 nm because it is highly sensitive to water [32]. The significant electrostatic and/or hydrophobic interactions between ANS and big macromolecules can lead to (1) a short-wavelength shift of maximum of ANS fluorescence emission, and (2) a significant increase in ANS fluorescence due to shielding of ANS from water

[33]. Based on the double fluorescent titration technique [33–35], one can estimate the constant of binding of ANS to a dendrimer and the number of dendrimer binding sites [35]. Since nucleic acids interact with dendrimers in a similar way, ANS can represent the provisional "monomer unit" of a nucleic acid for preliminary screening of a dendrimer. These authors found the binding constant of cationic phosphorus dendrimer of fourth generation for ANS to be 1–10×10^6 l/mol (in contrast to 10^4 l/mol in the case of cationic poly(amidoamine) fourth-generation dendrimers) [31]. The data can explain the stability of complexes between phosphorus dendrimers and nucleic acids in the presence of heparin (a highly sulfated glycosaminoglycan present in blood that has the highest negative charge density of known biological molecules) [36].

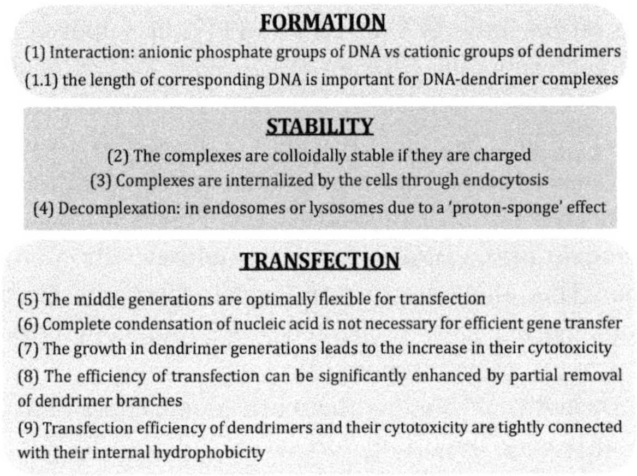

FORMATION
(1) Interaction: anionic phosphate groups of DNA vs cationic groups of dendrimers
(1.1) the length of corresponding DNA is important for DNA-dendrimer complexes

STABILITY
(2) The complexes are colloidally stable if they are charged
(3) Complexes are internalized by the cells through endocytosis
(4) Decomplexation: in endosomes or lysosomes due to a 'proton-sponge' effect

TRANSFECTION
(5) The middle generations are optimally flexible for transfection
(6) Complete condensation of nucleic acid is not necessary for efficient gene transfer
(7) The growth in dendrimer generations leads to the increase in their cytotoxicity
(8) The efficiency of transfection can be significantly enhanced by partial removal of dendrimer branches
(9) Transfection efficiency of dendrimers and their cytotoxicity are tightly connected with their internal hydrophobicity

Figure 8.4 The main mechanisms of interaction between dendrimers and nucleic acids, and their transfection into cells [10, 29, 30].

8.5 Phosphorus Dendrimers: Mediated Gene Delivery

Due to the aforementioned effective interaction, phosphorus dendrimers proved to be prominent gene carriers [16]. The first attempt, in 1999, to show cationic phosphorus dendrimers as excellent carriers for DNA was made by Loup *et al.* [38], who synthesized five different generations of CPD and examined them as transfecting agents of the luciferase gene in 3T3 cells. The most efficient representatives of this series of P-dendrimers had a transfection activity level comparable with linear PEI, with only five equivalents of tertiary amine per nucleotide. These dendrimers had a better transfection efficiency in serum than without it [38]. Maksimenko *et al.* [39] analyzed the mechanisms of the transfection efficiency of phosphorus and poly(amidoamine) dendrimers using anionic oligomers (oligonucleotides, dextran sulfate). Anionic oligomers significantly increased the capacity of the PAMAM and phosphorus dendrimers to deliver DNA into cells when they were mixed with plasmid DNA before adding the dendrimers. The efficiency of the DNA/dendrimer penetration depends on the size, structure, and charge of anionic oligomers [39].

Maszewska *et al.* [40] were the first to screen the transfection efficiency and cytotoxicity of phosphorus dendrimers in different cells. Phosphorus dendrimers showed rather moderate cytotoxicity toward HeLa, HEK 293, and HUVEC cells in a standard MTT assay in serum-containing medium, generally lower than lipofectin. Investigation of cellular uptake has shown the necessity for serum to be present for transfection with phosphorus dendrimers. These compounds efficiently delivered fluorescein-labeled oligodeoxyribonucleotide into HeLa cells in serum-containing medium, but failed to do so in HUVEC cells. The dendrimers were successful mediators of transfection of the HeLa cells with a DNA plasmid containing the functional gene of enhanced green fluorescent protein (EGFP) [40]. Summarizing these data, Caminade *et al.* [41] concluded that phosphorus dendrimers can be used: (1) as three-dimensional linkers for oligonucleotides, affording highly sensitive microarrays (biochips), and (2) as gene carriers due to the strong interaction of positively charged dendrimers with DNA. An additional benefit is the attachment of fluorescent marker to the phosphorus dendrimer core, as noted by Kazmierczak-Baranska *et al.* [42]. This dendrimer fluoresced brightly in CH_2Cl_2, but only weakly in water. The cytotoxicity of this conjugate was relatively low in HeLa and A549 cells, but less toxic after 48 h than 24 h. Association of this dendrimer with GFP plasmid analyzed by circular dichroism indicated a possible disturbing of the helical B-type structure of DNA [42]. The potential of phosphorus dendrimer to transfect stem cells was studied by Shakhbazau *et al.* [43], who found that, in contrast to linear PEI, the phosphorus dendrimer could deliver the neurotrophic factor, BDNF, in mesenchymal stem cells [43]. Shcharbin *et al.* [31] followed carefully phosphorus dendrimer of fourth generation as a drug and gene carrier. Cisplatin was used as the model drug and green fluorescent protein gene (pGFP) as the model gene. The combination of phosphorus dendrimers with cisplatin led to the significant enhancement of drug action on primary cultures of tumor cells (bioptates from craniospinal cancer of the fourth ventricle, IV stage) [31]. The second effect observed was the effective (40%) transfection of pGFP into HEK293 cells by phosphorus dendrimers [31], with only low cytotoxicity (10%). The effective delivery of small interfering RNAs (siRNA) and oligodeoxynucleotides (ODN) was initially shown by Briz *et al.* [44], who found that cationic phosphorus dendrimers of fourth generation formed stable complexes with ODNs or siRNAs, with very low cytotoxicity in Sup T1 cells and peripheral blood mononuclear cells. Functionality was validated by using specific siRNA against HIV-1 Nef, siNEF to interfere in HIV-1 replication. The dendriplex had a high efficiency in Nef silencing. In vitro treatment of HIV-infected peripheral blood mononuclear cells with the siNEF dendriplex also significantly reduced viral replication. The data showed how useful phosphorus-containing dendrimers can be in delivering and transfecting siRNA into CD4 T cells as a potential alternative therapy in HIV-1 infection [44].

8.6 Phosphorus Dendrimers as Vectors for Anti-cancer siRNA Delivery

Cancer accounted for 8.2 million deaths worldwide in 2012 according to the World Health Organization [45–47], and treatment includes surgery, chemotherapy, photodynamic therapy, and radiotherapy. Chemotherapy continues be of particular importance [45]. However, the non-selective nature and the lack of specific localization in the body of most of the therapeutic agents result in significant side effects that limit dose and/or frequency of administration. Another important limitation is the development of multidrug resistance. To overcome multidrug resistance at the genetic level, a combination of gene therapy and chemotherapy has a unique advantage of allowing increased efficacy due to additive or synergistic activity [45–47]. One of the new directions in gene therapy for treatment is the suppression of malignant transformation of normal cells [48, 49]. The regulation of apoptosis in cells is determined in part by the family of Bcl-2 proteins [50]. Suppression of the synthesis of anti-apoptotic proteins can be achieved using RNA interference (RNAi)—a process of selective gene silencing [48, 49, 51, 52]. A major limiting step for its success is the effective delivery and transfection of siRNA into the target cells [48, 49]. At present, complexes of nucleic acids with liposomes or cationic linear polymers are the popular non-viral systems. However, a better perspective for gene therapy is presented by nanomaterials and, foremost, dendrimers [45, 46, 48, 49]. Dendrimers are promising due to their functionality and ability to selectively target cancer- or tumor-initiating cells by different mechanisms. This helps overcome many dose-dependent side effects and restricted drug access, as well finally leading to overcoming multiple drug resistance and enhancing the effectiveness of chemotherapy [46, 47]. Ionov *et al.* [36, 53] proposed to use cationic phosphorus dendrimers of third and fourth generations as gene carriers for anti-cancer siRNA siBCL-2, siBCL-xL, siMCL-1, and their mixtures ("cocktails") to treat cancer cells. Their results indicated that siRNAs formed complexes with all the dendrimers. siRNAs were not released from dendriplexes by heparin, and the dendrimers were also effective in protecting siRNA from RNase A activity. A comparison of different dendrimers showed that phosphorus dendrimer-based complexes were taken up by cells most efficiently of all the selected siRNAs. However, the viability of cells depended on the nature of the dendrimer, phosphorus dendrimers being more cytotoxic than poly(amidoamine) and carbosilane ones. The higher generations proved more cytotoxic. However, phosphorus dendrimers were the most effective in delivering siRNA cocktails (100 μmol/l) into HeLa and HL-60 (human leukemia cells). These dendriplexes were the most promising cytotoxically (up to 8% of live HeLa cells for phosphorus G4 dendrimer). The main mechanism of action of siRNAs (siBCL-2, siBCL-xL, siMCL-1) is to induce apoptosis [50, 54]. In contrast, death of cells induced by pure phosphorus dendrimers is by necrosis [55], which means that synergy between several major mechanisms can enhance cell death to obtain a better anti-cancer result [56, 57].

8.7 Future Perspectives and Screening of New Dendrimers for Gene Therapy in Cancer

Thus, phosphorus dendrimers have a great potential in being used as prominent gene carriers. On the other hand, the still unresolved question is whether we should tune dendrimers to the DNA or RNA sequence to get the best results (Fig. 8.5).

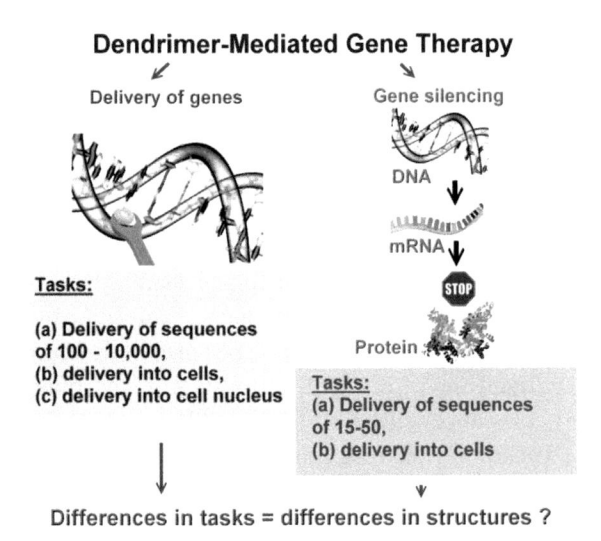

Figure 8.5 Different tasks for the different applications of dendrimers in gene therapy.

In the screening of phosphorus dendrimers for monocyte activation, Caminade *et al.* [58] found of pivotal importance the structure–function relationship for these dendrimers toward monocytes. Thirteen synthesized compounds possessing identical terminal groups, but different internal structures, differed markedly in activating monocytes [58]. This demonstrates how the scaffold of nanodrugs strongly influences their properties, in some ways reminiscent of the backbone of proteins.

To compare phosphorus dendrimers with other gene-delivery systems, several important points should be noted: (1) Viral vectors remain the most efficient system for DNA delivery, but they are highly immunogenic; there are high levels of pre-existing immunity, and the risk of insertional mutagenesis remains [5, 59]. (2) The requirement for the development of non-viral systems for gene delivery in clinical applications. In contrast, dendrimers are non-immunogenic [48] and have a relatively high efficiency of transfection compared to other non-viral systems, *e.g.*, liposomes, PLGA nanoparticles, chitosan, and linear PEI [47, 48]. They also do not pose any risk of insertional mutagenesis. Dendrimers may be potentially advantageous over viral vectors in delivering siRNAs into the cytosol of cells, but not the nucleus [47, 48]. The toxicity and cytotoxicity of dendrimers both *in vitro* and *in vivo* remain an important issue to be investigated (see above). There is little doubt that phosphorus dendrimers hold out much promise as candidates for gene delivery, but there is a long way to go before they can be effectively applied in human gene therapy.

Acknowledgments

This work was supported by the Belarusian Republican Foundation for Fundamental Research, Project No. M15CO-041, Project No. DEC-2012/04/M/NZ1/00059, and by a Marie Curie International Research Staff Exchange Scheme Fellowship within the 7th European Community Framework Programme, project No. PIRSES-GA-2012-316730 NANOGENE, co-financed by the Polish Ministry of Science and Higher Education.

References

1. Cyranoski, D. and Reardon, S. (2015). Chinese scientists genetically modify human embryos, 22 April 2015, *Nature News*. http://www.nature.com/news/chinese-scientists-genetically-modify-human-embryos-1.17378.

2. Naldini, L. (2015). Gene therapy returns to centre stage, *Nature*, **526**, pp. 351–360.

3. Lam, J. K. W., Chow, M. Y. T., Zhang, Y., and Leung, S. W. S. (2015). siRNA versus miRNA as therapeutics for gene silencing, *Mol. Ther. Nucl. Ac.*, **4**, pp. e252 (1–20).

4. Resnier, P., Montier, T., Mathieu, V., Benoit, J.-P., and Passirani, C. (2013). A review of the current status of siRNA nanomedicines in the treatment of cancer, *Biomaterials*, **34**, pp. 6429–6443.

5. Knight, S., Collins, M., and Takeuchi, Y. (2013). Insertional mutagenesis by retroviral vectors: Current concepts and methods of analysis, *Curr. Gene Ther.*, **13**, pp. 211–227.

6. Wirth, T., Parker, N., and Ylä-Herttuala, S. (2013). History of gene therapy, *Gene*, **525**, pp. 162–169.

7. Fire, A. Z. (2007). Gene silencing by double-stranded RNA (Nobel Lecture), *Angew. Chem. Int. Ed.*, **46**, pp. 6966–6984.

8. de Fougerolles, A., Vornlocher, H.-P., Maraganore, J., and Lieberman, J. (2007). Interfering with disease: A progress report on siRNA-based therapeutics, *Nat. Rev. Drug Discov.*, **6**, pp. 443–453.

9. Scholz, C. and Wagner, E. (2012). Therapeutic plasmid DNA versus siRNA delivery: Common and different tasks for synthetic carriers, *J. Control. Rel.*, **161**, pp. 554–565.

10. Shcharbin, D., Shakhbazau, A., and Bryszewska, M. (2013). Poly(amidoamine) dendrimer complexes as a platform for gene delivery, *Expert Opin. Drug Deliv.*, **10**, pp. 1687–1698.

11. Kim, B. Y. S., Rutka, J. T., and Chan, W. C. W. (2010). Nanomedicine, *New Engl. J. Med.*, **363**, pp. 2434–2443.

12. Zhang, L., Gu, F. X., Chan, J. M., Wang, A. Z., Langer, R. S., and Farokhzad, O. C. (2008). Nanoparticles in medicine: Therapeutic applications and developments, *Clin. Pharmacol. Ther.*, **83**, pp. 761–769.

13. Zhang, Y. and Wang, T. H. (2012). Quantum dot enabled molecular sensing and diagnostics, *Theranostics*, **2**, pp. 631–654.

14. Madani, S. Y., Naderi, N., Dissanayake, O., Tan, A., and Seifalian, A. M. (2011). A new era of cancer treatment: Carbon nanotubes as drug delivery tools, *Int. J. Nanomed.*, **6**, pp. 2963–2979.

15. Tomalia, D. A., Naylor, A. M., and Goddard III, W. A. (1990). Starburst dendrimers: Molecular-level control of size, shape, surface chemistry, topology, and flexibility from atoms to macroscopic matter, *Angew. Chem. Int. Ed.*, **29**, pp. 138–175.

16. Mignani, S., El Kazzouli, S., Bousmina, M. M., and Majoral, J.-P. (2014). Dendrimer space exploration: An assessment of dendrimers/dendritic scaffolding as inhibitors of protein–protein interactions, a potential new area of pharmaceutical development, *Chem. Rev.*, **114**, pp. 1327–1342.

17. Shcharbina, N., Shcharbin, D., and Bryszewska, M. (2013). Nanomaterials in stroke treatment: Perspectives, *Stroke*, **44**, pp. 2351–2355.

18. Krug, H. F. (2014). Nanosafety research: Are we on the right track? *Angew. Chem. Int. Ed.*, **53**, pp. 12304–12319.

19. Shcharbin, D., Shcharbina, N., Shakhbazau, A., Mignani, S., Majoral, J.-P., and Bryszewska, M. (2015). Phosphorus-containing nanoparticles: Biomedical patents review, *Expert Opin. Ther. Pat.*, **25**, pp. 539–548.

20. Shcharbin, D., Janaszewska, A., Klajnert-Maculewicz, B., Ziemba, B., Dzmitruk, V., Halets, I., Loznikova, S., Shcharbina, N., Milowska, K., Ionov, M., Shakhbazau, A., and Bryszewska, M. (2014). How to study dendrimers and dendriplexes III. Biodistribution, pharmacokinetics and toxicity *in vivo, J. Control. Rel.*, **181**, pp. 40–52.

21. Launay, N., Caminade, A.-M., Lahana, R., and Majoral, J.-P. (1994). A general synthetic strategy for neutral phosphorus-containing dendrimers, *Angew. Chem. Int. Ed.*, **33**, pp. 1589–1592.

22. Launay, N., Caminade, A.-M., and Majoral, J.-P. (1995). Synthesis and reactivity of unusual phosphorus dendrimers. A useful divergent growth approach up to the seventh generation, *J. Am. Chem. Soc.*, **117**, pp. 3282–3283.

23. Galliot, C., Prévoté, D., Caminade, A.-M., and Majoral, J.-P. (1995). Polyaminophosphines containing dendrimers. Syntheses and characterizations, *J. Am. Chem. Soc.*, **117**, pp. 5470–5476.

24. Solassol, J., Crozet, C., Perrier, V., Leclaire, J., Béranger, F., Caminade, A. M., Meunier, B., Dormont, D., Majoral, J. P., and Lehmann, S. (2004). Cationic phosphorus-containing dendrimers reduce prion replication both in cell culture and in mice infected with scrapie, *J. Gen. Virol.*, **85**, pp. 1791–1799.

25. Spataro, G., Malecaze, F., Turrin, C. O., Soler, V., Duhayon, C., Elena, P. P., Majoral, J. P., and Caminade, A. M. (2010). Designing dendrimers for ocular drug delivery, *Eur. J. Med. Chem.*, **45**, pp. 326–334.

26. Krishna, T. R., Parent, M., Werts, M. H. V., Moreaux, L., Gmouh, S., Charpak, S., Caminade, A.-M., Majoral, J.-P., and Blanchard-Desce, M. (2006). Water-soluble dendrimeric two-photon tracers for *in vivo* imaging, *Angew. Chem. Int. Ed.*, **45**, pp. 4645–4648.

27. Hayder, M., Poupot, M., Baron, M., Nigon, D., Turrin, C. O., Caminade, A. M., Majoral, J. P., Eisenberg, R. A., Fournié, J. J., Cantagrel, A., Poupot, R., and Davignon, J. L. (2011). A phosphorus-based dendrimer targets inflammation and osteoclastogenesis in experimental arthritis, *Sci. Transl. Med.*, **3**, pp. 81ra35.

28. Shakhbazau, A., Mishra, M., Chu, T. H., Brideau, C., Cummins, K., Tsutsui, S., Shcharbin, D., Majoral, J. P., Mignani, S., Blanchard-Desce,

M., Bryszewska, M., Yong, V. W., Stys, P. K., and van Minnen, J. (2015). Fluorescent phosphorus dendrimer as a spectral nanosensor for macrophage polarization and fate tracking in spinal cord injury, *Macromol. Biosci.*, **15**, pp. 1523–1534.

29. Tomalia, D., Christensen, J., and Boas, U. (2012). *Dendrimers, Dendrons and Dendritic Polymers: Discovery, Applications, the Future* (Cambridge University Press, USA).

30. Mandal, T., Kumar, M. V., and Maiti, P. K. (2014). DNA assisted self-assembly of PAMAM dendrimers, *J. Phys. Chem. B*, **118**, pp. 11805–11815.

31. Shcharbin, D., Dzmitruk, V., Shakhbazau, A., Goncharova, N., Seviaryn, I., Kosmacheva, S., Potapnev, M., Pedziwiatr-Werbicka, E., Bryszewska, M., Talabaev, M., Chernov, A., Kulchitsky, V., Caminade, A. M., and Majoral, J. P. (2011). Fourth generation phosphorus-containing dendrimers: Prospective drug and gene delivery carrier, *Pharmaceutics*, **3**, pp. 458–473.

32. Humphry-Baker, R., Grätzel, M., and Steiger, R. (1980). Drastic fluorescence enhancement and photochemical stabilization of cyanine dyes through micellar Systems, *J. Am. Chem. Soc.*, **102**, pp. 847–852.

33. Slavik, J. (1982). Anilinonaphthalene sulfonate as a probe of membrane composition and function, *Biochim. Biophys. Acta*, **694**, pp. 1–25.

34. Scatchard, G. (1949). The attractions of proteins for small molecules and ions, *Ann. N. Y. Acad. Sci.*, **51**, pp. 660–672.

35. Shcharbin, D., Szwedzka, M., and Bryszewska, M. (2007). Does fluorescence of ANS reflect its binding to PAMAM dendrimer? *Bioorg. Chem.*, **35**, pp. 170–174.

36. Ionov, M., Lazniewska, J., Dzmitruk, V., Halets, I., Loznikova, S., Novopashina, D., Apartsin, E., Krasheninina, O., Venyaminova, A., Milowska, K., Nowacka, O., Gomez-Ramirez, R., de la Mata, F. J., Majoral, J. P., Shcharbin, D., and Bryszewska, M. (2015). Anticancer siRNA cocktails as a novel tool to treat cancer cells. Part (A). Mechanisms of interaction, *Int. J. Pharm.*, **485**, pp. 261–269.

37. Kulchitsky, V. A., Alexandrova, R., Suziedelis, K., Paschkevich, S. G., and Potkin, V. I. (2014). Perspectives of fullerenes, dendrimers, and heterocyclic compounds application in tumor treatment, *Rec. Pat. Nanomed.*, **4**, pp. 82–89.

38. Loup, C., Zanta, M.-A., Caminade, A.-M., Majoral, J.-P., and Meunier, B. (1999). Preparation of water-soluble cationic phosphorus-containing

dendrimers as DNA transfecting agents, *Chem. A Eur. J.*, **5**, pp. 3644–3650.

39. Maksimenko, A. V. Mandrouguine, V. Gottikh, M. B., Bertrand, J.-R., Majoral, J.-P., and Malvy, C. (2003). Optimisation of dendrimer-mediated gene transfer by anionic oligomers, *J. Gene Med.*, **5**, pp. 61–71.

40. Maszewska, M., Leclaire, J., Cieslak, M., Nawrot, B., Okruszek, A., Caminade, A. M., and Majoral, J. P. (2003). Water-soluble polycationic dendrimers with a phosphoramidothioate backbone: Preliminary studies of cytotoxicity and oligonucleotide/plasmid delivery in human cell culture, *Oligonucleotides*, **13**, pp. 193–205.

41. Caminade, A. M., Turrin, C. O., and Majoral, J. P. (2008). Dendrimers and DNA: Combinations of two special topologies for nanomaterials and biology, *Chem. Eur. J.*, **14**, pp. 7422–7432.

42. Kazmierczak-Baranska, J., Pietkiewicz, A., Janicka, M., Wei, Y., Turrin, C.O., Majoral, J. P., Nawrot, B., and Caminade, A. M. (2010). Synthesis of a fluorescent cationic phosphorus dendrimer and preliminary biological studies of its interaction with DNA, *Nucleosid. Nucleotid. Nucl. Acids*, **29**, pp. 155–167.

43. Shakhbazau, A. V., Shcharbin, D. G., Goncharova, N. V., Seviaryn, I. N., Kosmacheva, S. M., Kartel, N. A., Bryszewska, M., Majoral, J. P., and Potapnev, M. P. (2011). Neurons and stromal stem cells as targets for polycation-mediated transfection, *Bull. Exp. Biol. Med.*, **151**, pp. 126–129.

44. Briz, V., Serramía, M. J., Madrid, R., Hameau, A., Caminade, A. M., Majoral, J. P., and Muñoz-Fernández, M. A. (2012). Validation of a generation 4 phosphorus-containing polycationic dendrimer for gene delivery against HIV-1, *Curr. Med. Chem.*, **19**, pp. 5044–5051.

45. Maeda, H. (2012). Macromolecular therapeutics in cancer treatment: The EPR effect and beyond, *J. Control. Rel.*, **164**, pp. 138–144.

46. Mignani, S., Bryszewska, M., Klajnert-Maculewicz, B., Zablocka, M., and Majoral, J. P. (2015). Advances in combination therapies based on nanoparticles for efficacious cancer treatment: An analytical report, *Biomacromolecules*, **16**, pp. 1–27.

47. Mignani, S., El Kazzouli, S., Bousmina, M. M., and Majoral, J. P. (2014). Dendrimer space exploration: An assessment of dendrimers/dendritic scaffolding as inhibitors of protein-protein interactions, a potential new area of pharmaceutical development, *Chem. Rev.*, **114**, pp. 1327–1342.

48. Biswas, S. and Torchilin, V. (2013). Dendrimers for siRNA delivery, *Pharmaceuticals*, **6**, pp. 161–183.

49. Resnier, P., Montier, T., Mathieu, V., Benoit, J.-P., and Passirani, C. (2013). A review of the current status of siRNA nanomedicines in the treatment of cancer, *Biomaterials*, **34**, pp. 6429–6443.

50. Burlacu, A. (2003). Regulation of apoptosis by Bcl-2 family proteins, *J. Cell. Mol. Med.*, **7**, pp. 249–257.

51. Milhavet, O., Gary, D. S., and Mattson, M. P. (2003). RNA interference in biology and medicine, *Pharmacol. Rev.*, **55**, pp. 629–648.

52. Tiemann, K., Höhn, B., Ehsani, A., Forman, S. J., Rossi, J. J., and Saetrom, P. (2010). Dual-targeting siRNAs, *RNA*, **16**, pp. 1275–1284.

53. Dzmitruk, V., Szulc. A., Shcharbin, D., Janaszewska, A., Shcharbina, N., Lazniewska, J., Novopashina, D., Buyanova, M., Ionov, M., Klajnert-Maculewicz, B., Gómez-Ramirez, R., Mignani, S., Majoral, J. P., Muñoz-Fernández, M. A., and Bryszewska M. (2015). Anticancer siRNA cocktails as a novel tool to treat cancer cells. Part (B). Efficiency of pharmacological action, *Int. J. Pharm.*, **485**, pp. 288–294.

54. Reed, J. C. (2011). Cancer. Priming cancer cells for death, *Science*, **334**, pp. 1075–1076.

55. Lazniewska, J., Milowska, K., Zablocka, M., Mignani, S., Caminade, A. M., Majoral, J. P., Bryszewska, M., and Gabryelak, T. (2013). Mechanism of cationic phosphorus dendrimer toxicity against murine neural cell lines, *Mol. Pharm.*, **10**, pp. 3484–3496.

56. Fulda, S. (2014). Therapeutic exploitation of necroptosis for cancer therapy, *Semin. Cell Dev. Biol.* **35**, pp. 51–56.

57. He, C., Liu, D., and Lin, W. (2015). Self-assembled core-shell nanoparticles for combined chemotherapy and photodynamic therapy of resistant head and neck cancers, *ACS Nano*, **9**, pp. 991–1003.

58. Caminade, A. M., Fruchon, S., Turrin, C. O., Poupot, M., Ouali, A., Maraval, A., Garzoni, M., Maly, M., Furer, V., Kovalenko, V., Majoral, J. P., Pavan, G. M., and Poupot, R. (2015). The key role of the scaffold on the efficiency of dendrimer nanodrugs, *Nature Commun.*, **6**, pp. 7722.

59. Vannucci, L., Lai, M., Chiuppesi, F., Ceccherini-Nelli, L., and Pistello, M. (2013). Viral vectors: A look back and ahead on gene transfer technology, *New Microbiol.*, **36**, pp. 1–22.

Chapter 9

First-in-Class Anti-cancer Nanoparticle Copper(II) Phosphorus Dendrimers as Pro-apoptotic Bax Activators

Serge Mignani,[a] Nabil El Brahmi,[b] Thierry Cresteil,[c] and Jean-Pierre Majoral[d]

[a]*Université Paris Descartes, PRES Sorbonne Paris Cité, CNRS UMR 860, Laboratoire de Chimie et de Biochimie pharmacologiques et toxicologique, 45, rue des Saints Pères, 75006 Paris, France*
[b]*Euromed Research Institute, Euro-Mediterranean University of Fes (UEMF), Route de Meknes, 30000, Fès, Morocco*
[c]*IPSIT, Faculté de Pharmacie, Université Paris Sud, 92290 Chatenay-Malabry, France*
[d]*Laboratoire de Chimie de Coordination du CNRS, 205 route de Narbonne, 31077 Toulouse Cedex 4, France*
serge.mignani@parisdescartes.fr

This chapter traces the design and construction of original multivalent Cu-conjugated phosphorus dendrimers, their anti-proliferative activities against various human cancer cell lines as well as their mode of action via Bax activation. Recently, we found multivalent Cu-conjugated phosphorus dendrimers with potent anti-proliferative activities. These activities are comparable in cell

Phosphorus Dendrimers in Biology and Nanomedicine: Synthesis, Characterization, and Properties
Edited by Anne-Marie Caminade, Cédric-Olivier Turrin, and Jean-Pierre Majoral
Copyright © 2018 Pan Stanford Publishing Pte. Ltd.
ISBN 978-981-4774-33-8 (Hardcover), 978-1-315-11085-1 (eBook)
www.panstanford.com

lines overexpressing the efflux pump ABC B1, while cross-resistance was observed in ovarian cancer cell lines resistant to cisplatin. To understand the mechanism of action of these dendrimer complexes, cell death pathways have been examined in human cancer cell lines. This study has shown that early apoptosis was followed by secondary necrosis after multivalent phosphorus dendrimers exposure. We now know that the multivalent plain phosphorus dendrimer moderately activated caspase-3 activity, while the multivalent Cu-conjugated phosphorus dendrimer strikingly reduced the caspase-3 content and activity.

In light of this fact, we thought that the potent apoptosis activation could be the result of a noticeable translocation of Bax to the mitochondria, causing the release of AIF into the cytosol, its translocation to the nucleus and a severe DNA fragmentation, without modulation of the cell cycle. We noticed that the multivalent Cu-conjugated phosphorus dendrimer is more efficient than its non-complexed analog to activate this pathway in close relationship with the higher anti-proliferative potency.

Therefore, the multivalent Cu-conjugated phosphorus dendri-mers represent new and promising first-in-class anti-proliferative agents with an original mechanism of action in nanomedicine. To our knowledge, it is the first example of nanoparticles in general and dendrimers in particular showing potent anti-cancer activity through Bax activation pathway inducing apoptosis tumor cell death.

9.1 Introduction and Strategy Used

Despite the considerable efforts dedicated to research on cancer (prevention, diagnosis, and treatment), it has increased over recent decades and is one of the most deadly diseases (with around 25 million cancer patients in the world today) [1]. Three different anti-cancer drug waves can be chronologically outlined as follows [2] (Fig. 9.1): (1) conventional chemotherapeutics; (2) anti-cancer drugs based on high molecular-targeting precision; and (3) anti-cancer drugs targeting cellular multicomponent machineries and effector systems. Unfortunately, all of these approaches, applied alone, have side effects. For example, with chemotherapy, these side effects vary largely depending on the individual, the cancer type, and the treatment used. Nevertheless, synergy between these different classes offers hope for the future in the design of drugs able to combat not only drug-resistant cancer cells on biological assays but also pre-existing drug resistance in cancer patients. As medicinal chemists, we think that the future in the oncology field will be the development of anti-cancer agents based nanomedicine, antibody drug conjugates, inhibitors of protein–protein interactions, and immunotherapy approach.

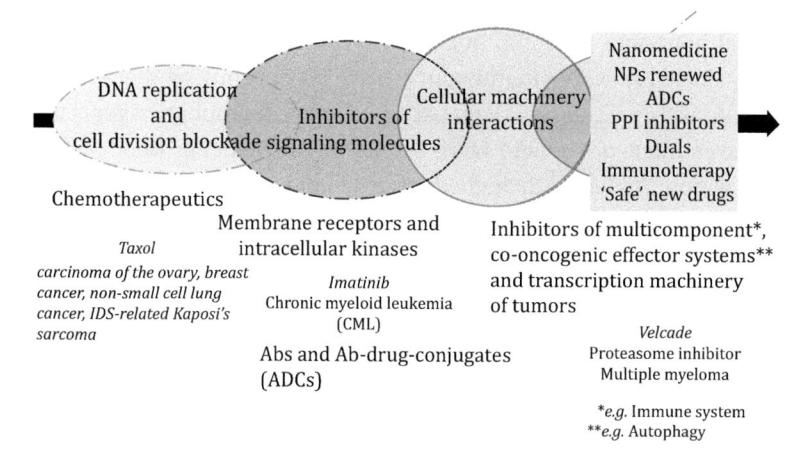

Figure 9.1 Schematic representation of the chronological waves of anti-cancer drugs.

The discovery of new anti-cancer drugs capable of killing or reprograming malignant cells with minimum side effects is a big challenge. Kamb, Wee, and Lengauer highlighted that various factors affect tumor formation and growth, especially, tumor heterogeneity and adaptability [3]. Both factors participate toward the resulting cancer phenotype as cardinal features (so named hallmarks of cancer).

For almost three decades, several fundamental questions have arisen concerning how best to solve the conundrum. These have included strategic choices between developing selective or multi-targeted anti-cancer agents, and between using classical phenotypic assay screening or target-based screening (hypothesis-driven approach) to reveal potential hits. Globally speaking, the oncology domain is rapidly moving from a one-size-fits-all approach (cytotoxic chemotherapy) to a more personalized medicine strategy used to select the right drug for a select patient population. So did the pharmaceutical industry invest in the right technologies? Unfortunately, no universal solution exists!

Nanomedicine, or the application of nanotechnology in medicine, is the monitoring, repair, construction as well as the control of human biological systems using engineered nanodevices. In recent years, much more attention has been paid to research in nanomedicine devoted to oncology and nowadays, it represents a real hope and potential means to tackle cancer progression and metastasis [4]. Noble metal nanoparticles as promising theranostic nanotools (dual role as a diagnostic and active therapeutic agent) for the treatment of cancers were intensively developed. Dendrimers are nanoparticles with high degree of molecular uniformity and perfectly controlled size (1–15 nm), shape, and surface chemistry [5]. Interestingly, because of their highly branched three-dimensional architecture and versatile surface functionalization, dendrimers have been engineered for use as nanodevices (either nanocarriers drug approaches or drugs *per se*). Nanoparticles such as dendrimers are used in two different manners for drug delivery: (1) encapsulation in the nanoparticles or (2) conjugation using specific stimuli-sensitive linkers. The highly branched three-dimensional architecture of dendrimers is characterized by homostructural layers between branching points and a compact spherical geometry in solution, which offers various opportunities to fine tune the drug design, helping to promote the development of novel, better suited biological nanodevices and of important alternative approaches to the delivery of biologically active compounds in oncology. The main successes of dendrimers in general have been due to their appropriate, reproducible, and optimized design parameters addressing the physicochemical limitations of classical drugs (*e.g.*, solubility, specificity, stability, biodistribution, and therapeutic efficiency) and overcoming biological obstacles to reaching the right target(s) (*e.g.*, first-pass effect, immune clearance, cell penetration, off-target interactions, etc.). Evidence supporting the high potential of dendrimers as nanocarriers for therapeutic use is first provided by the observed improvement in pharmacokinetics (PK) and pharmacodynamics (PD) of both drug–dendrimer conjugates and drug–dendrimer encapsulates *versus* plain drugs. Interestingly, reports have demonstrated their successful administration via intravenous, intraperitoneal, ocular, transdermal, oral, intranasal, pulmonary, and intravaginal routes for the treatment of life-threatening diseases [6].

Since several years, the objective of our multidisciplinary research group is to develop first-in-class anti-cancer drugs based on cellular phenotypic screening and phosphorus dendrimers as novel biologically active and promising chemotypes. Despite several analyses showing that more first-in-class drugs were discovered through target-based approaches (~2/3) than via phenotypic screening and chemocentric approaches (~1/3), we strongly believe neither strategy to be superior over the other. Indeed, phenotypic screening represents a good opportunity to find new mechanisms of action for both specific and non-specific drug effects, and also helps surmount the challenge faced revealing validated targets for translational medicine between bench to clinic or vice versa [7]. In addition, we believe that cellular models represent good starting point—but not universal—as therapeutically translatable cancer phenotypes. Several interesting applications of phosphorus dendrimers, active *per se*, developed in our laboratory were reported in the past: anti-prion [8] and anti-inflammatory properties [9], NK cells multiplication [10], effects on Alzheimer's and Parkinson's diseases [11], use for diagnosis [12], etc., allowing us to propose the dendrimer space concept, which should extend the possibilities to fight against several diseases.

9.2 Phenotypic Screening as Source of Potent Anti-cancer Agents Based on Multivalent Cu(II)-Conjugated Phosphorus Dendrimers

Recently, we reported the design and synthesis of biocompatible original multivalent Cu(II)-conjugated phosphorus dendrimers bearing a cyclotriphosphazene ring core as scaffold for original phosphorus dendrimers complexing metals such as copper(II). We reported also the synthesis of their corresponding mononuclear Cu(II) complexes [13]. Our objective was the preparation of multivalent Cu(II)-conjugated phosphorus dendrimers and the testing of their anti-proliferative activities against a representative panel of relevant human cancer cell lines. Based on a classical initial phenotypic screening, the anti-proliferative capacity of three different series of multivalent phosphorus dendrimers (generations 1–3, Fig. 9.2) was first evaluated against KB (epidermal carcinoma) and leukemia HL60 (promyelocytic) cells.

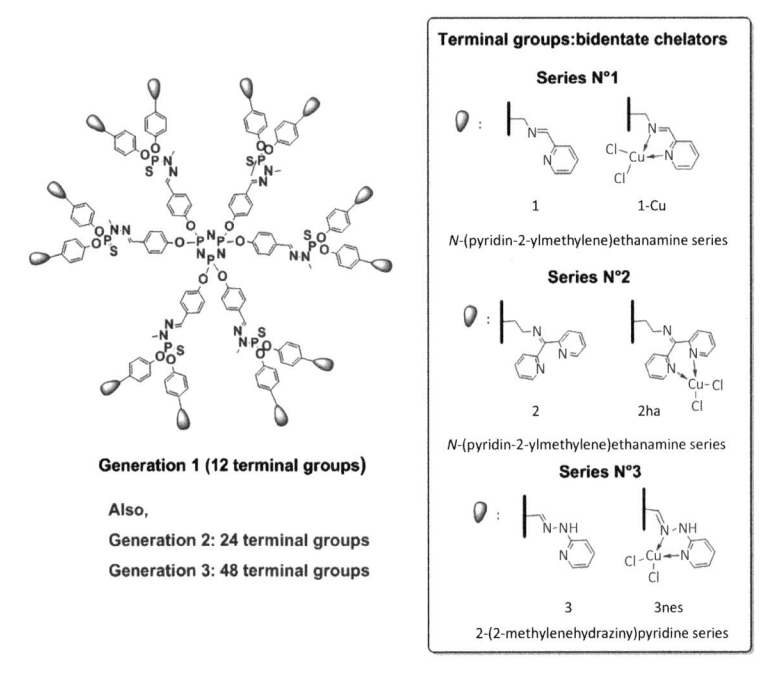

Figure 9.2 Two-dimensional schematic chemical structure of phosphorus dendrimers and corresponding multivalent copper-conjugated phosphorus dendrimers prepared.

Clearly, for each series, the first studies suggested the strong impact of the terminal moieties number and type (complexed or not) on the anti-proliferative activity. Generation 3 of dendrimers bearing an *N*-(pyridin-2-ylmethylene) ethanamine motif (first series) complexed or not with Cu(II) (named 1G3-Cu (Fig. 9.3) and 1G3, respectively) displayed the highest anti-proliferative efficiency against KB and HL60 cell lines with IC$_{50}$ ≈ 0.5–2 µM. Also, as shown in Fig. 9.3, the inhibition of cell proliferation (percentage inhibition at 1 µM) of 1G-Cu increased linearly for both KB and HL60 with the number of the terminal groups (1–48). The trend curve corresponds to the following equation: % inhibition = ~1.4 × (nbr terminal groups) = ~ 0.05 × (µg Cu/L). Consequently, each terminal group of 1G-Cu participates in the global activity.

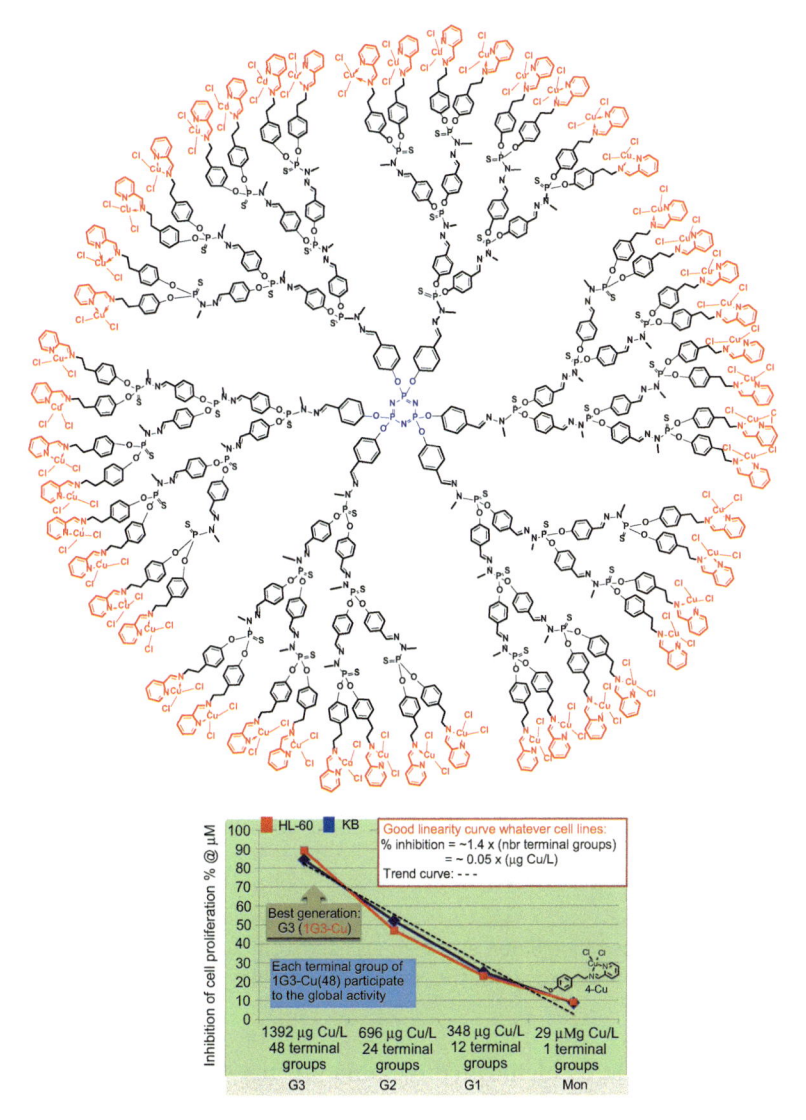

Figure 9.3 Two-dimensional schematic chemical structure of 1G3-Cu (top) and inhibition of cell proliferation *versus* number of terminal groups in KB and HL60 cell lines (bottom).

On a representative panel of tumor cell lines as well as non-cancer cells, 1G3 and 1G3-Cu were then tested. As shown in Fig. 9.4, around two- to fourfold improvement in the anti-proliferative inhibition of the Cu(II)-complexed dendrimer 1G3-Cu *versus* the plain dendrimer 1G3 was observed in KB and HL60 cell lines (IC_{50} 1.2–1.6 µM for 1G3 *versus* 0.4–0.6 µM for 1G3-Cu). The dendrimers 1G3 and 1G3-Cu displayed similar potency against HCT116 (human colon cancer), MCF7 (hormone-responsive breast cancer), and U87 (human glioblastoma-astrocytoma) cancer cells with IC_{50} ~0.2–0.8 µM). Remarkably, the complexation of the terminal ligands of G3 dendrimers by Cu(II) strongly increased the IC_{50} values (~4–10-fold) in non-cancer cell lines such as MCR5 (proliferative human lung fibroblasts, IC_{50} ~0.08 for 1G3 *versus* ≈0.8 for 1G3-Cu) and quiescent EPC cells (endothelial progenitor cells, Cyprinus carpio, IC_{50} ~0.36 for 1G3 *versus* 1.39 for 1G3-Cu), referred as "safety" cell lines.

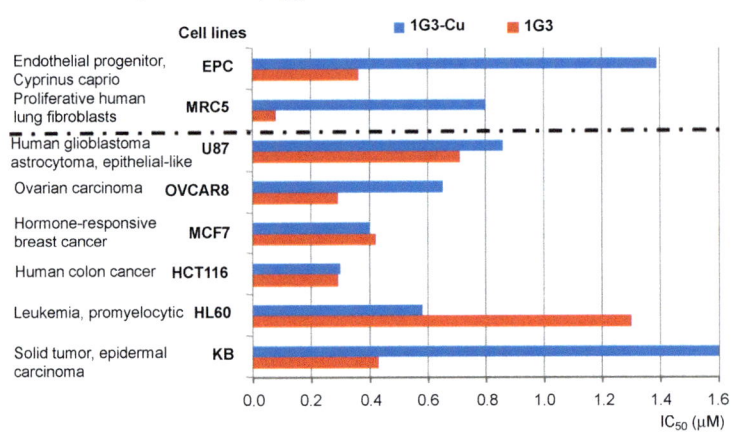

Concentrations of 1G3 and 1G3-Cu causing a half-maximum inhibition of cell proliferation (IC_{50})

Figure 9.4 Growth inhibition effects of 1G3 and 1G3-Cu upon a panel of cell lines. The dotted line separates the non-cancer cell lines from the cancer cell lines.

Importantly, as highlighted in Table 9.1, the stronger cytotoxic effect of 1G3-Cu and 1G3 *versus* cisplatin (~13- to 35-fold) in KB and HL60 cells was also noticed in cisplatin-sensitive ovarian carcinoma cell lines A2780 and OVCAR8, as well as in their cisplatin-resistant counterparts. In this case, cisplatin has been selected as a "classical" organometallic competitor.

Table 9.1 Cytotoxic activities of 1G3 and 1G3-Cu against cisplatin-sensitive and cisplatin-resistant cell lines

IC_{50} (μM)	KB	HL60	A2780	A2780 resistant	OVCAR8	SK-OV-3	
cisplatin	6.3	11.6	4.0	8.5	1.8	4.3	
$1G_3$	1.6	1.3	>10	NI	NI	NI	X 13
$1G_3$-Cu(II)	0.47	0.58	0.12	0.24	0.13	0.24	- 35

X 2 X 2

NI: not inhibitory

9.3 Mechanism of Action of 1G3 and 1G3-Cu

On the basis of our encouraging preliminary results, we decided to investigate the mechanism of action of phosphorus dendrimers 1G3 and 1G3-Cu, by exploring the programmed cell death pathway (PCD) and the alternative caspase-independent PCD and necrosis processes.

In the first and global approach, the biological activity of dendrimers was evaluated by flow cytometry (FACS) analysis: KB and HL60 cells were treated with dendrimers 1G3 and 1G3-Cu for 24 h before being examined by flow cytometry, allowing the discrimination between intact cells and cells entering apoptosis or dead cells. As illustrated in Fig. 9.5, 1G3 induced rapidly the entry of cells in early apoptosis, while 1G3-Cu induced a massive apoptosis at the same concentration. The release of LDH from cells is a hallmark of necrosis, a redundant process involved in cell death promoted by chemicals. In cells treated with 1G3 and 1G3-Cu, no activation of the direct necrotic process was noticed (data not shown). Therefore, it can be concluded that dendrimers induced cell death through the activation of the apoptotic process.

Caspase-3 is believed to be the terminal effector of the apoptotic cascade. Many chemicals have been reported to activate caspase-3, thus initiating DNA degradation and cell death [14]. Therefore, an activation of caspase-3 could be expected in cells entering in an active apoptotic process after being treated with 1G3 and 1G3-Cu.

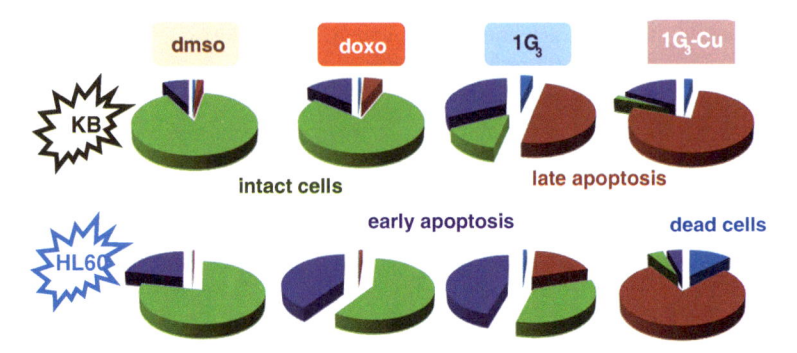

Figure 9.5 FACS analysis of KB and HL60 cells treated for 24 h with 5 µM 1G3 and 1G3-Cu.

If 1G3 was a potent activator of caspase-3, 1G3-Cu surprisingly reduced caspase-3 activity in KB and HL60 cells (Fig. 9.6). This unexpected effect was not related to the presence of the copper atom, since copper chloride had no or moderate inhibitory effect on caspase-3 activity in cells treated for 48 h with $CuCl_2$ or when caspase-3 activity was monitored in the presence of $CuCl_2$.

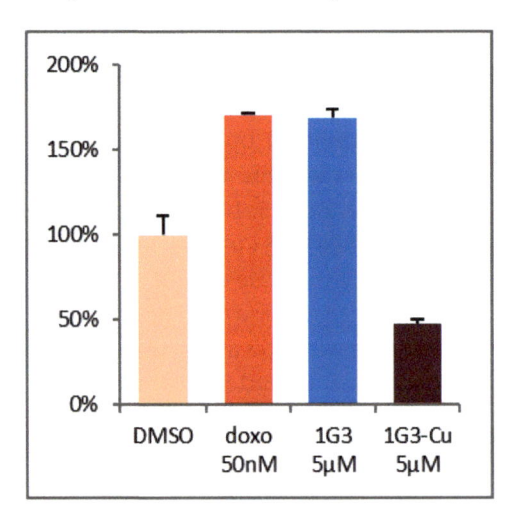

Figure 9.6 Caspase-3 activation in KB cells treated for 48 h with 1G3 and 1G3-Cu.

Additionally, the presence of caspase-3 protein was investigated by immunochemistry in the cytosol of KB cells: basically caspase-3 was synthesized as its inactive 32 kDa form before being cleaved into its 17 kDa active form by cellular proteases. As shown in Fig. 9.7A, 1G3 promoted the conversion of the inactive procaspase-3 into its active form, whereas 1G3-Cu reduced the content in both active and inactive forms, in line with the lower activity reported in Fig. 9.6. Therefore, it is possible to conclude that apoptosis induced by 1G3-Cu does not involve the caspase-dependent pathway, in contrast with the activation of caspase-3-dependent apoptosis by 1G3.

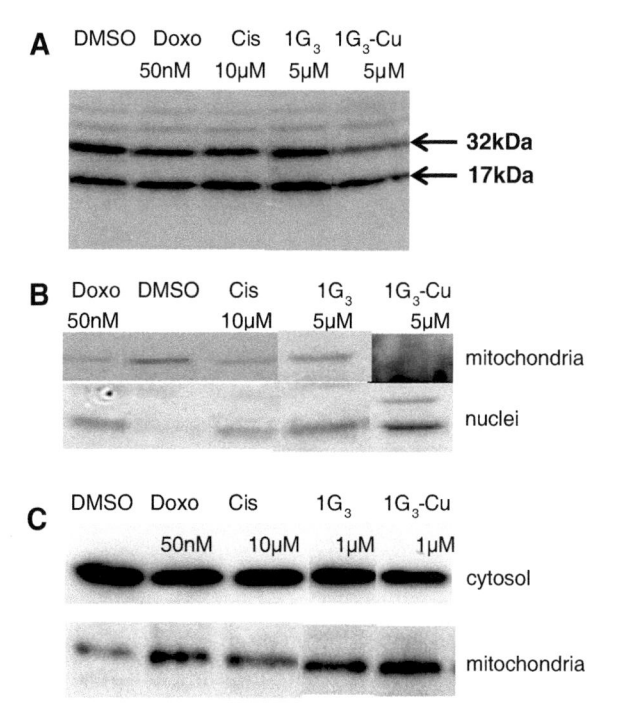

Figure 9.7 Immunochemical determination of caspase-3 (A), AIF (B), and Bax (C) in subcellular fractions isolated from KB and HL60 cells treated with 1G3 and 1G3-Cu.

An alternative caspase-independent apoptosis pathway involves the release of apoptosis inducing factor (AIF) from the mitochondria and its translocation to the nucleus. To assess this possible mechanism, cells were treated with 1G3 and 1G3-Cu, and mitochondrial, nuclear, and cytosolic subfractions were prepared and used for immunochemical determinations. In cells treated with the vehicle, AIF was mostly detected in the mitochondrial compartment. Following exposure to doxorubicin and cisplatin, the AIF content was strikingly reduced in the mitochondria and concomitantly increased in the cytosol (not shown) and nuclei (Fig. 9.7B). With 1G3, the AIF mitochondrial content was moderately reduced while increased in nuclei on a dose-dependent basis. A similar dose-dependent translocation was noticed with 1G3-Cu but with a higher efficiency resulting in an almost complete transfer of AIF from mitochondria to nuclei.

The release of mitochondrial proteins was regulated by the opening of mitochondrial pores. A major contributor for the opening of these pores is Bax, a pro-apoptotic member of the Bcl2 protein family. Under apoptotic stimuli, Bax is activated and translocated from the cytosol to mitochondria to lower the mitochondrial membrane potential and finally favor the release of AIF. To validate its involvement into the apoptotic process elicited by 1G3-Cu, the Bax content was estimated by immunochemistry in cytosol and mitochondria (Fig. 9.7C). With 1G3, the mitochondrial Bax content was moderately enriched in detriment to the cytosolic compartment. A similar evolution was noticed with 1G3-Cu but with a much higher efficiency. Thus, 1G3-Cu actively translocates Bax to the mitochondria, promotes the AIF release, and finally induces apoptosis.

The mode of action of cisplatin and other platinum-containing chemicals has been attributed to the formation of stable adducts between chemicals and DNA, through either intra- or inter-strand cross-links, resulting in DNA fragmentation and preventing DNA reparation and replication. The existence of DNA fragments can be demonstrated by dUTP nick-end labeling (TUNEL): Alteration of the DNA integrity by chemicals generated small DNA fragments, which can be labeled with Br-dUTP, detected with fluorescent antibodies, and visualized by FACS. The fragmentation of DNA induced by 1G3 and 1G3-Cu was evaluated and compared with those promoted by cisplatin and doxorubicin (Table 9.2).

Table 9.2 DNA fragmentation in KB and HL60 cells following 24 h exposure to 1G3 and 1G3-Cu

Cells	KB (%)	HL60 (%)
DMSO	4.1	9.9
doxo 50 nM	24.8	23.4
Cisplatin 5 µM	3.9	23.0
1G3 5 µM	52.9	16.8
1G3-Cu 5 µM	86.2	78.7
$CuCl_2$ 5 µM	2.6	nd

The proportion of cells containing fragmented DNA was extremely low in cells treated with DMSO and was increased after cisplatin or doxorubicin exposure [15]. Copper chloride had no effect, but a considerable augmentation in the number of cells containing fragmented DNA was observable with 1G3 and even more with 1G3-Cu. It can be concluded that the apoptotic progression initiated by 1G3 and 1G3-Cu results in a striking DNA alteration.

Basically, cytotoxic anti-cancer agents elicited cell cycle arrests in specific DNA replication phases, according to their mode of action and cellular target. We addressed the question whether or not DNA was more susceptible to fragmentation induced by 1G3 and 1G3-Cu. After DNA staining and analysis in flow cytometry, healthy cells were separated by their relative content in DNA: either 2n chromosomes (phase G0/G1), 4n chromosomes (phase G2/M), or intermediate (phase S) with apoptotic cells containing fragmented DNA (phase sub-G1). By contrast with doxorubicin, which accumulated cells in phase G2/M, 1G3 and 1G3-Cu did not substantially modify the distribution of cells in the different cell cycle phases of living cells, but as previously stated considerably enlarged the number of apoptotic cells containing fragmented DNA. Therefore, it can be concluded that 1G3 and 1G3-Cu had no effect in the control of cell cycle (Table 9.3).

Information collected in these studies suggested that, very interestingly, the pro-apoptotic Bax protein, a central death regulator, was actively translocated to the mitochondrial compartment, allowing the release of apoptosis inducing factor and finally the activation of the caspase-independent apoptotic pathway.

Table 9.3 Cell cycle analysis of KB cells treated for 24 h with DMSO (A), doxorubicin (B), 1G3 (C), or 1G3-Cu (D)

	DMSO	Doxo 50 nM	1G3 5 µM	1G3-Cu 5 µM
G2/M (%)	9.1	46.1	3.7	4.2
S Phase (%)	35.5	45.1	32.1	27.0
G0/G1 (%)	51.4	4.9	34.0	24.2
Sub G1 (%)	4.0	3.5	30.2	44.6

To the best of our knowledge, few anti-cancer small molecules and copper complexes were described as Bax activators. Thus, based on NMR and biochemical analyses, Gavathiotis et al. [16] described the direct and selective small pyrazolone derivative BAM7, which activates pro-apoptotic Bax (Fig. 9.8). Using Glide 4.0, the authors generated a diverse in silico compilation of 750,000 small molecules from commercially available libraries and docked the database of three-dimensional molecules on average minimized Bax structures (standard precision and then extraprecision docking mode). BAM7 showed an IC_{50} of 3.3 µM in a competitive FPA involving FITC-BIM SAHB and Bax construction. BAM7 binds to BH3-binding groove at the *N*-terminal face of Bax and induces Bax-dependent cell death. Then, a lead optimization of BAM7 has been recently reported by Stornaiuolo, Marinelli, and their coworkers [17]. This study led to BTC-8 as Bax activator exhibiting higher affinity for Bax than Bcl-2 (~15-fold, µM range). This means that BTC-8 is both more active and more selective for Bax than BAM7. The ability of BTC-8 to induce apoptosis was evaluated on MEF knock-out cells. BTC-8 displayed an EC_{50} = 1.1 µM lower than BAM7 (~7-fold). BTC-8 activates Bax and induced mitochondrial outer membrane permeabilization (MOMP).

In another recent report, three chemically diverse small-molecule agonists of Bax have been reported, as follows: Compounds SMBA1, SMBA2, and SMBA3 have been discovered by screening of the National Cancer Institute (NCI) library database of approximately 300,000 small molecules based computational modelling analysis of the pocket around S^{184} using DOCK program [18]. These three compounds bind to Bax protein with high affinities (Ki ~ 50 nM) and led to the activation of Bax by specific binding to the pocket at S^{184}, blocking the serine phosphorylation and allowing Bax oligomerization in mitochondria. Importantly, SMBA1 suppressed dose-dependently growth against A549 lung tumor xenograft models in Nu/Nu mice at the dose of 40 and 60 mg/kg per day, intraperitoneally, during 10 days. This suppression of lung cancer occurs through apoptosis in lung tumor tissues through the activation of caspase-3 based on immunohistochemistry technique.

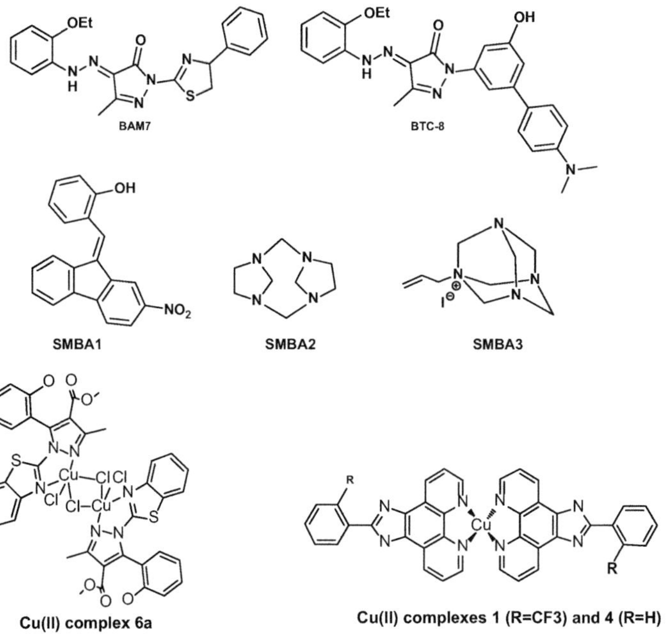

Figure 9.8 Chemical structures of small-molecule and copper-complex activators of Bax.

In addition, several original solid complexes containing Pt(II) and Cu(II) as the central atom were prepared by Budzisz et al. [19]. Among these complexes, the copper(II) complex **6a** (Fig. 9.8) displayed moderate cytotoxic activities toward human promyelocytic leukemia cells (HL60), human acute lymphoblastic leukemia (NALM-6), and human malignant melanoma (WM-115) with $IC_{50}s$ ~20–50 µM and ~8–12 µM, respectively. Complex **6a** showed comparable cytotoxicity than cisplatin, whereas

8a displayed two times more potency than cisplatin. Additionally, the copper(II) complex **6a** induced overexpression of Bax after 5 h of exposure, while various patterns of Bax and p53 gene expressions were observed in melanoma cells.

Then, Zhao et al. reported the anti-proliferative activities of Cu(II)-benzoimidazole complexes against four human tumor cell lines [20]. Later Li et al. [21] reported that the Cu(II) compound induced apoptosis by release of cytochrome c, cleavage of procaspase-3 and -9 and ADP-ribose polymerase (PARP), as well the activation of Bcl-2 and Bax in SGC-7901 cell line. Interestingly, this Cu(II)-complex, injected intra-peritoneally, significantly suppressed tumor growth in S180 bearing mice after a treatment of 10 mg/kg.

Very recently, Nagababu designed and developed novel Cu(II) polypyridyl complexes as anti-cancer agents. The Cu(II) complexes **1** and **4** exhibited cytotoxicity against several cancer cell lines such as B16F10 melanoma cells, SK-OV-3 ovarian cells, A549 lung cancer and invasive ductal carcinoma MDA-MB-231 cells with IC_{50}s $\sim$0.1–2.1 µM. Interestingly, these two complexes displayed anti-proliferative activity toward endothelial cells (HUVECs) resulting on their antiangiogenic properties with IC_{50}s in µM range. Additionally, excessive formation of intracellular ROS and upregulation of Bax protein may be the plausible mechanism behind their anti-cancer activities [22].

9.4 Conclusion

In summary, we paved the synthesis and the antitumor activities of the original copper-conjugated phosphorus dendrimers and corresponding monomers. The most potent compound is the 1G3-Cu dendrimer. We showed that 1G3-Cu represents a new and promising first-in-class anti-proliferative agent with an original mechanism of action in the nanomedicine field. Very interestingly, the pro-apoptotic Bax protein, a central death regulator, was actively translocated by 1G3-Cu to the mitochondrial compartment allowing the release of apoptosis inducing factor and finally the activation of the caspase-independent apoptotic pathway. To our knowledge, it is the first example of nanoparticles in general and dendrimers in particular displaying potent anti-cancer activity through Bax protein activation pathway inducing tumor cell death. We show that 1G3-Cu represents a new and promising first-in-class anti-proliferative agent with an original mechanism of action in the nanomedicine field. The study of the anti-cancer properties of other dendritic complexes, in particular of gold complexes, is underway [23].

Acknowledgments

Thanks are due to the CNRS and CEFIPRA (Project number 5303-2) for financial support.

References

1. Jemal, A., Bray, F., Center, M. M., Ferlay, J., Ward, E., and Forman, D. (2011). Gobal cancer statistics, *Cancer. J. Clin.*, **61**, pp. 69–90.

2. Dobbelstein, M. and Moll, U. (2014). Targeting tumour-supportive cellular machineries in anti-cancer drug development, *Nat. Rev. Drug Discov.*, **13**, pp. 179–196.

3. Kamb, A., Wee, S., and Lengauer, C. (2007). Why is cancer drug discovery so difficult, *Nat. Rev. Drug Discov.*, **6**, pp. 115–120.

4. Pillai, G. (2014). Nanomedicines for cancer therapy: An update of FDA approved and those under various stages of development, *SOJ Pharm. Pharmaceut. Sci.*, **1**, 13.

5. (a) Lee, C. C., Mackay, J. A., Frechet, J. M. J., and Szoka, F. C. (2005). Designing dendrimers for biological applications, *Nat. Biotechnol.*, **23**, pp. 1517–1526. (b) Svenson, S. and Tomalia, D. A. (2005). Commentary: Dendrimers in biomedical applications reflections on the field, *Adv. Drug Deliv. Rev.*, **57**, pp. 2106–2129.

6. (a) Gillies, E. R. and Fréchet, J. M. (2005). Dendrimers and dendritic polymers in drug delivery, *Drug Discov. Today*, **10**, pp. 35–43. (b) Caminade, A.-M. and Majoral, J. P. (2005). Water-soluble phosphorus-containing dendrimers, *Prog. Polym. Sci.*, **30**, pp. 491–505. (c) McCarthy, T. D., Karellas, P., Henderson, S. A., Giannis, M., O'Keefe, D. F., Heery, G., Paull, J. R. A., Matthews, B. R., and Holan, G. (2005). Dendrimers as drugs: Discovery and preclinical and clinical development of dendrimer-based microbicides for HIV and STI prevention, *Mol.*

Pharm., **2**, pp. 312–318. (d) Griffe, L., Poupot, M., Marchand, P., Maraval, A., Turrin, C. O., Rolland, O., Metivier, P., Bacquet, G. Fournie, J. J., Caminade, A.-M., Poupot, R., and Majoral, J.-P. (2008). Tailored control and optimization of the number of phosphonic acid termini on phosphorus-containing dendrimers for the *ex vivo* activation of human monocytes, *Chem. Eur. J.*, **14**, pp. 4836–4850. (e) Wolinsky, J. B., Mark, W., and Grinstaff, M. (2008). Advanced therapeutic and diagnostic applications of dendrimers for cancer treatment, *Adv. Drug Deliv. Rev.*, **60**, pp. 1037–1055. (f) Mintzer, M. A. and Grinstaff, M. W. (2010). Biomedical applications of dendrimers: A tutorial, *Chem. Soc. Rev.*, **40**, pp. 173–190. (g) Astruc, D., Boisselier, E., and Omelas, C. (2010). Dendrimer designed for functions: From physical, and supramolecular properties to applications in sensing, catalysis, molecular electronic, photonics, and nanomedicine, *Chem. Rev.*, **110**, pp. 1857–1959. (h) Menjoge, A. R., Kannan, R. M., and Tomalia, D. A. (2010). Dendrimer-based drug and imaging conjugates: Design considerations for nanomedical applications, *Drug Discov. Today*, **15**, pp. 171–185. (i) Maksimenko, A. V., Mandrouguine, V., Gottikh, M. B., Bertrand, J. R., Majoral, J.-P., and Malvy, C. (2003). Optimisation of dendrimer-mediated gene transfer by anionic oligomers, *J. Gene Med.*, **5**, pp. 61–71. (j) Spataro, G., Malecaze, F., Turrin, C. O., Soler, V., Duhayon, C., Elena, P. P., Majoral, J.-P., and Caminade, A.-M. (2010). Designing dendrimers for ocular drug delivery, *Eur. J. Med. Chem.*, **45**, pp. 326–334. (k) El Kazzouli, S., Mignani, S., Bousmina, M., and Majoral, J.-P. (2012). Dendrimer therapeutics: Covalent and ionic attachments, *New. J. Chem.*, **36**, pp. 227–240. (l) Khandare, J., Calderon, M., Dagia, N. M., and Haag, R. (2012). Multifunctional dendritic polymers in nanomedicine: Opportunities and challenges, *Chem. Soc. Rev.*, **41**, pp. 2824–2848.

7. (a) Mignani, S., Huber, S., Tomás H., Rodrigues, J., and Majoral, J.-P. (2016). Compound high-quality criteria: A new vision to guide the development of drugs, current situation, *Drug Discov. Today*, **21**, pp. 573–584. (b) Mignani, S., Huber, S., Tomás H., Rodrigues, J., and Majoral, J.-P. (2015). Why and how have drug discovery strategies in pharma changed? What are the new mindsets?, *Drug Discov. Today*, **21**, pp. 239–249.

8. Solassol, J., Crozet, C., Perrier, V., Leclaire, J., Béranger, F., Caminade, A. M., Meunier, B., Dormon, D., Majoral, J. P., and Lehmann, S. (2004). Cationic phosphorous-containing dendrimers reduce prion replication both in cell cultures and in mice infected with scrapie, *J. Gen. Virol.*, **85**, pp. 1791–1799.

9. (a) Poupot, M., Griffe, L., Marchand, P., Maraval, A., Rolland, O., Martinet, L., L'Faqihi-Olive, F. E., Turrin, C. O., Caminade, A. M., Fournié, J. J., Majoral, J. P., and Poupot, R. (2006). Design of phosphorylated dendritic architectures to promote human monocyte activation, *FASEB J.*, **20**, pp. 2339–2351. (b) Hayder, M., Poupot, M., Baron, M., Nigon, D., Turrin, C. O., Caminade, A. M., Majoral, J. P., Eisenberg, R. A., Fournié, J. J., Cantagrel, A., Poupot, R., and Davignon, J. L. (2011). Phosphorus-based dendrimer as nanotherapeutics targeting both inflammation and osteoclastogenesis in experimental arthritis, *Sci. Transl. Med.*, **3**, pp. 81ra35.

10. Griffe, L., Poupot, M., Marchand, P., Maraval, A., Turrin, C. O., Rolland, O., Métivier, P., Bacquet, G., Fournié, J. J., Caminade, A. M., Poupot, R., and Majoral, J. P. (2007). Multiplication of human natural killer cells by nanosized phosphonate-capped dendrimers, *Angew. Chem. Int. Ed.*, **46**, pp. 2523–2526.

11. Mignani, S., Bryszewska, M., Zablocka, M., Klajnert-Maculewicz, B., Cladera, J, Shcharbin, D., and Majoral, J. P. (2017). Can dendrimer-based nanoparticles fight neurodegenerative diseases? Current situation *versus* other established approaches, *Prog. Polym. Sci.*, **64**, 23–51.

12. (a) Le Berre, V., Trévisiol, E., Dagkessamanskaia, A., Sokol, S., Caminade, A. M., Majoral, J. P., Meunier, B., and François, J. (2003). Dendrimeric coating of glass slides for sensitive DNA microarrays analysis, *Nucleic Acids Res.*, **31**, pp. e88. (b) Trévisiol, E., Leberre-Anton, V., Leclaire, J., Pratviel, G., Caminade, A. M., Majoral, J. P., François, J. M., and Meunier, B. (2003). Dendrislides, dendrichips: A simple chemical functionalization of glass slides with phosphorus dendrimers as an effective mean for the preparation of biochips, *New. J. Chem.*, **27**, pp. 1713–1719.

13. El Brahmi, N., El Kazzouli, S., Mignani, S., el Essassi, M., Aubert, G., Laurent, R., Caminade, A-M., Bousmina, M. M., Cresteil, T., and Majoral, J. P. (2013). Original multivalent copper(II)-conjugated phosphorus dendrimers and corresponding mononuclear copper(II) complexes with antitumoral activities, *Mol. Pharm.*, **10**, pp. 1459–1464.

14. Janicke, R. U., Sprengart, M. L., Wati, M. R., and Porter, A. G. (1998). Caspase-3 is required for DNA fragmentation and morphological changes associated with apoptosis, *J. Biol. Chem.*, **273**, pp. 9357–9360.

15. Chtchigrovsky, M., Eloy, L., Jullien, H., Saker, L., Ségal-Bendirdjian, E., Poupon, J., Bombard, S., Cresteil, T., Retailleau, P., and Marinetti, A. (2013). Antitumor trans-N-heterocyclic carbene-amine-Pt(II) complexes: Synthesis of dinuclear species and exploratory

investigations of DNA binding and cytotoxicity mechanisms, *J. Med. Chem.*, **56**, pp. 2074–2086.

16. Gavathiotis, E., Reyna, D. E., Bellair, J. A., Leshchiner, E. S., and Wallenski, L. D. (2012). Direct and selective small-molecule activation of proapoptotic Bax, *Nat. Chem. Bio.*, **8**, pp. 639–645.

17. Stornaiulo, M., La Regina, G., Passacantilli, S., Grassia, G., Coluccia, A., La Pietra, V., Giustiniano, M., Cassese, M., Di Maro, S., Brancaccio, D., Taliani, S., Ialenti, A., Silvestri, R., Martini, C., Novellino, E., and Marinelli, L. (2015). Structure-based lead optimization and biological evaluation of Bax direct activators as novel potential anti-cancer agents, *J. Med. Chem.*, **58**, pp. 2135–2148.

18. Xin, M., Li, R., Xie, M., Park, D., Owoniloko, T. K., Sica, G., Corsino, P. E., Zhou, J., Ding, C., White, M. A., Magis, A. T., Ramalingam, S. S., Curran, W. J., Khuri, F. R., and Deng, X. (2014). Small-molecule Bax agonists for cancer therapy, *Nature Comm.*, Article number: 4935. Doi:10.1038/ncomms5935.

19. Budzisz, E., Miernika, M., Lorenz, I. P., Mayer, P., Balcerzak, E., Krajewska, U., and Rozalski, M. (2010). Synthesis, X-ray structures and cytotoxic activity of platinum(II), palladium(II) and copper(II) complexes with chelating ligands, *Eur. J. Med. Chem.*, **45**, pp. 2613–2621.

20. Zhao, J. A., Li, S., Zhao, D., Chen, S., and Hu, J. (2013). Metal and structure tuned *in vitro* antitumor activity of benzimidazole-based copper and zinc complexes, *J. Coord. Chem.*, **66**, pp. 1650–1660.

21. Li, R., Cui, B., Li, Y., Zhao, C., Jia, N., Wang, C., Wu, Y., and Wen, A. (2014). A new synthetic Cu(II) compound, $[Cu_3(p\text{-}3\text{-}bmb)_2Cl_4 \cdot (CH_3OH)_2]_n$, inhibits tumor growth *in vivo* and *in vitro*, *Eur. J. Pharm.*, **724**, pp. 77–85.

22. Nagababu, P., Barui, A. K., Thulasiram, B., Devi, C. S., Satyanarayana, S., Patra, C. R., and Sreedhar, B. (2015). Antiangiogenic activity of mononuclear copper(II) polypyridyl complexes for the treatment of cancers, *J. Med. Chem.*, **58**, pp. 5226–5241.

23. Mignani, S., El Brahmi, N., El Kazzouli, S., Laurent, R., Ladeira, S., Caminade, A. M., Pedziwiatr-Werbicka, E., Szewczyk, E., Bryszewska, M., Bousmina, M., Cresteil, T., Majoral, J. P. (2017). Original multivalent Gold (III) and dual Gold(III)-Copper(II) conjugated phosphorus dendrimers as potent antitumoral and antimicrobial agents, *Mol. Pharm.*, **14**, pp. 4087–4097.

Chapter 10

Rational Design of Mannodendrimers Targeting Human C-type Lectin Receptors to Prevent Lung Inflammation

Jérôme Nigou,[a] Jacques Prandi,[a] Emilyne Blattes,[a] Sandro Silva-Gomes,[a] Anne-Marie Caminade,[b] Alain Vercellone,[a] and Germain Puzo[a]

[a]*Institut de Pharmacologie et de Biologie Structurale, Université de Toulouse, CNRS, UPS Toulouse, France*
[b]*Laboratoire de Chimie de Coordination, Université de Toulouse, CNRS, UPS Toulouse, France*
jerome.nigou@ipbs.fr

The human pathogen *Mycobacterium tuberculosis* produces a lipoglycan, namely mannose-capped lipoarabinomannan, which displays anti-inflammatory properties by targeting specific C-type lectin receptors on the surface of immune cells. We designed and synthesized poly(phosphorhydrazone) dendrimers grafted with mannose residues, called mannodendrimers, to mimic the bioactive supramolecular structure of mannose-capped lipoarabinomannan, with the objective of developing innovative anti-inflammatory molecules.

Phosphorus Dendrimers in Biology and Nanomedicine: Synthesis, Characterization, and Properties
Edited by Anne-Marie Caminade, Cédric-Olivier Turrin, and Jean-Pierre Majoral
Copyright © 2018 Pan Stanford Publishing Pte. Ltd.
ISBN 978-981-4774-33-8 (Hardcover), 978-1-315-11085-1 (eBook)
www.panstanford.com

10.1   Introduction

Bacterial intracellular pathogens have evolved multiple molecular mechanisms to alter immune responses, thereby securing their colonization and survival inside the host. *Mycobacterium tuberculosis* (Mtb), the causative agent of human tuberculosis, survives within host phagocytic cells, including alveolar macrophages and dendritic cells (DCs) [1], which it manipulates to down-regulate the inflammatory response [2].

Inflammation is a natural process of defense against infection. In this way, the pro-inflammatory cytokines TNF-α and IL-12, and the axis formed between the latter and IFN-γ, play an essential role to protect individuals against mycobacterial infections [3–5]. Cytokine production in the lung upon Mtb infection is mediated and modulated by innate immune receptors, namely pattern recognition receptors (PRRs), such as toll-like receptors (TLRs) and C-type lectin-like receptors (CLRs), which are expressed by alveolar macrophages and DCs. By targeting TLRs and CLRs, most particularly via the abundant glycolipids and lipoglycans exposed at its cell envelope surface, Mtb qualitatively and quantitatively controls the inflammatory response at the site of infection. Lipomannan (LM) and phosphatidyl-*myo*-inositol mannosides (PIMs), via recognition by TLR2/TLR1 (for reviews, see Refs. [6, 7]), and trehalose-6,6′-dimycolate (TDM or cord-factor), via binding to the CLR Mincle [8], induce the production of pro-inflammatory cytokines. In contrast, mannose-capped lipoarabinomannan (ManLAM) recognition by the CLR Dectin-2 induces the production of the anti-inflammatory cytokine IL-10 [9]. In addition, ManLAM binds two other CLRs, namely DC-SIGN (dendritic cell-specific intracellular adhesion molecule grabbing non-integrin) [10–13] and MR (mannose receptor) [14, 15]. ManLAM binding to DC-SIGN inhibits the pro-inflammatory cytokine IL-12 and TNF-α [16–18] and increases the anti-inflammatory cytokine IL-10 [10] production by LPS (lipopolysaccharide)-stimulated human DCs. Although MR is expressed on DCs, ManLAM only binds DC-SIGN on these cells [10]. However, MR also triggers an anti-inflammatory signal [16, 19, 20], which is likely to mediate ManLAM immunosuppressive effects in macrophages [7].

ManLAMs are complex amphipatic macromolecules with an average molecular weight of around 17 kDa. Their structure is composed of three domains: (i) a mannosyl-phosphatidyl-*myo*-inositol (MPI) anchor, (ii) a heteropolysaccharidic core of D-mannan linked to D-arabinan, and (iii) mannose caps made of mono-, $\alpha(1\rightarrow2)$-di-, and $\alpha(1\rightarrow2)$-tri-mannosides substituting the end of the D-arabinan side chains [21, 22]. Anti-inflammatory activity of ManLAM mediated by its binding to DC-SIGN, MR, or Dectin-2 requires both the mannose caps and the fatty acyl residues borne by the MPI anchor [9, 14, 16, 18]. ManLAM bioactivity is associated, not to its monomeric, but to a supramolecular structure resulting from a highly ordered organization of ManLAM in aqueous solution induced by the presence of the fatty acyl appendages [23]. This 30 nm spherical structure is composed of around 450 ManLAM molecules, with the mannose caps exposed to the surface. It allows ManLAM multipoint attachment, via the mannose caps, to multimeric and/or clustered CLRs expressed at the surface of phagocytic cells, thereby ensuring high affinity binding and triggering of intracellular signaling for the modulation of pro-/anti-inflammatory cytokine production [7, 18, 22, 23].

Uncovering the molecular mechanisms underlying ManLAM ability to down-regulate the host inflammatory response by targeting CLRs has opened avenues for the rational design of innovative classes of anti-inflammatory molecules [17]. Indeed, new targets need to be proposed to control inflammation, because classical therapeutic strategies to fight inflammation, such as corticosteroids, are non-specific, immunosuppressive, and can be deleterious in prolonged or high-dose therapy [24, 25]. We thus undertook to synthesize ManLAM analogs that would mimic its bioactive supramolecular structure in terms of architecture and multivalence. The task required development of a spherical backbone or scaffold and then functionalization of this scaffold by mannooligosaccharide caps.

Dendrimers are compounds of choice to generate three-dimensional structures; they are monodispersed, polyfunctionalized and hyperbranched macromolecules whose nanometer size, multivalent character, and molecular weight can be controlled rigorously during synthesis, contrary to polymers [26]. Dendrimers can adopt a spherical conformation and are particularly suitable for the surface attachment of multiple copies of epitopes closely packed leading to a high density of ligands and consequently to synthetic molecules with both high valency and avidity for CLRs [27, 28]. The first glycodendrimers bearing covalently bound α-D-mannopyrannoside reported in the literature were synthesized from commercially available dendrimers, *i.e.*, poly(L-lysine) [29] and poly(amidoamine) scaffolds [30]. More recently, poly(glycerol) dendrimers [31] and poly(peptide) dendrimers [32] were also used as scaffolds for the same purpose. We used poly(phosphorhydrazone) (PPH) dendrimers for their known biocompatibility, easy preparation, and the possibility to introduce various chemical groups at the end of the branches [33]. Indeed, PPH dendrimers variously functionalized at their termini have been shown to display numerous biological properties [34–37].

Here we review the design and synthesis of mannosylated PPH dendrimers (hereafter referred to as mannodendrimers) that mimic the bioactive supramolecular structure of ManLAM, efficiently target the CLR DC-SIGN on human DCs, and display anti-inflammatory properties *in vivo* in a mouse model of acute lung inflammation [17].

10.2 Chemical Synthesis of Mannodendrimers

Mannodendrimers were synthesized by grafting synthetic mono-, $\alpha(1{\rightarrow}2)$-di-, or $\alpha(1{\rightarrow}2)$-tri-mannopyranosides (M, D, and T, respectively; Fig. 10.1A,B) found in ManLAM caps to the surface of PPH dendrimers.

10.2.1 Synthesis of the Dendrimer Core

PPH dendrimers with an NH_2-derivatized surface [38] were obtained by reaction of the growing dendrimer (generations 1 to 4 with $P(S)Cl_2$ surface) with the alcohol function of N-BOC tyramine (Scheme 10.1). The progress of the reaction was monitored by ^{31}P NMR spectroscopy of the crude reaction mixture. For the four generations of PPH dendrimers analyzed by ^{31}P NMR, the resonance of phosphorus atoms of the core and branches showed similar chemical shifts at 8.5 ppm and approximately 62.5 ppm, respectively. Deprotection of the BOC group under acidic conditions produced the required dendrimers with NH_3^+ groups on their surface.

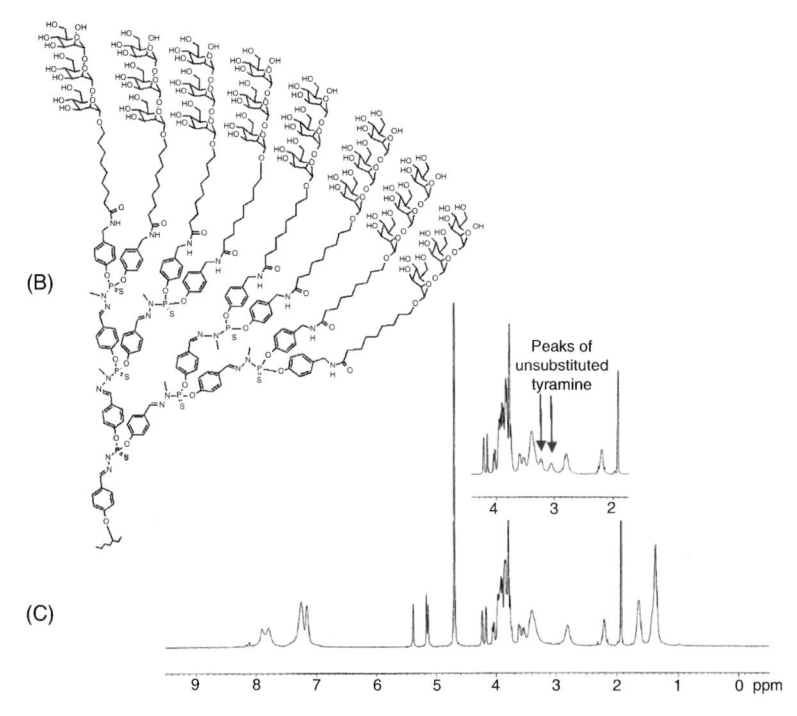

Name	1M	2M	3M	1D	2D	3D	4D	3T
Generation	1	2	3	1	2	3	4	3
Number of caps	12	24	48	12	24	48	96	48
Mannoside	mono	mono	mono	di	di	di	di	tri
Molecular weight (g.mol⁻¹)	5846.7	12825.7	26639.3	8658.1	18448.6	37993.4	76999.1	48118.2

Figure 10.1 (A) Name and characteristics of mannodendrimers. (B) Partial view of the structure of mannodendrimer 3T; only one out of six identical branches on the N_3P_3 core is represented. (C) ^1H NMR spectrum of 3T; in the upper panel, spectrum of a partially mannosylated dendrimer.

10.2.2 Synthesis of Oligomannosides

The $\alpha(1\rightarrow2)$ linkages, which are the only ones present in the caps of ManLAM, were elaborated using a linear sequence of glycosylation/deprotection [39]. To secure the stereochemical outcome of the glycosylation reactions as α, a participating group was introduced on the 2-position of the mannosyl donors (**2**) and (**3**), while positions 3, 4, and 6 were protected by permanent protecting groups during all the synthesis. The mannosidic glycosyl donor carried either a thiomannoside or a trichloroacetimidate groups as activable groups on the anomeric position (compounds **2** and **3**, Scheme 10.1A). These mannosyl donors **2** and **3** were obtained in one or two steps from orthoester (**1**), available in good overall yield in five steps from D-mannose using optimized procedures [40].

For efficient interaction of the oligomannosides at the surface of the dendrimer with clustered DC-SIGN on the cell surface, some flexibility of the glycosidic ligands in solution is needed; for that, we chose to introduce a nine-carbon-long linker between the end groups of the dendrimer and the oligomannosides. According to these guidelines, oligomannosides, mono- (**5**), di- (**7**), and tri-mannosides (**8**) were then elaborated and they were fully deprotected in two steps before coupling to the dendrimer.

10.2.3 Coupling Step and Structural Characterization

Our first attempt to prepare a mannosylated dendrimer was the coupling of hydrazide (**10**) with a dendrimer carrying aldehyde groups at its surface. The chemical efficiency of this process was very high, and the total substitution of the surface groups of the dendrimer was obtained in one step with only a small excess of the oligomannoside moiety. However, after purification of the reaction mixture, the product was found to be totally insoluble in water, which is mandatory for biological evaluation of the mannodendrimers. To overcome this solubility problem, we chose to use a more classical coupling reaction, well documented for the preparation of modified proteins [41, 42], and we replaced the acyl hydrazone function by an amide bond. The mannosyl hydrazine was activated as the acylazide (**11**), which was coupled on a dendrimer presenting primary amine functions at its surface. This procedure proved to be much less efficient than the previous one, but we were able to obtain satisfactory yields of mannodendrimers after repeating the coupling reaction three times.

Total substitution of the dendrimer was ascertained by ^{1}H NMR by disappearance of the signals corresponding to unsubstituted tyramine at 3.05 and 3.25 ppm (Fig. 10.1C) and mostly, these mannodendrimers were very soluble in water.

All products were purified by size-exclusion chromatography and were characterized by ^{1}H, ^{13}C, and ^{31}P NMR (see Fig. 10.1C for a typical ^{1}H NMR spectrum). The availability of mono-, di-, and tri-mannosidic building blocks, together with dendrimers of various generations (from 1 to 4) gave a whole family of mannodendrimers, differing by their overall size, the length of the oligosaccharide, the number and the density of the oligomannosides at their surface. Mannodendrimers were named for simplification purposes according to their generation (1 to 4) and to the structure of the caps: mono- (M), di- (D), or tri- (T) mannosides (Fig. 10.1A). The dendrimer of third generation substituted by tri-mannosides was called 3T; its partial structure is depicted in Fig. 10.1B, and its ^{1}H NMR spectrum is shown in Fig. 10.1C. Homogeneity and polydispersity of the mannodendrimers could be assessed using analytical size-exclusion chromatography with multi-angle light-scattering detection. Using this technique, mannodendrimer 3T was found to be pure and its measured polydispersity to be 1.17 ± 0.33 [17].

Fluorescent dyes could be easily introduced on the dendrimer during the synthesis (Scheme 10.1B), and these modifications can be carried out at different steps of the preparation of the mannodendrimers. Julolidine, a useful dye for *in vitro* studies, was introduced directly on the phosphorus backbone of the dendrimer; 5–10% of the tyramines were replaced by julolidine-substituted phenol (**12**) during the last step of the dendrimeric core synthesis (Scheme 10.1B) [43]. Deprotection of the amine groups and mannosylation of the dendrimer as usual proceeded smoothly and gave fluorescent mannosylated dendrimers. Another general way to tag the dendrimers is to bind the fluorophore to the amine groups at the surface of the dendrimer. To illustrate this, VivoTag® 680 XL Fluorochrome (PerkinElmer), a near-infrared fluorescent probe, which is suitable for *in vivo* observations in small animals, was introduced on amine groups at the surface of the dendrimer before mannosylation. Trouble-free mannosylation of the surface was then carried out and gave another kind of fluorescent mannodendrimer.

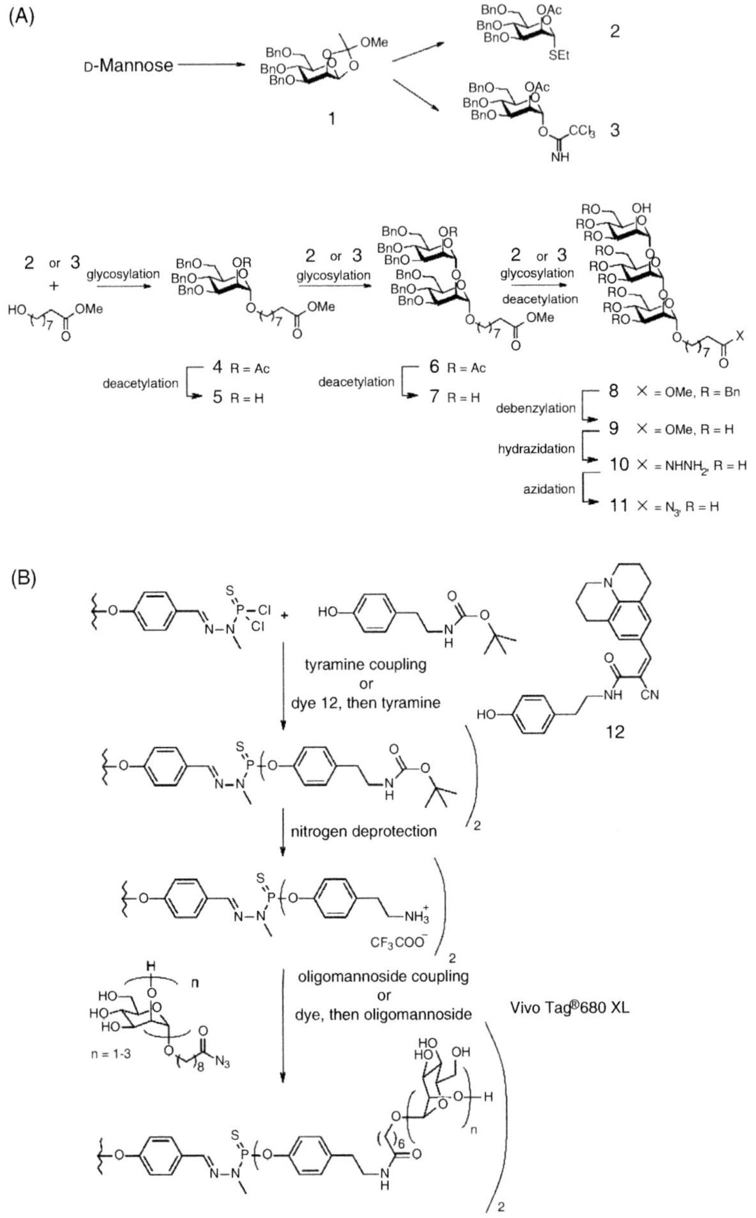

Scheme 10.1 (A) Synthesis of mono-, di-, and tri-mannosides. (B) Elaboration of mannodendrimers and fluorescent mannodendrimers.

10.3 Mannodendrimer Binding to DC-SIGN and Human DCs

The synthesis of mannodendrimers was oriented toward the most active molecules as identified by a series of bio-assays with increasing stringency [17]: ability to (i) bind a recombinant soluble tetrameric form of DC-SIGN (sDC-SIGN), (ii) bind the full-length membrane-expressed DC-SIGN receptor (mDC-SIGN) using stably transfected HEK cells, (iii) bind DC-SIGN on the surface of human monocyte-derived DCs, and finally (iv) inhibit pro-inflammatory cytokine production by LPS-stimulated DCs.

10.3.1 Mannodendrimer Binding to a Soluble Form of DC-SIGN

The ability of the synthesized mannodendrimers (Fig. 10.1) to bind DC-SIGN was first evaluated from the IC_{50} values determined using an inhibition binding assay with a recombinant soluble tetrameric form of the human DC-SIGN protein (sDC-SIGN) and ManLAM-coated microplates (Fig. 10.2A). All the mannodendrimers synthesized were able to bind sDC-SIGN, but as expected, binding efficiency was strongly dependent on the dendrimer generation that determines both the size of the molecule and the number of mannose caps at the surface. Indeed, IC_{50} values slightly decreased from 2.0 ± 0.3 μM for 1M to 1.4 ± 0.3 μM for 2M, but more drastically to 105 ± 14 nM for the 3M mannodendrimer. Mannodendrimer avidity thus increased from the first-generation 1M characterized by a scaffold size of ~2 nm [44] and 12 mannose caps to the third-generation 3M with a scaffold size of ~6 nm [44] capped of 48 mono-mannoside units. A similar effect was also observed for di-mannosylated dendrimers. Indeed, 1D and 2D mannodendrimers showed a similar IC_{50} value of 220 ± 35 nM and 260 ± 40 nM, respectively, but this value decreased to 53 ± 8 nM for 3D. In addition to the scaffold size, mannodendrimer binding efficiency was also affected, although to a much lesser extent, by the length of the mannose caps. An increase in the avidity was particularly observed between the dendrimers capped with single mannosides (1M, 2M, and 3M) and the dendrimers capped by di-mannosides (1D, 2D, and 3D), as illustrated by the IC_{50} values of 105 ± 14 nM for 3M compared to 53 ± 8 nM for the 3D.

Altogether these data revealed that efficient mannodendrimer binding to sDC-SIGN requires at least a third-generation mannodendrimer, regardless of the cap length. Interestingly, among the mannodendrimers synthesized, 3M, 3D, 3T, and 4D showed a binding efficiency to sDC-SIGN similar to that of ManLAM (Fig. 10.2A).

10.3.2 Mannodendrimer Binding to Membrane-Expressed DC-SIGN

The binding of mannodendrimers to DC-SIGN was further evaluated using a more relevant form of the receptor, *i.e.*, a full-length receptor in a cell membrane context (mDC-SIGN), using HEK293 transfected cells expressing the wild-type DC-SIGN protein fused at its *N*-terminal end with the green fluorescent protein GFP (HEK::DC-SIGN cells). The bioassay consisted in evaluating the capacity of the mannodendrimers to inhibit the mDC-SIGN-dependent binding of HEK::DC-SIGN cells to mannan-coated microplates (Fig. 10.2B). IC_{50} values were determined for all the mannodendrimers (Fig. 10.2B), except 1M that was poorly inhibitory with an IC_{50} value estimated over 1mM. Again, the dendrimer generation was critical, with IC_{50} values decreasing from 5 ± 2 μM for 2M to 1.1 ± 0.3 μM for 3M; and from 490 ± 170 nM for 1D to 166 ± 88 nM for 2D and to 3.0 ± 0.5 nM for 3D. However, the cap length was also a determinant parameter for binding to this more relevant form of the receptor. The IC_{50} value decreased from 5 ± 2 μM for 2M to 166 ± 88 nM for 2D; and from 1.1 ± 0.3 μM for 3M to 3 ± 0.5 and 5 ± 2 nM for 3D and 3T, respectively. These data are in agreement with the crystal structure of the DC-SIGN CRD in complex with an oligomannoside showing that this domain preferentially binds an internal rather than a terminal mannosyl residue, via coordination linkages between the calcium cation and the equatorial hydroxyls 3 and 4 [27, 45], thus supporting a higher affinity for di- *versus* mono-mannosides, but a similar affinity between tri- and di-mannosides. In addition, DC-SIGN is a transmembrane protein that is organized as tetramers [27] and distributed as clustered patches at the cell surface [46]. Therefore, the high functionalization of third-generation dendrimers with 48 mannosylated caps leads to efficient multipoint attachment to the receptor; this degree of attachment seems optimum since avidity was not improved by a fourth-generation scaffold (96 mannosylated caps).

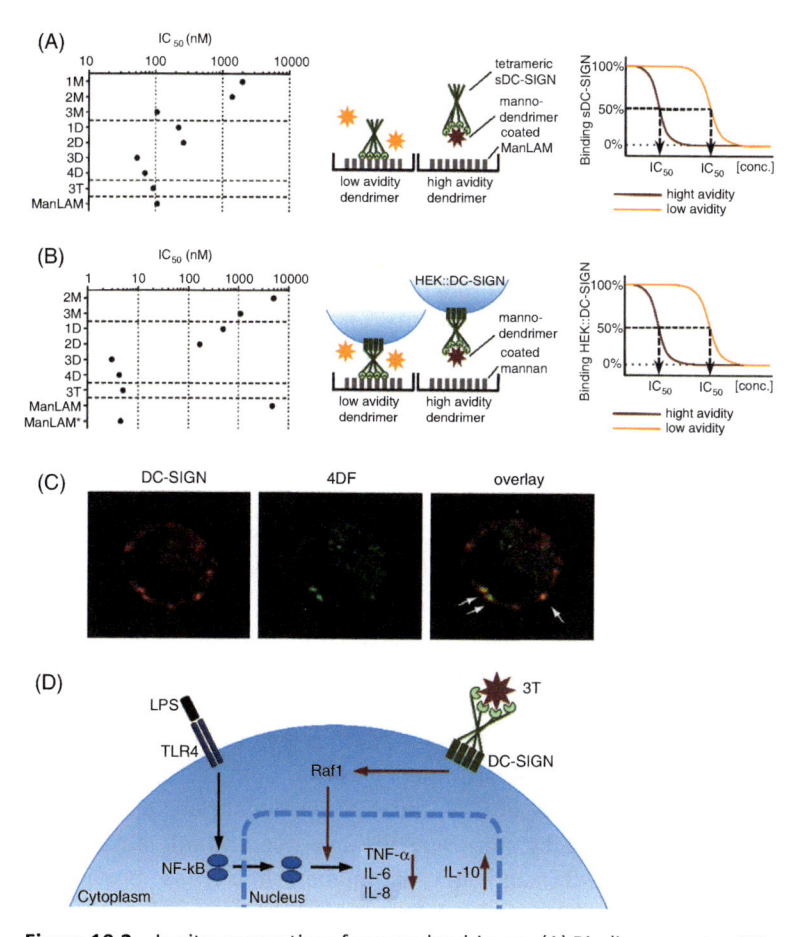

Figure 10.2   In vitro properties of mannodendrimers. (A) Binding assay to sDC-SIGN. (B) Binding assay to mDC-SIGN. (C) Confocal microscopy analysis showing the colocalization of fluorescent mannodendrimers (4DF, in green) with DC-SIGN (in red) at the surface of human DCs. (D) 3T reduces the production of the pro-inflammatory cytokines TNF-α, IL-6, and IL-8 and increases the production of the anti-inflammatory cytokine IL-10 by LPS-stimulated DCs, in a DC-SIGN- and Raf-1-dependent manner.

Interestingly, 3D, 3T, and 4D, with IC_{50} values of ~5 nM, bound mDC-SIGN as efficiently as the ManLAM bioactive particle (ManLAM*) (Fig. 10.2B). However, ManLAM molecule statically bears ~8 mannose caps, mainly di-mannosides (~6) [21, 47]. So ManLAM particles, which are composed of ~450 ManLAM monomers and exhibit a size of 30 nm [23], are capped by ~2700 di-mannoside units. A mannodendrimer with a scaffold of ~6 nm capped with 48 di-mannosides (3D) was thus sufficient to obtain a molecule with the same avidity for DC-SIGN than the ManLAM particle.

10.3.3 Mannodendrimers Selectively Bind DC-SIGN on Human DCs

Human DCs play a pivotal role in the initiation of the inflammatory response following infection [48], via the recognition of PAMPs (pathogen-associated molecular patterns) by PRRs [49], including TLRs and CLRs. Among the CLRs recognizing ManLAM, human monocyte-derived DCs express DC-SIGN and MR, but not Dectin-2. To investigate the direct binding of mannodendrimers to the surface of human DCs by flow cytometry, we prepared fluorescent derivatives of 3T and 4D (3TF and 4DF, respectively) by statistical labeling with the julolidine dye (Section 10.2.3). We first established that the grafting of the fluorescent dye did not affect the binding of the mannodendrimers, as demonstrated by unchanged IC_{50} values toward sDC-SIGN. In addition, we found that 3TF and 4DF bound, as efficiently as fluorescently labeled ManLAM [11, 14, 15], DC-SIGN or MR expressed by artificial cell lines, as well as human DCs [17]. 3T and 4D, as ManLAM, are thus ligands of both DC-SIGN and MR. However, the binding of 3TF and 4DF on the surface of DCs was partially inhibited by anti-DC-SIGN but not anti-MR antibodies, indicating that 3T and 4D mannodendrimers, as previously reported for ManLAM [10], selectively bind DC-SIGN on human DCs. Accordingly, confocal microscopy analysis indicated that fluorescent mannodendrimers co-localized with DC-SIGN at the surface of human DCs (Fig. 10.2C). The selectivity of mannodendrimers for DC-SIGN on DCs is not clearly understood but might be explained by different reasons: (i) a higher avidity for DC-SIGN *versus* MR, as a result of binding mechanisms involving, on the one hand, recognition by the CRD of two *versus* one mannosyl residues [45], and on the other hand, clusters of DC-SIGN tetramers [27, 46] *versus* randomly distributed MR; and (ii) DC-SIGN CRDs spike up from the cell surface [50] and might thus be encountered by the ligands before the MR.

10.4 *In Vitro* and *In Vivo* Anti-inflammatory Activities of Mannodendrimers

The most active mannodendrimers identified on the basis of their ability to bind DC-SIGN (Section 10.3) were tested for their capacity to modulate cytokine production by LPS-stimulated human DCs *in vitro*. Then, the most potent one, 3T, was evaluated for its potency *in vivo*, using a mouse model of lung acute inflammation.

10.4.1 Modulation of Cytokine Production by Human DCs

3D, 4D, and 3T mannodendrimers, which exhibited the lowest IC_{50} values, were tested for the ability to modulate cytokine production *in vitro*. 3T and 4D, at sub-micromolar concentrations, reduced TNF-α production by LPS-stimulated human DCs in a dose-dependent manner. Surprisingly, 3D mannodendrimer failed to inhibit cytokine production, although it exhibited a similar IC_{50} value in the mDC-SIGN binding assay (Fig. 10.2B). As expected, 2D mannodendrimer, exhibiting a ~50-fold higher IC_{50} value (Fig. 10.2B), showed no inhibitory activity. Although the inhibitory activity of mannodendrimers was mediated by DC-SIGN, as determined by the use of an anti-DC-SIGN antibody, the avidity of mannodendrimers for DC-SIGN was not sufficient to predict their capacity to inhibit pro-inflammatory cytokine production. It seems that a scaffold size of third- or fourth-generation substituted by tri- and di-mannosides, respectively, was required for signaling via DC-SIGN [17].

3T mannodendrimer was selected to further study its anti-inflammatory properties. Interestingly, it reduced the production of the pro-inflammatory cytokines IL-6 and IL-8 and increased the production of the anti-inflammatory cytokine IL-10 by LPS-stimulated DCs (Fig. 10.2D). The signaling pathway involved was next investigated. DC-SIGN triggering on human DCs was previously found to activate the phosphorylation of the serine and threonine kinase Raf-1, which, upon activation of TLR4 signaling, subsequently leads to acetylation of the NF-κB subunit p65 [51]. As expected, 3T induced Raf-1 phosphorylation after LPS stimulation [17]. Altogether the data indicated that 3T mannodendrimer modulates LPS-induced TLR4 signaling in a DC-SIGN and Raf-1-dependent manner.

10.4.2 Mannodendrimers Prevent Acute Lung Inflammation in Mice

To test the anti-inflammatory activity of mannodendrimers *in vivo*, we used a model of acute lung inflammation, which involved exposure of mice to aerosolized LPS [17]. It is characterized by an influx of neutrophils and the production of chemokines and cytokines, including TNF-α, into the lung alveoli. Neutrophil sequestration into the lungs and associated inflammatory damage are believed to contribute to the pathogenesis of diverse lung diseases, including acute lung injury, the acute respiratory distress syndrome, chronic obstructive lung disease, and cystic fibrosis [52]. Our most potent mannodendrimer, 3T, was thus tested for its ability to reduce the inflammation using two readouts: the number of neutrophils and the cytokines concentration in the bronchoalveolar lavage (BAL). Mice were dosed orally by gavage with 3T once daily for 15 days at 1 mg/kg/day, then exposed to aerosolized LPS. The path of 3T through the animal stomach and gut (Fig. 10.3A) could be followed by using a mannodendrimer tagged with the near-infrared fluorescent probe VivoTag® 680 XL (Section 10.2.3). BALs were collected 3 h or 18 h after LPS exposure for cytokine dosage or neutrophils count, respectively. Treatment with 3T was found to significantly reduce neutrophil recruitment and TNF-α production in mice exposed to aerosolized LPS. This anti-inflammatory activity of 3T mannodendrimer was dependent on the murine DC-SIGN homolog SIGNR1 [53, 54], as demonstrated by the use of *Signr1*-deficient mice [17], and was supported by lung histopathology analysis showing reduction of alveolar wall thickening and inflammatory cell infiltration (Fig. 10.3B).

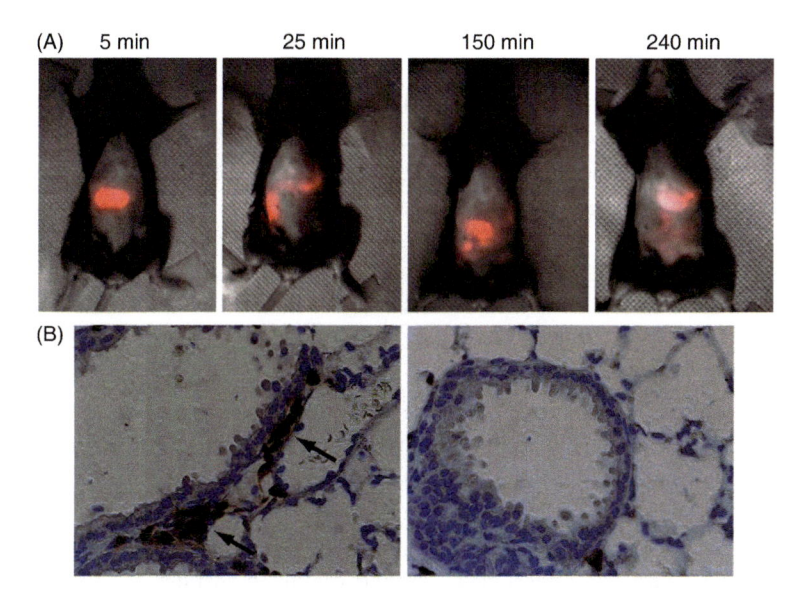

Figure 10.3 In vivo anti-inflammatory activity of the 3T mannodendrimer. (A) In vivo imaging of 3T labeled with the near-infrared fluorescent probe VivoTag 680 XL (PerkinElmer). Mice received by gavage 300 µg of the fluorescent mannodendrimer and were observed at the indicated time points using a Fluobeam® system (Fluoptics). (B) 3T inhibits lung neutrophil recruitment. Lung sections of mice submitted to an LPS challenge and treated (right) or not (left; neutrophils stained in black are indicated by an arrow) with 3T.

10.5 Conclusion and Perspectives

By mimicking the strategy used by Mtb to down-regulate the host inflammatory response, we have been able to rationally design mannodendrimer 3T, which is a novel type of fully synthetic powerful anti-inflammatory molecule. Its mode of action is original and different from that of corticosteroids, which are classically used to fight inflammation, but are non-specific, immunosuppressive, and can be deleterious during prolonged or high-dose therapy [24]. Mannodendrimer 3T should now be tested in different pathological models to determine the broader applicability of its therapeutic use.

Acknowledgments

This work was supported by CNRS, Université de Toulouse, and the Fondation pour la Recherche Médicale (FRM). We gratefully acknowledge Dr Muriel Golzio (IPBS, Toulouse) for her help with the experiment using the Fluobeam system.

References

1. Russell, D. G. (2007). Who puts the tubercle in tuberculosis? *Nat. Rev. Microbiol.*, **5**, pp. 39–47.

2. Nau, G. J., Richmond, J. F., Schlesinger, A., Jennings, E. G., Lander, E. S., and Young, R. A. (2002). Human macrophage activation programs induced by bacterial pathogens, *Proc. Natl. Acad. Sci. U.S.A.*, **99**, pp. 1503–1508.

3. Jouanguy, E., Doffinger, R., Dupuis, S., Pallier, A., Altare, F., and Casanova, J. L. (1999). IL-12 and IFN-gamma in host defense against mycobacteria and salmonella in mice and men, *Curr. Opin. Immunol.*, **11**, pp. 346–351.

4. Casanova, J. L. and Abel, L. (2002). Genetic dissection of immunity to mycobacteria: The human model, *Annu. Rev. Immunol.*, **20**, pp. 581–620.

5. Keane, J., Gershon, S., Wise, R. P., Mirabile-Levens, E., Kasznica, J., Schwieterman, W. D., Siegel, J. N., and Braun, M. M. (2001). Tuberculosis associated with infliximab, a tumor necrosis factor alpha-neutralizing agent, *N. Engl. J. Med.*, **345**, pp. 1098–1104.

6. Ray, A., Cot, M., Puzo, G., Gilleron, M., and Nigou, J. (2013). Bacterial cell wall macroamphiphiles: Pathogen-/microbe-associated molecular patterns detected by mammalian innate immune system, *Biochimie*, **95**, pp. 33–42.

7. Vergne, I., Gilleron, M., and Nigou, J. (2015). Manipulation of the endocytic pathway and phagocyte functions by *Mycobacterium tuberculosis* lipoarabinomannan, *Front. Cell. Infect. Microbiol.*, **4**, pp. 187.

8. Ishikawa, E., Ishikawa, T., Morita, Y. S., Toyonaga, K., Yamada, H., Takeuchi, O., Kinoshita, T., Akira, S., Yoshikai, Y., and Yamasaki, S. (2009). Direct recognition of the mycobacterial glycolipid, trehalose dimycolate, by C-type lectin Mincle, *J. Exp. Med.*, **206**, pp. 2879–2888.

9. Yonekawa, A., Saijo, S., Hoshino, Y., Miyake, Y., Ishikawa, E., Suzukawa, M., Inoue, H., Tanaka, M., Yoneyama, M., Oh-Hora, M., Akashi, K., and

Yamasaki, S. (2014). Dectin-2 is a direct receptor for mannose-capped lipoarabinomannan of mycobacteria, *Immunity*, **41**, pp. 402–413.

10. Geijtenbeek, T. B., Van Vliet, S. J., Koppel, E. A., Sanchez-Hernandez, M., Vandenbroucke-Grauls, C. M., Appelmelk, B., and Van Kooyk, Y. (2003). Mycobacteria target DC-SIGN to suppress dendritic cell function, *J. Exp. Med.*, **197**, pp. 7–17.

11. Pitarque, S., Herrmann, J. L., Duteyrat, J. L., Jackson, M., Stewart, G. R., Lecointe, F., Payre, B., Schwartz, O., Young, D. B., Marchal, G., Lagrange, P. H., Puzo, G., Gicquel, B., Nigou, J., and Neyrolles, O. (2005). Deciphering the molecular bases of *Mycobacterium tuberculosis* binding to the lectin DC-SIGN reveals an underestimated complexity, *Biochem. J.*, **392**, pp. 615–624.

12. Maeda, N., Nigou, J., Herrmann, J. L., Jackson, M., Amara, A., Lagrange, P. H., Puzo, G., Gicquel, B., and Neyrolles, O. (2003). The cell surface receptor DC-SIGN discriminates between Mycobacterium species through selective recognition of the mannose caps on lipoarabinomannan, *J. Biol. Chem.*, **278**, pp. 5513–5516.

13. Tailleux, L., Schwartz, O., Herrmann, J. L., Pivert, E., Jackson, M., Amara, A., Legres, L., Dreher, D., Nicod, L. P., Gluckman, J. C., Lagrange, P. H., Gicquel, B., and Neyrolles, O. (2003). DC-SIGN is the major *Mycobacterium tuberculosis* receptor on human dendritic cells, *J. Exp. Med.*, **197**, pp. 121–127.

14. Venisse, A., Fournie, J. J., and Puzo, G. (1995). Mannosylated lipoarabinomannan interacts with phagocytes, *Eur. J. Biochem.*, **231**, pp. 440–447.

15. Schlesinger, L. S., Hull, S. R., and Kaufman, T. M. (1994). Binding of the terminal mannosyl units of lipoarabinomannan from a virulent strain of Mycobacterium tuberculosis to human macrophages, *J. Immunol.*, **152**, pp. 4070–4079.

16. Nigou, J., Zelle-Rieser, C., Gilleron, M., Thurnher, M., and Puzo, G. (2001). Mannosylated lipoarabinomannans inhibit IL-12 production by human dendritic cells: Evidence for a negative signal delivered through the mannose receptor, *J. Immunol.*, **166**, pp. 7477–7485.

17. Blattes, E., Vercellone, A., Eutamene, H., Turrin, C. O., Theodorou, V., Majoral, J. P., Caminade, A. M., Prandi, J., Nigou, J., and Puzo, G. (2013). Mannodendrimers prevent acute lung inflammation by inhibiting neutrophil recruitment, *Proc. Natl. Acad. Sci. U.S.A.*, **110**, pp. 8795–8800.

18. Nigou, J., Gilleron, M., Rojas, M., Garcia, L. F., Thurnher, M., and Puzo, G. (2002). Mycobacterial lipoarabinomannans: Modulators of dendritic

cell function and the apoptotic response, *Microbes Infect.*, **4**, pp. 945–953.

19. Chieppa, M., Bianchi, G., Doni, A., Del Prete, A., Sironi, M., Laskarin, G., Monti, P., Piemonti, L., Biondi, A., Mantovani, A., Introna, M., and Allavena, P. (2003). Cross-linking of the mannose receptor on monocyte-derived dendritic cells activates an anti-inflammatory immunosuppressive program, *J. Immunol.*, **171**, pp. 4552–4560.

20. Zhang, J., Tachado, S. D., Patel, N., Zhu, J., Imrich, A., Manfruelli, P., Cushion, M., Kinane, T. B., and Koziel, H. (2005). Negative regulatory role of mannose receptors on human alveolar macrophage proinflammatory cytokine release *in vitro*, *J. Leukoc. Biol.*, **78**, pp. 665–674.

21. Nigou, J., Gilleron, M., and Puzo, G. (2003). Lipoarabinomannans: From structure to biosynthesis, *Biochimie*, **85**, pp. 153–166.

22. Gilleron, M., Jackson, M., Nigou, J., and Puzo, G. (2008). Structure, biosynthesis, and activities of the phosphatidyl-myo-inositol-based lipoglycans, in: *The Mycobacterial Cell Envelope*, Daffe, M. and Reyrat, J. (eds.), ASM Press, Washington DC, pp. 75–105.

23. Riviere, M., Moisand, A., Lopez, A., and Puzo, G. (2004). Highly ordered supra-molecular organization of the mycobacterial lipoarabinomannans in solution. Evidence of a relationship between supra-molecular organization and biological activity, *J. Mol. Biol.*, **344**, pp. 907–918.

24. Barnes, P. J. (2011). Glucocorticosteroids: Current and future directions, *Br. J. Pharmacol.*, **163**, pp. 29–43.

25. Rhen, T. and Cidlowski, J. A. (2005). Antiinflammatory action of glucocorticoids: New mechanisms for old drugs, *N. Engl. J. Med.*, **353**, pp. 1711–1723.

26. Caminade, A. M., Turrin, C. O., Laurent, R., Ouali, A., and Delavaut-Nicot, B. (2011) *Dendrimers: Towards Catalytic, Material and Biomedical uses*, John Wiley & Sons, Chichester.

27. Mitchell, D. A., Fadden, A. J., and Drickamer, K. (2001). A novel mechanism of carbohydrate recognition by the C-type lectins DC-SIGN and DC-SIGNR. Subunit organization and binding to multivalent ligands, *J. Biol. Chem.*, **276**, pp. 28939–28945.

28. Taylor, M. E. and Drickamer, K. (1993). Structural requirements for high affinity binding of complex ligands by the macrophage mannose receptor, *J. Biol. Chem.*, **268**, pp. 399–404.

29. Grandjean, C., Rommens, C., Gras-Masse, H., and Melnyk, O. (2000). One-pot synthesis of antigen-bearing, lysine-based cluster mannosides

using two orthogonal chemoselective ligation reactions, *Angew. Chem. Int. Ed. Engl.*, **39**, pp. 1068–1072.

30. Page, D. and Roy, R. (1997). Synthesis and biological properties of mannosylated starburst poly(amidoamine) dendrimers, *Bioconjug. Chem.*, **8**, pp. 714–723.

31. Elsner, K., Boysen, M. M., and Lindhorst, T. K. (2007). Synthesis of new polyether glycodendrons as oligosaccharide mimetics, *Carbohydr. Res.*, **342**, pp. 1715–1725.

32. Euzen, R. and Reymond, J. L. (2011). Synthesis of glycopeptide dendrimers, dimerization and affinity for Concanavalin A, *Bioorg. Med. Chem.*, **19**, pp. 2879–2887.

33. Caminade, A.-M., Laurent, R., Zablocka, M., and Majoral, J.-P. (2012). Organophosphorus chemistry for the synthesis of dendrimers, *Molecules*, **17**, pp. 13605–13621.

34. Hayder, M., Poupot, M., Baron, M., Nigon, D., Turrin, C. O., Caminade, A. M., Majoral, J. P., Eisenberg, R. A., Fournie, J. J., Cantagrel, A., Poupot, R., and Davignon, J. L. (2011). A phosphorus-based dendrimer targets inflammation and osteoclastogenesis in experimental arthritis, *Sci. Transl. Med.*, **3**, pp. 81ra35.

35. Hayder, M., Varilh, M., Turrin, C. O., Saoudi, A., Caminade, A. M., Poupot, R., and Liblau, R. S. (2015). Phosphorus-based dendrimer ABP treats neuroinflammation by promoting IL-10-producing CD4(+) T cells, *Biomacromolecules*, **16**, pp. 3425–3433.

36. Griffe, L., Poupot, M., Marchand, P., Maraval, A., Turrin, C. O., Rolland, O., Metivier, P., Bacquet, G., Fournie, J. J., Caminade, A. M., Poupot, R., and Majoral, J. P. (2007). Multiplication of human natural killer cells by nanosized phosphonate-capped dendrimers, *Angew. Chem. Int. Ed. Engl.*, **46**, pp. 2523–2526.

37. Blanzat, M., Turrin, C. O., Aubertin, A. M., Couturier-Vidal, C., Caminade, A. M., Majoral, J. P., Rico-Lattes, I., and Lattes, A. (2005). Dendritic catanionic assemblies: In vitro anti-HIV activity of phosphorus-containing dendrimers bearing galbeta1cer analogues, *Chembiochem*, **6**, pp. 2207–2213.

38. Launay, N., Caminade, A. M., and Majoral, J. P. (1997). Synthesis of bowl-shaped dendrimers from generation 1 to generation 8, *J. Organomet. Chem.*, **529**, pp. 51–58.

39. Peters, T. (1991). Synthesis and conformational analysis of methyl 2-O-(α-D-mannopyranosyl)-α-D-mannopyranoside, *Liebigs Ann. Chem.*, **1991**, pp. 135–141.

40. Franks, N. E. and Montgomery, R. (1968). Stereoselective ring-opening of β-D-mannopyranose 1,2-(alkyl orthoacetates), *Carbohydr. Res.*, **6**, pp. 286–298.

41. Inman, J. K., Merchant, B., Claflin, L., and Tacey, S. E. (1973). Coupling of large haptens to proteins and cell surfaces: Preparation of stable, optimally sensitized erythrocytes for hapten-specific, hemolytic plaque assays, *Immunochemistry*, **10**, pp. 165–174.

42. Lemieux, R. U., Bundle, D. R., and Baker, D. A. (1975). The properties of a "synthetic" antigen related to the human blood-group Lewis a, *J. Am. Chem. Soc.*, **97**, pp. 4076–4083.

43. Rolland, O., Griffe, L., Poupot, M., Maraval, A., Ouali, A., Coppel, Y., Fournie, J. J., Bacquet, G., Turrin, C. O., Caminade, A. M., Majoral, J. P., and Poupot, R. (2008). Tailored control and optimisation of the number of phosphonic acid termini on phosphorus-containing dendrimers for the ex-vivo activation of human monocytes, *Chem. Eur. J.*, **14**, pp. 4836–4850.

44. Leclaire, J., Coppel, Y., Caminade, A. M., and Majoral, J. P. (2004). Nanometric sponges made of water-soluble hydrophobic dendrimers, *J. Am. Chem. Soc.*, **126**, pp. 2304–2305.

45. Feinberg, H., Mitchell, D. A., Drickamer, K., and Weis, W. I. (2001). Structural basis for selective recognition of oligosaccharides by DC-SIGN and DC-SIGNR, *Science*, **294**, pp. 2163–2166.

46. Cambi, A., de Lange, F., van Maarseveen, N. M., Nijhuis, M., Joosten, B., van Dijk, E. M., de Bakker, B. I., Fransen, J. A., Bovee-Geurts, P. H., van Leeuwen, F. N., Van Hulst, N. F., and Figdor, C. G. (2004). Microdomains of the C-type lectin DC-SIGN are portals for virus entry into dendritic cells, *J. Cell. Biol.*, **164**, pp. 145–155.

47. Nigou, J., Vercellone, A., and Puzo, G. (2000). New structural insights into the molecular deciphering of mycobacterial lipoglycan binding to C-type lectins: Lipoarabinomannan glycoform characterization and quantification by capillary electrophoresis at the subnanomole level, *J. Mol. Biol.*, **299**, pp. 1353–1362.

48. Banchereau, J. and Steinman, R. M. (1998). Dendritic cells and the control of immunity, *Nature*, **392**, pp. 245–252.

49. Takeuchi, O. and Akira, S. (2010). Pattern recognition receptors and inflammation, *Cell*, **140**, pp. 805–820.

50. Tabarani, G., Thepaut, M., Stroebel, D., Ebel, C., Vives, C., Vachette, P., Durand, D., and Fieschi, F. (2009). DC-SIGN neck domain is a pH-sensor controlling oligomerization: SAXS and hydrodynamic studies of extracellular domain, *J. Biol. Chem.*, **284**, pp. 21229–21240.

51. Gringhuis, S. I., den Dunnen, J., Litjens, M., van Het Hof, B., van Kooyk, Y., and Geijtenbeek, T. B. (2007). C-type lectin DC-SIGN modulates Toll-like receptor signaling via Raf-1 kinase-dependent acetylation of transcription factor NF-κB, *Immunity*, **26**, pp. 605–616.

52. Zemans, R. L., Colgan, S. P., and Downey, G. P. (2009). Transepithelial migration of neutrophils: Mechanisms and implications for acute lung injury, *Am. J. Respir. Cell. Mol. Biol.*, **40**, pp. 519–535.

53. Powlesland, A. S., Ward, E. M., Sadhu, S. K., Guo, Y., Taylor, M. E., and Drickamer, K. (2006). Widely divergent biochemical properties of the complete set of mouse DC-SIGN-related proteins, *J. Biol. Chem.*, **281**, pp. 20440–20449.

54. Tanne, A., Ma, B., Boudou, F., Tailleux, L., Botella, H., Badell, E., Levillain, F., Taylor, M. E., Drickamer, K., Nigou, J., Dobos, K. M., Puzo, G., Vestweber, D., Wild, M. K., Marcinko, M., Sobieszczuk, P., Stewart, L., Lebus, D., Gicquel, B., and Neyrolles, O. (2009). A murine DC-SIGN homologue contributes to early host defense against *Mycobacterium tuberculosis*, *J. Exp. Med.*, **206**, pp. 2205–2220.

Chapter 11

Phosphorus-Containing Dendrimers Against Diseases of the Central Nervous System

Anne-Marie Caminade, Cédric-Olivier Turrin, and Jean-Pierre Majoral
Laboratoire de Chimie de Coordination, CNRS, 205 Route de Narbonne, BP 44099, 31077 Toulouse Cedex 4, France
anne-marie.caminade@lcc-toulouse.fr

11.1 Introduction

The central nervous system (CNS) is constituted of the brain and the spinal cord. Diseases of the CNS comprise many neurological disorders, practically all of them being presently incurable, and their causes are generally poorly understood. Some of these diseases concern both parts of the CNS, such as multiple sclerosis (MS). MS is a demyelinating disease in which the damage to the insulating cover of nerve cells in the brain and the spinal cord disrupts their ability to communicate. MS is the most common autoimmune disorder affecting the CNS [1], with about 2.3 million people affected globally [2]. Neurodegenerative diseases concern the progressive loss of structure and function of neurons in the brain, inducing death of neurons. They are major causes of impaired quality of life, morbidity, and mortality. Many neurodegenerative diseases are associated with the aggregation of misfolded proteins. In particular, Alzheimer's disease is characterized by the accumulation in the brain of the misfolded β-amyloid and hyperphosphorylated tau proteins in senile plaques [3]. It is the cause of 60% to 70% of dementia. In 2015, about 48 million people worldwide were suffering from Alzheimer's disease [4]. Parkinson's disease is the second most common neurodegenerative disorder, after Alzheimer's disease, with about 5.9 million people affected [2]. It is characterized by the abnormal accumulation of the α-synuclein protein bound to ubiquitin to form insoluble fibrils [5]. Transmissible spongiform encephalopathies affect the brain and the nervous system. The infectious agent is the misfolded, insoluble, prion protein, called the scrapie form (PrP^{Sc}) [6]. The most known prion diseases are the Creutzfeldt–Jakob disease, and its new variant (nvCJD), a human disorder caused by the bovine spongiform encephalopathy.

All these diseases of the CNS have no cure to date. They are characterized by progressive and severe decline of the activities of daily living, with psychological and physical consequences. These consequences at the "macro" level are due to events that occur at the molecular level, in particular the transformation of proteins to a misfolded form and/or their aggregation, leading to brain cells dysfunction, then death. Thus, it is necessary to find potential drugs that could fight at the molecular and macromolecular levels against these diseases. Several types of dendrimers have been already tested with this aim [7]. In this chapter, we will present the potential role of several types of phosphorus-containing dendrimers to fight against diverse diseases of the CNS, including prion, Alzheimer's, Parkinson's, and MS diseases.

11.2 Properties of Poly(phosphorhydrazone) Dendrimers bearing Ammonium End Groups

The most important poly(phosphorhydrazone) (PPH) dendrimer used up to now against diverse neurodegenerative diseases is the generation 4, built from a cyclotriphosphazene core, and covered by ammonium terminal functions, shown in Fig. 11.1 [8]. This dendrimer will be used in all paragraphs under this heading, as well as generations 2, 3, and 5 of the same series in some cases.

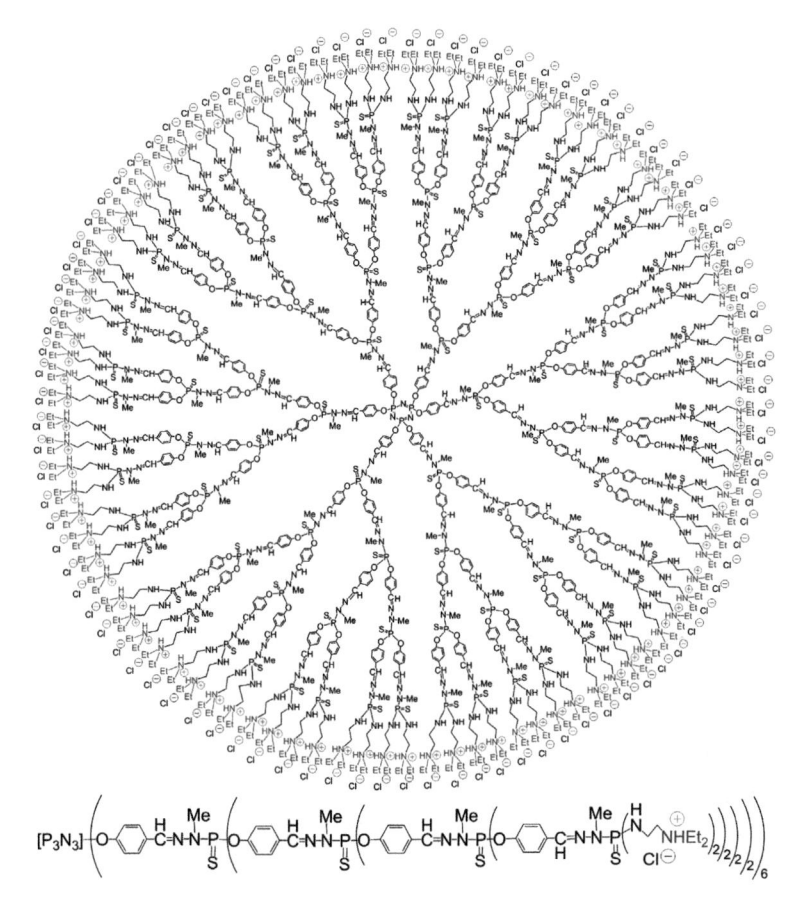

Figure 11.1 Generation 4 (G4) of poly(phosphorhydrazone) dendrimer ended by ammonium groups (full structure and linear structure with parentheses).

11.2.1 Preliminary Experiments

The compound shown in Fig. 11.1 was obtained straightforward by reaction of *N,N*-diethylethylenediamine with the $P(S)Cl_2$ terminal functions of PPH dendrimers. This reaction generates HCl, which is directly trapped by the tertiary amine terminal groups to generate the tertiary ammonium groups. Generation 4 is the most widely used, but all generations from 1 to 5 (G1 to G5) were also synthesized. The corresponding methylated dendrimers (Me instead of H on the NEt_2 terminal functions) were also synthesized. All these dendrimers were used first as carriers of the plasmid luciferase, for *in vitro* transfection experiments. Transfection concerns the deliberate introduction of genetic materials (nucleic acids, plasmid DNA, siRNA, etc.) inside cells. As genetic materials are generally negatively charged, the carrier is generally positively charged, and this association is able to cross the cell membrane. The use of dendrimers for such purpose has been recognized very early [9]. In the case of PPH dendrimers, the transfected cells were 3T3 (mammalian) cells. The methylated (quaternary ammoniums) series was found very toxic and had poor transfection efficiency, which decreased when the generation of the dendrimer increased. On the contrary, the protonated series (tertiary ammoniums) was found by far less toxic toward 3T3 cells and displayed good transfection efficiencies, increasing as the generation increased, up to G4, and a plateau was reached for G5 [8].

It was deduced from this seminal work that the generation 4 with tertiary ammonium group was the most interesting compound of the series. Other types of terminal functions were also used as terminal functions of PPH dendrimers but were found generally less efficient [10]. Other examples of use of these dendrimers as carriers of diverse biological entities (DNA, siRNa, etc.), for gene therapy in cancer and for immunotherapies against HIV-1 infection, can be seen in Chapters 8 and 7, respectively.

11.2.2 Assays against Prion, Alzheimer's, and Parkinson's Diseases

Prions are proteins constituted of 209 amino acids in humans. The infectious isoform of prions, the scrapie form (PrP^{Sc}), is rich in β-structure, because the unordered and helical regions in the non-pathologic form of the prion protein are modified. In a seminal work, Prusiner *et al.* reported that branched polyamines, in particular poly(ethyleneimine) (PEI), and dendrimers of type poly(amidoamine) (PAMAM) and poly(propylenimine) (PPI), were able to eliminate the scrapie (abnormal) form of the prion protein (PrP^{Sc}) from scrapie-infected neuroblastoma (ScN2a) cells in culture. PrP^{Sc} was undetectable after 1 week of exposure to dendrimers, and this condition persisted for 3 weeks. For both families of dendrimers, the best results (IC_{50} at 80 ng/mL) were obtained with the generation 4 of PAMAM and PPI dendrimers, having 64 and 32 primary amine terminal functions, respectively. The structure of both dendrimers is shown in Fig. 11.2. However, this experiment could not be generalized to several strains of prions, as the G4 PPI dendrimer has no clear activity against PrP^{Sc} from Sc237-infected Syrian hamster brain homogenates [11].

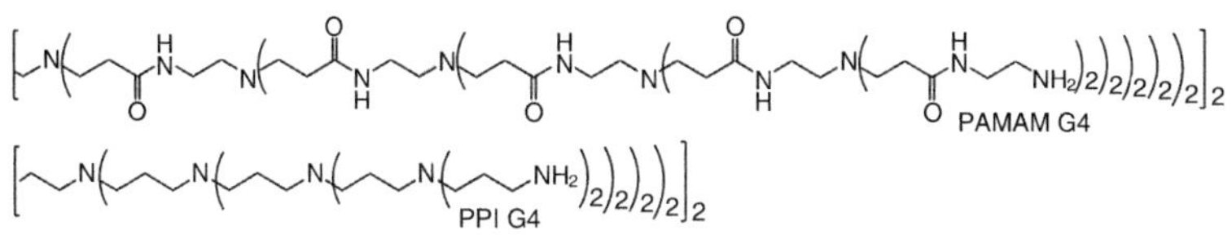

Figure 11.2 Linear representation of generation 4 of PAMAM and PPI dendrimers. At physiological pH, most amine functions are protonated.

Generations 3 to 5 of PPH dendrimers ended by tertiary ammonium groups (Fig. 11.1) were also tested against prion diseases, using ScN2a-infected cells. The IC_{50} values (concentration at which 50% of PrP^{Sc} replication was inhibited) were 600 nM (10 µg/mL) for generation 3, 45 nM (1.5 µg/mL) for generation 4, and 75 nM (5 µg/mL) for generation 5, illustrating here also the best efficiency with generation 4 (Fig. 11.3, left). No difference in cell behavior was noted in the presence of the dendrimers; a significant cytotoxicity was observed only for concentrations above 25 µg/mL. In order to check the time-course of action of the G4 PPH dendrimer, it was added in ScN2a-infected cells at the concentration of 10 µg/mL. A significant decrease in PrP^{Sc} levels was already observed after 4 h (Fig. 11.3, right). Once cured, the cells were cultured in the absence of dendrimers for 3 weeks; neither PrP^{Sc} reappearance, nor cell-to-cell transmission of infectivity was observed [12].

The G4 dendrimer was then tested toward a series of different prion strains from scrapie homogenates, in particular 22L, Chandler, BSE (bovine spongiform encephalopathies, also called "mad cow" disease), and 263K. A significant decrease in the PrP^{Sc} levels was observed in all cases when treated with the G4 PPH dendrimer. In view of these excellent results on cells, this dendrimer was tested *in vivo*. C57BL/6 mice were infected with scrapie brain homogenate derived from terminally ill C506M3 mice. A group of mice was treated with 50 or 100 µg of G4 dendrimer per mice, every 2 days, by intra-peritoneal injection, from day 2 to day 30 post-infection. Control group received only the vehicle (saline). Treatment with the G4 dendrimer inhibited significantly the accumulation of PrP^{Sc} in mice spleen, up to 66% when using 50 µg of dendrimer, or up to 88% with 100 µg [12]. This was really an important feature, as it is known that PrP^{Sc} accumulates in spleen a long time before it reaches the CNS [13].

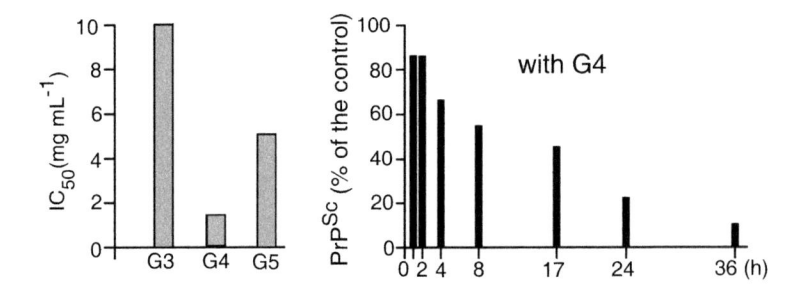

Figure 11.3 Left: IC$_{50}$, concentration at which 50% of PrP^{Sc} is inhibited by the dendrimers, depending on the generation. Right: Time-course of action of dendrimer G4 at 10 µg/mL in ScN2a-infected cells.

It is known that PrP^{Sc} forms spontaneously fibril–amyloid-like structures, due to the presence of β-forms, which accumulate in the CNS, finally leading to death. To investigate the interaction between dendrimers and prions, it appeared interesting to use not the full structure of the prion, but some sequences of their constituents, which are known to play a crucial role, in particular in the early steps of the formation of fibrils. The accumulation of amyloid fibrils can be monitored by changes in the fluorescence of thioflavine T (ThT), which displays an enhanced fluorescence and a red shift in the presence of β-sheet rich structures. Circular dichroism and infrared spectroscopy are also usable to follow the transformation of secondary structures into β-forms, characteristic for aggregates. The prion peptide PrP 185-208 was chosen for the first experiments, as it easily forms fibrils (in the presence of heparin at pH 5.5).

Furthermore, its structure has an analogous sphingolipid-binding domain to that of Alzheimer's peptide 1-28 [14]. The aggregation process of the prion peptide PrP 185-208 was studied in the presence of the G4 PPH dendrimer (dendrimer/peptide ratio = 0.002). The dendrimer clearly interferes with the aggregation process, as shown in particular by modification of the ThT fluorescence. The cationic G4 PPH dendrimer was both able to slow down the formation of aggregates by decreasing the nucleation rate, and to lower the final amount of amyloid fibrils [15].

Another approach to determine the influence of the dendrimer on the aggregation process consisted in studying its interaction with heparin. Indeed, heparin is a highly negatively charged glycosaminoglycan (GAG), which has many medical applications, in particular as anti-coagulant. However, it has been shown that heparin (as well as other polyanionic GAGs) can also induce the formation of β-sheet and of fibril–amyloid-like structures [16]. Thus, it appeared interesting to check the influence of heparin-dendrimers interactions, on aggregation of the prion peptide PrP 185-208, as heparin was present in the previous study of PrP 185-208 aggregation.

It was first shown that PrP 185-208 aggregates in the presence of 0.04 mg/mL of heparin, but concentrations 10 times lower or higher did not induce aggregation. Then the direct interaction of several dendrimers with heparin was studied. The dendrimers used were PPI dendrimer (16 terminal groups), PAMAM dendrimer (64 terminal groups) (see structure of both families in Fig. 11.2), and the G4 PPH dendrimer (96 terminal groups) (Fig. 11.1). In all cases, the interaction is essentially electrostatic. Several methods were used for studying the interaction, in particular EPR (electron paramagnetic resonance), using 4-trimethylammonium, 2,2,6,6-tetramethylpiperidine-1-oxyl bromide (CAT1) as spin probe. Other example of the utility of this technique for analyzing biological events can be seen in Chapter 3. It was shown here that the PPH dendrimers strongly interact with heparin, although a part of heparin was left free, whereas in the case of PAMAM dendrimers, no free heparin was detected. Furthermore, it was shown, using the ThT probe, that fluorescence was observed only for the PPH G4–heparin complex, not in the presence of PPH G4 alone, and not in the presence of heparin alone. Such phenomenon was observed only with the PPH G4, and not with the other dendrimers (PAMAM and PPI). This fluorescence assay is in agreement with the EPR data, which indicated a strong PPH G4–heparin interaction, as ThT is fluorescent only when it is immobilized. Studies using heparin, the prion peptide PrP 185-208, and the dendrimers, in diverse proportions demonstrated that dendrimers and PrP compete for interaction with heparin. Thus, interactions between dendrimers and heparin are indirectly responsible for the inhibition or enhancement of PrP fibril formation. At high dendrimer concentration (1 μM), they directly inhibit fibril formation, whereas at low concentration (0.01 μM), they indirectly impede fibril formation by sequestering a part of the heparin (data obtained with PAMAM dendrimers) [17].

These three families of dendrimers were also used for EPR study of their interaction with the prion peptide PrP 106-126 (also able to form amyloid aggregates) and Alzheimer's peptide 1-28 (Aβ 1-28). It was shown that the interaction with Aβ 1-28 is essentially dipolar, the strongest interaction being observed with the PAMAM dendrimers. The interactions of the dendrimers with PrP 106-126 were weaker than with Aβ 1-28. The interactions arose from polar and low polar groups, and the PAMAM dendrimers showed a relatively stronger binding efficiency [18]. More recently, the interaction of the G4 PPH dendrimer with the prion peptide PrP 185-208 were also analyzed by EPR, using nitroxide spin probes. These studies confirmed that the dendrimers interact with the amyloid monomers, thus preventing the formation of fibrils [19].

Alzheimer's disease is characterized by two hallmarks in the brain: the accumulation of β-amyloid, a low molecular weight peptide, which aggregates into fibrils then plaques, and the accumulation of hyperphosphorylated MAP-tau protein into neurofibrillar tangles. As indicated in the previous paragraphs, the prion peptide PrP 185-208 has an analogous sphingolipid-binding domain to that of Alzheimer's peptide 1-28; thus, the interaction between Alzheimer's peptide 1-28 (Aβ_{1-28}) and positively charged poly(phosphorhydrazone) (PPH) dendrimers (generations 3 and 4) was also studied. As for the previous experiments, the aggregation process into fibrils was monitored in particular using the fluorescence of Thioflavin T (ThT) as a fluorescent probe. The experiments were carried out from $t = 0$ to $t = 180$ min. In all cases, a plateau was reached after about 150 min. A nonlinear effect of concentration in dendrimers was observed on the occurrence of the amyloid fibril formation. At very low concentration in dendrimer G3 or G4 (0.01 μM), acceleration of the fibril formation was observed. The plateau was reached only after 60 min, and the final amount of fibrils was significantly higher than for the control (without dendrimer). On the contrary, at high concentrations (1 and 10 μM), both dendrimers completely inhibited the aggregation process of $A\beta_{1-28}$ (Fig. 11.4). The results were confirmed by transmission electron microscopy images. Moreover, it was observed that the PPH dendrimers significantly reduced the toxicity caused by the aggregated forms of $A\beta_{1-28}$ toward mouse neuroblastoma cell line (N2a) [20].

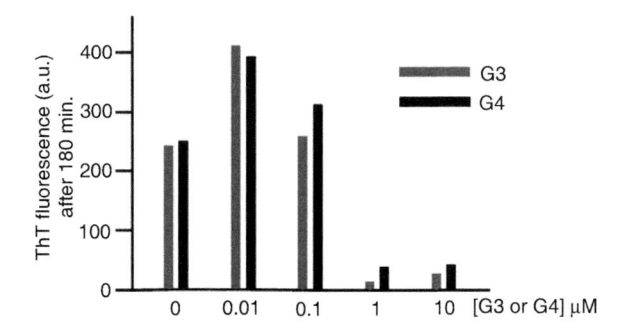

Figure 11.4 Formation of fibrils detected by the fluorescence of ThT, in the presence of $A\beta_{1-28}$ (50 μM), heparin (0.041 mg/mL), and diverse concentrations of positively charged PPH dendrimers G3 and G4. Fluorescence measured after 180 min, at pH 5.5 and 37°C.

Analogous experiments were carried out in the case of the MAP-tau protein, and monitored by the fluorescence of Thioflavin S. In the absence of dendrimer (control), or in concentration ratio MAP-tau/dendrimer 1/0.15, the fluorescence intensity increased, due to the aggregation. When increasing tenfold the dendrimer concentration (ratio 1/1.5), both dendrimers significantly inhibited the aggregation process [20].

The aggregation process of β-amyloid peptide ($A\beta$) and of MAP-tau is neurotoxic. Even if the mechanism of neurotoxicity is unclear, the involvement of decreased acetylcholinesterase (AChE) activity, oxidative stress (reactive oxidative species, ROS), and neuroinflammation is associated to Alzheimer's disease. In view of the influence of the positively charged PPH dendrimers on the decrease in the aggregation processes, it was important to check if they could also have an influence on the aforementioned problems. Diverse experiments, varying the concentration in dendrimers, were carried out to check the influence on these three points (AChE, ROS, inflammation).

Acetylcholinesterase is a major enzyme involved in acetylcholine-mediated neurotransmission. Several mechanisms in Alzheimer's disease induce the decrease or disruption of cholinergic neurotransmission. Thus, there is a need for AChE inhibitors for blocking the AcH hydrolysis, and promoting the cholinergic function. The cationic PPH dendrimers have almost no activity on AChE and induced an increase in the hydrolysis rate only at high concentrations (10 µM), that is 10 times more than what is needed to block amyloid fibril formation. These dendrimers are not inhibitors of AChE, but they are not antagonistic to AChE inhibitors [21].

The antioxidant properties of the cationic PPH dendrimers were measured using two methods: scavenging of the stable radical DPPH (2,2-dipheny-1-picrylhydrazyl) and ability to reduce ferric ions to ferrous ions (FRAP). Both PPH dendrimers were able to reduce the amount of DPPH, but there was no correlation between the quantity of dendrimer and the efficiency in scavenging the radicals (Fig. 11.5, left). On the contrary, for both generations used, there was an exponential in the reduction of Fe^{3+} when the concentration in dendrimer increased (Fig. 11.5, right). Thus, both generations of PPH dendrimers display a weak antioxidant activity [21].

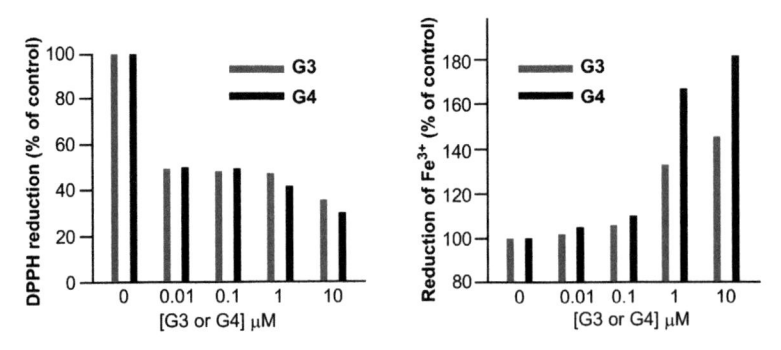

Figure 11.5 Antioxidant properties of G3 and G4 cationic PPH dendrimers. Left: for DPPH reduction; right: for Fe^{3+} reduction.

Microglia are cells that function as macrophages in the CNS. They show neurotoxic activity in the presence of abnormal amounts of pro-inflammatory and pro-apoptotic mediators, such as IL-1β, IL-6, IL-12, and TNF-α (a cytokine involved in systemic inflammations). The influence of the cationic PPH dendrimers on the secretion of TNF-α was measured in the mouse microglia cell line BV-2. These cells were incubated with bacterial lipopolysaccharide (LPS) to induce an immune response, in particular a twofold increase in the level of TNF-α secreted. The level of TNF-α in the presence of the PPH dendrimers (0.05 µM) was reduced and comparable to values observed for inactive microglia [21].

In view of the anti-aggregation properties of cationic PPH dendrimers toward prion and Alzheimer's peptides, it was tempting to test these dendrimers against other neurodegenerative diseases induced by the formation of fibrils. α-sinuclein (ASN) is a cytosolic protein, essentially found in the parts of the presynaptic nerve endings, in the CNS. Modification of the conformation (increase in β-sheet) and aggregation of the proteins disrupt their physiological function and have toxic effects on neurons. Disorders in the ASN structure are involved in the pathogenesis of synucleinopathies, particularly in Parkinson's disease. The influence of different concentrations of generations 3 and 4 of PPH dendrimers on fibrillation of ASN was analyzed. It was shown that both generations of dendrimers used in low concentration (ASN/dendrimer 1:0.1 and 1:0.5) inhibited the β-sheet formation, G3 being more efficient than G4. However, at higher concentrations (ASN/dendrimer 1:1 and 1:2), these dendrimers did not inhibit the fibril formation process [22].

In view of the positive properties of these PPH dendrimers against neurodegenerative diseases (mainly *in vitro*), it was impor-tant to measure the cytotoxicity against neural cells. It was shown by MTT assays performed on murine neuroblastoma cell line (N2a) that IC_{50} of G3 and G4 PPH dendrimers was ca. 1 µM [20]. A deeper insight on the mechanism of toxicity was carried out with genera-tions 2 and 3 PPH dendrimers toward two types of mouse neuronal cells: murine embryonic hippocampal cells (mHippoE-18, normal cells), and N2a (cancerous cells). It was shown that G2 and G3 PPH dendrimers ended by tertiary ammonium groups induce a rapid breakdown of cellular processes, leading to cell death, when used above the concentration of 1 µM. However, below the concentration of ca. 1 µM, these dendrimers are "safe" to both normal and cancerous mouse neuronal cells [23].

11.3 Properties of Viologen-Phosphorus Dendrimers

The properties of cationic poly(phosphorhydrazone) PPH dendrimers against neurodegenerative diseases have been extensively presented in the previous sections. These compounds have an internal neutral structure and positive charges only on the surface. Very recently, a new family of phosphorus-containing dendrimers has been synthesized, based on viologen (bialkylated 4,4′-bipyridine) units in the branches (see Chapter 1). This new family of dendrimers has intrinsically positive charges inside the structure, and generally a neutral surface, in contrast to PPH dendrimers. In most cases, these compounds are of low generations (0 or 1) and built from either trifunctional $P(S)Cl_3$ or hexafunctional $N_3P_3Cl_6$ core. Figure 11.6 displays the viologen dendrimers that have been used for biological experiments, but many others were synthesized [24].

Viologens are toxic compounds, inducing strong generation of ROS in organisms, and are also responsible for severe human poisoning, and may play a role in Parkinson's diseases [25]. Thus, it appears particularly important for safety reasons to perform several tests concerning the toxicity of the viologen-containing dendrimers.

The first biological properties tested with these new dendrimers concerned the cytotoxicity, hemotoxicity, and the antimicrobial and antifungal activities. Human erythrocytes were used for studying the hemotoxicity, measured by the release of hemoglobin. Tests were carried out after 2, 8, 13, and 24 h, and with dendrimer concentrations of 1, 5, 10, and 20 µM. Figure 11.7 displays the results for the eight dendrimers shown in Fig. 11.6, used at concentrations 1 and 20 µM, and after 24 h. At 1 µM, most dendrimers are not hemotoxic, with the notable exception of the dendrimers having the largest number of positive charges (18 and 36). At 20 µM, only two compounds have almost no hemotoxicity, the smallest G0 dendrimer PSG_0PO_3, and the largest G0 dendrimer, with poly(ethylene glycol) (PEG) terminal functions, $N_3P_3G_0PEG$ [26].

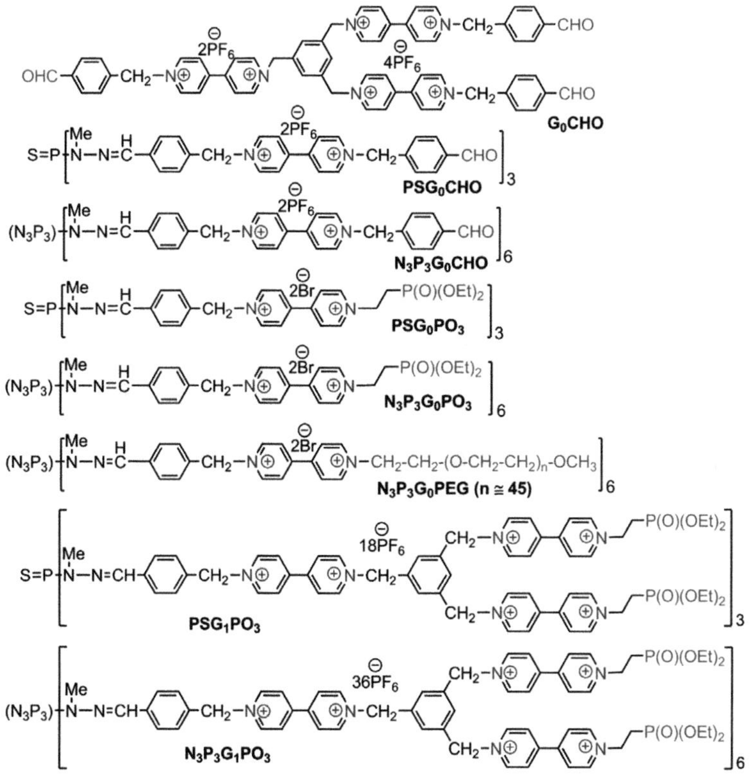

Figure 11.6 Chemical structure of phosphorus dendrimers bearing viologen units.

In vitro cytotoxicity was assayed with B14 Chinese hamster peritoneal fibroblast and N2a mouse neuroblastoma cell lines. Cell viability was determined by MTT assays. The results are shown in Fig. 11.8 for the highest concentration in dendrimer (20 µM). No clear tendency could be inferred from these data, but it is interesting to note that the PEGylated dendrimer, which was not hemotoxic, was not toxic toward the B14 (normal) cells, but was toxic against the N2a (cancerous) cells. A compound that is harmless to normal cells but highly toxic to cancer cells may open exciting perspectives in oncology [26].

The antimicrobial activity of the viologen dendrimers (concentrations ranging from 0.1 µM to 20 µM) was evaluated against one Gram-positive bacterium (*Staphylococcus aureus* ATCC

6538), three Gram-negative bacteria (*Escherichia coli* ATCC25922, *Proteus vulgaris* ATCC 13315, and *Pseudomonas aeruginosa* ATCC 15442), and yeast (*Candida albicans* ATCC 10231). It is known that chemicals containing viologen units present excellent anti-bacterial activities against *S. aureus* and *E. coli* [27]. The PEGylated dendrimer had no activity, even at the highest concentration. On the contrary, the dendrimers incorporating the largest number of viologen units had the highest anti-bacterial activity. They were able to reduce the growth of *S. aureus*, *E. coli*, and *P. vulgaris* [26].

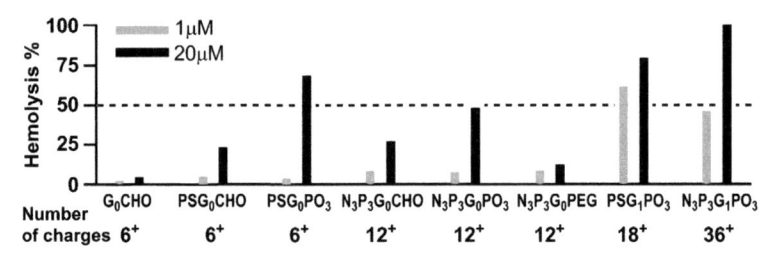

Figure 11.7 Hemotoxicity after 24 h induced by viologen dendrimers (1 or 20 μM), shown in Fig. 11.6.

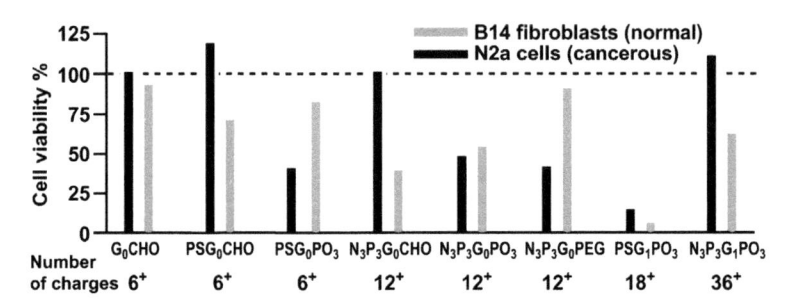

Figure 11.8 Cell viability after 24 h for cultures in the presence of 20 μM of the viologen dendrimers shown in Fig. 11.6.

As a preliminary work to study the interaction of these new dendrimers with protein, human serum albumin (HSA) was chosen as a classical model. HSA possesses one tryptophane residue, particularly suitable to monitor by fluorescence the possible interactions with the dendrimers. The fluorescence intensity of tryptophane in HSA decreased with successive addition of the viologen dendrimers, indicating a direct interaction. The viologen dendrimers with aldehyde terminal functions quenched the HSA fluorescence and additionnaly changed the secondary structure of albumin. Dendrimers with either phosphonate or PEG terminal functions strongly quenched HSA fluorescence, but did not change the secondary structure [28].

Cholinesterase inhibitors are the most commonly used drugs for treating neurodegenerative diseases; thus, it was interesting to test the influence of some viologen dendrimers on the activity of acetylcholinesterase (AChE) and butyrylcholinesterase (BChE). Indeed, both cholinesterases are deeply implicated in neurodegenerative diseases. They colocalize with $A\beta$ peptide plaques in Alzheimer's disease and accelerate the assembly of amyloid-β peptides into fibrils. Only two small dendrimers were tested: G_0CHO and $N_3P_3G_0PO_3$ (see structure in Fig. 11.6). Both dendrimers inhibited the activity of both enzymes [29].

Further studies were performed also with two dendrimers, both having the same number of internal charges, but different terminal functions: $N_3P_3G_0PO_3$ (phosphonates) and $N_3P_3G_0PEG$ (PEG) (see structure in Fig. 11.6). The interaction of both dendrimers with α-sinuclein (ASN) was carried out with the same aim than for the dendrimers with ammonium terminal functions, *i.e.*, against Parkinson's disease. It was first shown that both dendrimers interact with ASN by quenching its fluorescence, but they did not change the secondary structure of ASN [30]. More importantly, it was shown that this interaction resulted in the inhibition of ASN fibrils formation, with a high efficiency, even with a low ratio of these dendrimers. Figure 11.9 shows the comparison of both viologen dendrimers with the G3 and G4 PPH dendrimers ended by ammonium groups (Fig. 11.1), and with the G4 PAMAM dendrimer (Fig. 11.2). It is clear from Fig. 11.9 that the viologen dendrimers are the most efficient for the inhibition of ASN fibril formation, despite their very small size and reduced number of positive charges [31].

In view of these excellent results in the inhibition of ASN fibrils, the toxicity of two viologen dendrimers (PSG_0PO_3, and $N_3P_3G_0PO_3$, Fig. 11.6) was tested against neuronal cells. The chosen cells were the murine hippocampal cell line (mHippoE-18). Both tested dendrimers did not induce a strong cellular response, and only a low level of apoptosis was measured. Both dendrimers also induced a small decrease in the ROS level, a slight increase in catalase activity, but did not alter the level of antioxidant GSH (glutathione) [32]. This work was further developed in the presence of rotenone, a pesticide that induces an increased risk of Parkinson's diseases. It induces, in particular, an increase in the amount of ROS in neurons, α-synuclein aggregation, and activation of microglia. One viologen dendrimer ($N_3P_3G_0PO_3$), two PPH dendrimers with ammonium terminal groups (G3 and G4), and two PAMAM dendrimers (G3 and G4) were tested on mHippoE-18 cell line in the presence of rotenone (Fig. 11.10). All dendrimers (0.1 µM) increased cell viability in the presence of rotenone (1 µM) compared to rotenone alone. In the same conditions, the level of ROS was dramatically decreased, especially with PPH and viologen dendrimers. A favorable effect on mitochondrial system was observed mainly with the viologen dendrimer $N_3P_3G_0PO_3$ (Fig. 11.10, right). All these data demonstrate that despite being composed of potentially highly toxic viologen units, this family of dendrimers may have a large potential of biological uses [33].

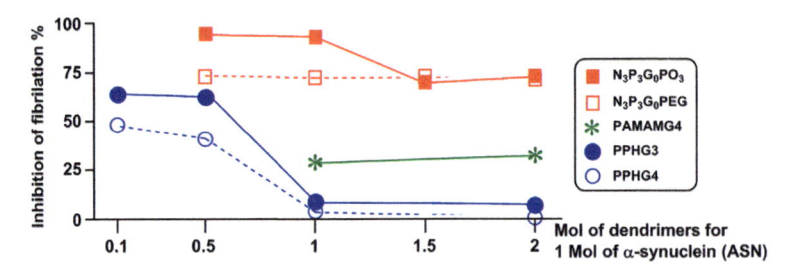

Figure 11.9 Inhibition of ASN fibril formation, depending on the ratio ASN/dendrimer (1:X, with X from 0.1 to 2), and the type of dendrimer.

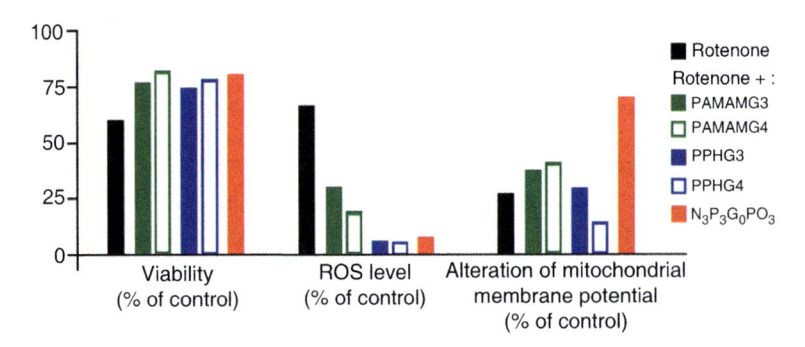

Figure 11.10 Three experiments carried out with mHippoE-18 cells, in the presence of rotenone (1 µM) in all cases. Influence of various dendrimers (0.1 µM) on cells viability (left), ROS levels (middle), and mitochondrial membrane potential (right), compared to control cell cultures (without rotenone, and without dendrimer).

11.4 Properties of Poly(phosphorhydrazone) Dendrimers Functionalized by Azabisphosphonate Groups

All the dendrimers shown in the previous paragraphs used for studying their potential against diseases of the CNS are positively charged, either on their terminal groups, or inside their structure. However, a negatively charged dendrimer was also tested for this purpose. Its structure is shown in Fig. 11.11. It is a first-generation PPH dendrimer functionalized on the periphery by azabisphosphonic sodium salts (called ABP). This compound has many biological properties toward the human immune system [34], as well as unique anti-inflammatory properties [35] *in vitro* and *in vivo* [36], which are emphasized in Chapter 12. In this chapter, we will focus on a single aspect of the biological properties of the ABP dendrimer, against inflammation of the CNS, which occurs particularly in the case of MS. The inflammation of the CNS in MS leads to the destruction of the myelin sheath surrounding the axons, resulting in impaired nerve conduction. As this dendrimer ABP has anti-inflammatory properties, it has been tested against MS with a classical mouse model of MOG_{35-55} induced experimental autoimmune encephalomyelities (EAE). Dendrimer ABP is able both to prevent the development of induced EAE and to inhibit established disease. Several cellular mechanisms operating *in vivo* in the mouse model were related to the observed effects. The ABP dendrimer drove the cytokine production by splenocytes from an inflammatory pattern to an anti-inflammatory one. It redirected myelin-specific CD4+ T-cell response toward IL-10 production (an anti-inflammatory cytokine). The dendrimer ABP had also an anti-inflammatory action on APCs (antigen presenting cells) [37].

More recently, the biological properties of dendrimer ABP toward the immortalized murine microglial cell line BV-2 have been tested. Microglia are resident macrophage cells located particularly in the brain. They are the first and main immune defense in the CNS. It was shown that the dendrimer ABP bound to BV-2 cells and drove them toward an anti-inflammatory state. This result strengthens the potential of dendrimer ABP for the treatment of chronic inflammatory diseases of the CNS [38].

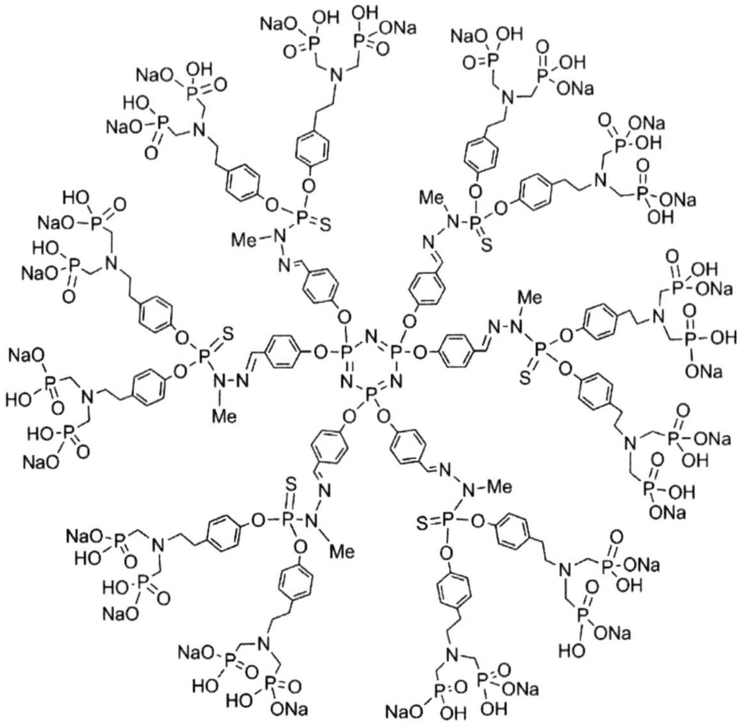

Figure 11.11 Chemical structure of a generation 1 PPH dendrimer ended by azabisphosphonic salts (ABP).

11.5 Conclusion

We have shown in this chapter the potential of several types of phosphorus-containing dendrimers to be drugs *per se*, to fight against different diseases of the CNS, at the molecular and macromolecular levels. Most of these experiments were carried out *in vitro*, but two of them have been transferred *in vivo*, with mice. These examples concern the prion disease, using a cationic G4 PPH dendrimer [12], and the model of the MS disease, using an anionic G1 PPH dendrimer [37]. In both cases, the dendrimers were injected intravenously with no special formulation, using only saline as vehicle. In both cases, the dendrimers were well tolerated by the mice, and a dramatic improvement compared to untreated mice was observed.

Despite these very positive results *in vivo*, these data do not clearly demonstrate if these dendrimers are able to cross the blood–brain barrier (BBB) or not. This is certainly a domain that should urgently be tested. For classical drugs, it is known that only 2% of CNS drugs cross the BBB and reach their therapeutic target in the brain, but several strategies already exist to overcome this problem, and might be applied to dendrimers [7].

References

1. Berer, K. and Krishnamoorthy, G. (2014). Microbial view of central nervous system autoimmunity, *FEBS Lett.*, **588**, pp. 4207–4213.

2. Global Burden of Disease Study 2013 Collaborators (2015). Global, regional, and national incidence, prevalence, and years lived with disability for 301 acute and chronic diseases and injuries in 188 countries, 1990-2013: A systematic analysis for the Global Burden of Disease Study 2013, *Lancet*, **386**, pp. 743–800.

3. Hashimoto, M., Rockenstein, E., Crews, L., and Masliah, E. (2003). Role of protein aggregation in mitochondrial dysfunction and neurodegeneration in Alzheimer's and Parkinson's diseases, *NeuroMolecular Med.*, **4**, pp. 21–35.

4. https://web.archive.org/web/20150318030901/http://www.who.int/mediacentre/factsheets/fs362/en.

5. Kalia, L. V. and Lang, A. E. (2015). Parkinson's disease, *Lancet*, **386**, pp. 896–912.

6. Clarke, A. R., Jackson, G. S., and Collinge, J. (2001). The molecular biology of prion propagation, *Phil. Trans. R. Soc. Lond. B*, **356**, pp. 185–195.

7. Mignani, S., Bryszewska, M., Zablocka, M., Klajnert-Maculewicz, B., Cladera, J., Shcharbin, D., and Majoral, J. P. (2017). Can dendrimer based nanoparticles fight neurodegenerative diseases? Current situation versus other established approaches, *Prog. Polym. Sci.*, **64**, pp. 23–51.

8. Loup, C., Zanta, M. A., Caminade, A. M., Majoral, J. P., and Meunier, B. (1999). Preparation of water-soluble cationic phosphorus-containing dendrimers as DNA transfecting agents, *Chem. Eur. J.*, **5**, pp. 3644–3650.

9. Haensler, J. and Szoka, F. C. (1993). Polyamidoamine cascade polymers mediate efficient transfection of cells in culture, *Bioconjugate Chem.*, **4**, pp. 372–379.

10. Padie, C., Maszewska, M., Majchrzak, K., Nawrot, B., Caminade, A. M., and Majoral, J. P. (2009). Polycationic phosphorus dendrimers: Synthesis, characterization, study of cytotoxicity, complexation of DNA, and transfection experiments, *New J. Chem.*, **33**, pp. 318–326.

11. Supattapone, S., Wille, H., Uyechi, L., Safar, J., Tremblay, P., Szoka, F. C., Cohen, F. E., Prusiner, S. B., and Scott, M. R. (2001). Branched polyamines cure prion-infected neuroblastoma cells, *J. Virol.*, **75**, pp. 3453–3461.

12. Solassol, J., Crozet, C., Perrier, V., Leclaire, J., Beranger, F., Caminade, A. M., Meunier, B., Dormont, D., Majoral, J. P., and Lehmann, S. (2004). Cationic phosphorus-containing dendrimers reduce prion replication both in cell culture and in mice infected with scrapie, *J. Gen. Virol.*, **85**, pp. 1791–1799.

13. Lasmezas, C. I., Cesbron, J. Y., Deslys, J. P., Demaimay, R., Anjou, K. T., Rioux, R., Lemaire, C., Locht, C., and Dormont, D. (1996). Immune system-dependent and -independent replication of the scrapie agent, *J. Virol.*, **70**, pp. 1292–1295.

14. Mahfoud, R., Garmy, N., Maresca, M., Yahi, N., Puigserver, A., and Fantini, J. (2002). Identification of a common sphingolipid-binding domain in Alzheimer, prion, and HIV-1 proteins, *J. Biol. Chem.*, **277**, pp. 11292–11296.

15. Klajnert, B., Cortijo-Arellano, M., Cladera, J., Majoral, J. P., Caminade, A. M., and Bryszewska, M. (2007). Influence of phosphorus dendrimers on the aggregation of the prion peptide PrP 185-208, *Biochem. Biophys. Res. Commun.*, **364**, pp. 20–25.

16. Gellermann, G. P., Ullrich, K., Unger, C., Fandrich, M., Sauter, S., and Diekmann, S. (2007). Identification of molecular compounds critical to Alzheimer's-like plaque formation, *J. Neurosci. Res.*, **85**, pp. 2037–2044.

17. Klajnert, B., Cangiotti, M., Calici, S., Ionov, M., Majoral, J. P., Caminade, A. M., Cladera, J., Bryszewska, M., and Ottaviani, M. F. (2009). Interactions between dendrimers and heparin and their implications for the anti-prion activity of dendrimers, *New J. Chem.*, **33**, pp. 1087–1093.

18. Klajnert, B., Cangiotti, M., Calici, S., Majoral, J. P., Caminade, A. M., Cladera, J., Bryszewska, M., and Ottaviani, M. F. (2007). EPR study

of the interactions between dendrimers and peptides involved in Alzheimer's and prion diseases, *Macromol. Biosci.*, **7**, pp. 1065–1074.

19. Ottaviani, M. F., Mazzeo, R., Cangiotti, M., Fiorani, L., Majoral, J. P., Caminade, A. M., Pedziwiatr, E., Bryszewska, M., and Klajnert, B. (2010). Time evolution of the aggregation process of peptides involved in neurodegenerative diseases and preventing aggregation effect of phosphorus dendrimers studied by EPR, *Biomacromolecules*, **11**, pp. 3014–3021.

20. Wasiak, T., Ionov, M., Nieznanski, K., Nieznanska, H., Klementieva, O., Granell, M., Cladera, J., Majoral, J. P., Caminade, A. M., and Klajnert, B. (2012). Phosphorus dendrimers affect Alzheimer's (A beta(1-28)) peptide and MAP-tau protein aggregation, *Mol. Pharm.*, **9**, pp. 458–469.

21. Wasiak, T., Marcinkowska, M., Pieszynski, I., Zablocka, M., Caminade, A. M., Majoral, J. P., and Klajnert-Maculewicz, B. (2015). Cationic phosphorus dendrimers and therapy for Alzheimer's disease, *New. J. Chem.*, **39**, pp. 4852–4859.

22. Milowska, K., Gabryelak, T., Bryszewska, M., Caminade, A. M., and Majoral, J. P. (2012). Phosphorus-containing dendrimers against alpha-synuclein fibril formation, *Int. J. Biol. Macromol.*, **50**, pp. 1138–1143.

23. Lazniewska, J., Milowska, K., Zablocka, M., Mignani, S., Caminade, A. M., Majoral, J. P., Bryszewska, M., and Gabryelak, T. (2013). Mechanism of cationic phosphorus dendrimer toxicity against murine neural cell lines, *Mol. Pharm.*, **10**, pp. 3484–3496.

24. Katir, N., Majoral, J. P., El Kadib, A., Caminade, A. M., and Bousmina, M. (2012). Molecular and macromolecular engineering with viologens as building blocks: Rational design of phosphorus-viologen dendritic structures, *Eur. J. Org. Chem.*, pp. 269–273.

25. Tanner, C. M., Kamel, F., Ross, G. W., Hoppin, J. A., Goldman, S. M., Korell, M., Marras, C., Bhudhikanok, G. S., Kasten, M., Chade A. R., Comyns, K., Richards, M. B., Meng, C., Priestley, B., Fernandez, H. H., Cambi, F., Umbach, D. M., Blair, A., Sandler, D. P., and Langston, J. W. (2011). Rotenone, paraquat, and Parkinson's disease, *Environ. Health. Perspect.*, **119**, pp. 866–872.

26. Ciepluch, K., Katir, N., El Kadib, A., Felczak, A., Zawadzka, K., Weber, M., Klajnert, B., Lisowska, K., Caminade, A. M., Bousmina, M., Bryszewska, M., and Majoral, J. P. (2012). Biological properties of new viologen-phosphorus dendrimers, *Mol. Pharm.*, **9**, pp. 448–457.

27. Ganesh Kumar, V., Govindaraju, K., Singaravelu, G., and Adhikesavalu, D. (2009). Antibacterial activity of viologen pendant indole stabilized silver nanoparticles, *J. Biopestic.*, **2**, pp. 217–221.

28. Ciepluch, K., Katir, N., El Kadib, A., Weber, M., Caminade, A. M., Bousmina, M., Majoral, J. P., and Bryszewska, M. (2012). Photo-physical and structural interactions between viologen phosphorus-based dendrimers and human serum albumin, *J. Lumin.*, **132**, pp. 1553–1563.

29. Ciepluch, K., Weber, M., Katir, N., Caminade, A. M., El Kadib, A., Klajnert, B., Majoral, J. P., and Bryszewska, M. (2013). Effect of viologen-phosphorus dendrimers on acetylcholinesterase and butyrylcholinesterase activities, *Int. J. Biol. Macromol.*, **54**, pp. 119–124.

30. Milowska, K., Grochowina, J., Katir, N., El Kadib, A., Majoral, J. P., Bryszewska, M., and Gabryelak, T. (2013). Interaction between viologen-phosphorus dendrimers and alpha-synuclein, *J. Lumin.*, **134**, pp. 132–137.

31. Milowska, K., Grochowina, J., Katir, N., El Kadib, A., Majoral, J. P., Bryszewska, M., and Gabryelak, T. (2013). Viologen-phosphorus dendrimers inhibit alpha-synuclein fibrillation, *Mol. Pharm.*, **10**, pp. 1131–1137.

32. Lazniewska, J., Janaszewska, A., Milowska, K., Caminade, A. M., Mignani, S., Katir, N., El Kadib, A., Bryszewska, M., Majoral, J. P., Gabryelak, T., and Klajnert-Maculewicz, B. (2013). Promising low-toxicity of viologen-phosphorus dendrimers against embryonic mouse hippocampal cells, *Molecules*, **18**, pp. 12222–12240.

33. Milowska, K., Szwed, A., Zablocka, M., Caminade, A. M., Majoral, J. P., Mignani, S., Gabryelak, T., and Bryszewska, M. (2014). In vitro PAMAM, phosphorus and viologen-phosphorus dendrimers prevent rotenone-induced cell damage, *Int. J. Pharm.*, **474**, pp. 42–49.

34. Griffe, L., Poupot, M., Marchand, P., Maraval, A., Turrin, C. O., Rolland, O., Metivier, P., Bacquet, G., Fournie, J. J., Caminade, A. M., Poupot, R., and Majoral, J. P. (2007). Multiplication of human natural killer cells by nanosized phosphonate-capped dendrimers, *Angew. Chem. Int. Ed.*, **46**, pp. 2523–2526.

35. Caminade, A. M., Fruchon, S., Turrin, C. O., Poupot, M., Ouali, A., Maraval, A., Garzoni, M., Maly, M., Furer, V., Kovalenko, V., Majoral, J. P., Pavan, G. M., and Poupot, R. (2015). The key role of the scaffold on the efficiency of dendrimer nanodrugs, *Nature Comm.*, **6**, 7722.

36. Hayder, M., Poupot, M., Baron, M., Nigon, D., Turrin, C. O., Caminade, A. M., Majoral, J. P., Eisenberg, R. A., Fournie, J. J., Cantagrel, A., Poupot, R., and Davignon, J. L. (2011). A phosphorus-based dendrimer targets inflammation and osteoclastogenesis in experimental arthritis, *Sci. Transl. Med.*, **3**, 11.

37. Hayder, M., Varilh, M., Turrin, C. O., Saoudi, A., Caminade, A. M., Poupot, R., and Liblau, R. S. (2015). Phosphorus-based dendrimer ABP treats neuroinflammation by promoting IL-10-producing CD4(+) T cells, *Biomacromolecules*, **16**, pp. 3425–3433.

38. Fruchon, S., Caminade, A. M., Turrin, C., and Poupot, R. (2015). A phosphorus-based dendrimer with anti-inflammatory properties towards microglia, *Glia*, **63**, pp. E329–E329.

Chapter 12

The ABP Dendrimer Saga

Rémy Poupot, Jérémy Ledall, and Séverine Fruchon
Centre de Physiopathologie de Toulouse-Purpan, Université de Toulouse,
CNRS, INSERM, UPS, France
remy.poupot@inserm.fr

12.1 Why Are Dendrimers So Attractive to Biologists?

Very soon after the pioneering synthesis of dendrimers [1], this new family of molecules has generated lots of attention for their uses in biological and medical applications. Four main features of dendrimers underlie their successful emergence in the biomedical field.

12.1.1 Single-Molecule Compounds

Due to their sequential process of synthesis, either divergent or convergent, dendrimers have perfectly defined structure and molecular weight. Their synthesis provides consistent isomolecular batches of product with a monodisperse size. This specific

Phosphorus Dendrimers in Biology and Nanomedicine: Synthesis, Characterization, and Properties
Edited by Anne-Marie Caminade, Cédric-Olivier Turrin, and Jean-Pierre Majoral
Copyright © 2018 Pan Stanford Publishing Pte. Ltd.
ISBN 978-981-4774-33-8 (Hardcover), 978-1-315-11085-1 (eBook)
www.panstanford.com

characteristic differentiates dendrimers both from linear polymers and other types of nanoparticles whose polymerization cannot be accurately controlled. These are key points for the fate of dendrimers in biomedical applications with respect to regulatory requirements, for the advent of new dendrimer-based therapeutics, and imaging and diagnostic tools.

12.1.2 Supramolecular Properties

Since their earliest syntheses, the supramolecular properties of dendrimers have been strongly involved in their uses. Indeed, at the very beginning, dendrimers, and their "octopus" mother molecules, were intended to extract organic compounds solubilized in water solution [2] and to solubilize hydrophilic salts in aprotic organic solvents [3], respectively. Later on, supramolecular interactions with guest molecules inside the dendrimer, and supramolecular interactions at the periphery of the dendrimer with substrates, molecular and/or cellular targets have been the rationale for biological and biomedical applications of dendrimers. Loading drugs in biocompatible carriers is a way to enhance water solubility, to increase half-life, but also to decrease potential toxicity. Dendrimers have been extensively used for such purposes, either as covalent conjugates or as encapsulating nanodevices [4]. Polycationic dendrimers have undergone a long-lasting exploitation as transfecting agents bearing DNA at their periphery [5]. More recently, and based on the same physico-chemical rationale, dendrimers emerged as promising non-viral supramolecular platforms to deliver small interfering RNA (siRNA) in interference-based therapies [6].

12.1.3 Nanometer Size

The nanometer size and globular shape of dendrimers are comparable to those of biomolecules (such as nucleic acids and proteins) and supramolecular biostructures (such as biological membranes and viruses). One can assume that the size of a first-generation (generation 1) dendrimer begins at 2 or 3 nm and that, more or less, 1 nm in size is gained with each supplemental generation. Hence, generation 1 dendrimers have approximately the size of human insulin (a small protein of 51 amino acids, with a molecular weight of 5800 Da). Toward the other end of the scale, generation 6 dendrimers are expected with a size of 7 to 8 nm, close to the one of human serum albumin (610 amino acids, with a molecular weight of 65,000 Da). The largest dendrimers ever synthesized are generation 13 compounds with a size of ≈30 nm and a molecular weight of ≈8.4 MDa, in the range of small viruses [7]. Therefore, dendrimers undoubtedly pertain to the nanoworld [8]. Together with their supramolecular properties, these structural characteristics make dendrimers perfect biomimics and carriers of biomolecules.

12.1.4 Multivalency

The multivalency of dendrimers is reminiscent to that of biological systems [9], and the majority of biological molecular interactions occur through polyvalent bindings [9, 10]. The multivalency of dendrimers enables their polyvalent interactions with biotargets. The valency of a ligand corresponds to the number of separate cognate interactions of the same kind, which can be established with its receptor(s). The strength of a single cognate interaction between a ligand and a receptor is called "affinity." Natural ligands with multiple receptor binding sites (multivalent ligands) or multivalent engineered nanodevices interact through polyvalent interactions with their partner receptors. The strength of these polyvalent cognate interactions is named "avidity" (also called "functional affinity"), and is much higher than the simple sum of the strengths of the single interactions. Thus, from monovalent to oligovalent, and then polyvalent ligands, there is a strong enhancement in the intensity and duration of the stimulating signal delivered to a cell through a ligand–receptor interaction. From this point of view, dendrimers are perfect nanoplatforms to enable polyvalent interactions involving ligands, which are originally monovalent and therefore, to alter a biological process [10, 11]. Although interactions between cells and nanostructures need to be refined [12], appropriately designed dendrimers are potential therapeutics to activate a protective physiological response or to efficiently inhibit a deleterious pathological disorder.

12.2 Where Does the ABP Dendrimer Come from?

12.2.1 A Rational Design

Peripheral blood mononuclear cells (PBMCs, *i.e.*, white blood cells) can be easily prepared from a blood sample. They represent a convenient way to access human primary immune cells. PBMCs comprise several kinds of cells. On the one hand, natural killer (NK) cells, monocytes, and dendritic cells (DC) are part of the innate immunity: they provide immediate defense against malignant cells and infections. On the other hand, B- and T-lymphocytes are part of the adaptive immunity: they require a prior sensitization to be active and provide long-lasting protection. At the end of the 1990s, we were studying a particular subpopulation of peripheral blood T cells, the so-called Vγ9Vδ2 T-lymphocytes [13]. These cells have an antitumor cytotoxic activity, which makes them potential effectors in cellular anti-cancer therapies [14]. They are stimulated by small pyrophosphorylated molecules [15], and we have shown that the pyrophosphate group is crucial for the bioactivity of these molecules [16]. Therefore, we proposed to call them phosphoantigens.

In line with the concept that polyvalent ligands should enable higher functional affinity, and finally stronger activation of target cells, as already evoked above, we proposed to Caminade's group in Toulouse to prepare phosphorus-based dendrimers bearing pyrophosphates groups at their surface. In more details, these phosphorus-based dendrimers are poly(phosphorhydrazone) (PPH) dendrimers based on a cyclo-triphosphazene (N_3P_3) core bearing phenoxymethyl-methylhydrazone (PPMH) branches. They can be ended by different surface groups, expectedly the intended pyrophosphate groups to specifically activate the Vγ9Vδ2 T-lymphocytes. This rational design failed on the instability of pyrophosphates in acidic environment, which makes the prospected synthesis random. Instead, the first dendrimer provided by Caminade's group was a generation 1 PPH dendrimer bearing 12 azabisphosphonate groups (ABP dendrimer, MW = 5820 Da, Fig. 12.1) [17].

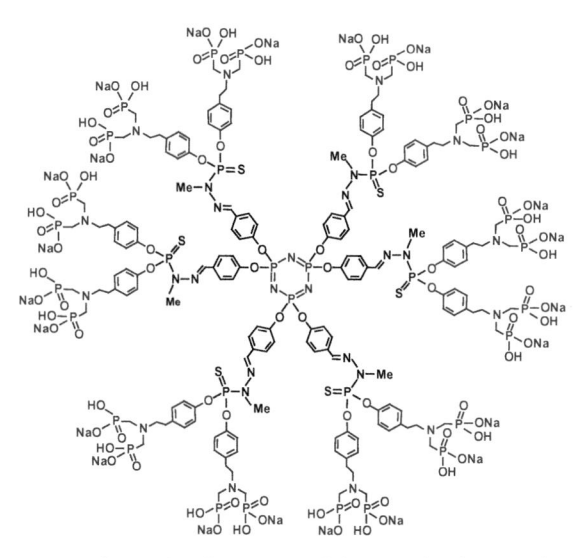

Figure 12.1 Two-dimensional structure of the ABP dendrimer: The N_3P_3 core, the PMMH branches, and the azabisphosphonate end groups (as mono-sodium salts) borne by tyramine.

It rapidly appeared that the ABP dendrimer had only a poor effect on the activation of $V\gamma 9V\delta 2$ T-lymphocytes, neither had the followers in the series with different azamono- and azabisphosphonate end groups. However, twists and turns of research led us to discover that some of the synthesized dendrimers have unprecedented immuno-modulatory effects on the human immune system.

12.2.2   Serendipity in Action

To track the ABP dendrimer in culture with human PBMCs, a fluorescein isothiocyanate (FITC)-conjugated analog of the molecule had been synthesized. Therein, an FITC group replaces statistically one of the 12 azabisphosphonate groups at the outer shell of the dendrimer. FITC is the most common fluorophore used in flow cytometry. By co-incubating the FITC-labelled ABP dendrimer with PBMCs in culture for a few minutes, we discovered that the primary cellular target of the compound is the monocyte subpopulation [17]. We have shown that at early time points of co-incubation, the fluorescent ABP dendrimer is bound to the cell surface of monocytes and can be displaced by competing with the ABP dendrimer. However, at later time points, the cellular localization of the fluorescent dendrimer, analyzed by confocal microscopy, progressively switches from the cell surface to intracellular compartments, indicating internalization. Within 3 to 6 days' culture, monocytes in culture with the ABP dendrimer at 20 μM undergo morphological and phenotypical changes and exhibit increased phagocytic activity toward bacteria. These monocytes in culture with the ABP dendrimer are also less apoptotic and thus remain viable over longer periods than control monocytes without dendrimer [17].

Surprisingly, when co-cultures of PBMCs with the ABP dendrimer at 20 μM are maintained during 2–3 weeks, we observe that the monocytes disappear from the cultures, and then a selective amplification of NK is observed, leading to cultures with more than 70% of NK cells [18]. Interestingly, NK cells and Vγ9Vδ2 T-lymphocytes share profiles of gene expression [19], and also some biological features.

Hence, at least two subpopulations of human immune cells are targeted by the ABP dendrimer, namely monocytes and NK cells, paving the way to different biomedical applications.

12.3 NK Cell–Based Anti-cancer Immunotherapies

NK cells are essentially cytotoxic effectors implicated in early immune responses against viral [20], bacterial [21], and parasitic infections [22, 23], as they specifically recognize and efficiently kill infected cells in the body. NK cells are also able to detect and kill abnormal, transformed cells generated daily in a human body [24, 25]. The cytotoxicity of NK cells is activated after integration of activating and inhibitory signals by a series of surface-specific receptors [26]. The activating signals can be delivered by stress-induced ligands such as pathogen-expressed molecules and abnormal host molecules, and transformed cells. Inhibitory signals are surface molecules expressed by the normal cells of the organism. These inhibitory signals prevent NK cells from killing autologous normal cells (this is the "self-recognition" process). On the contrary, infected and cancer cells usually down-regulate the expression of the inhibitory signals, which, together with the appearance and expression of activating signals, leads to the activation of the cytotoxicity of the NK cells (this is the "non-self-recognition"). Therefore, NK cells are of particular interest for immunocellular therapies, especially for cancer treatments, provided their production in batches compliant with their use in human therapy, both from a quantitative and qualitative point of view [25]. Indeed, these cellular therapies need billions of NK cells to iterate infusions after engraftment, but till now, the selective proliferation of human NK cells is tedious to achieve *ex vivo*. It usually relies upon long cultures of monocyte- and T-cell-depleted PBMCs in medium supplemented with cocktails of cytokines, mitogens, and irradiated feeder cells [27]. Unfortunately, such techniques do not represent economically realistic means for production of large batches of polyclonal NK cells, limiting the development of NK cell–based anti-cancer immunotherapies.

We have shown that the ABP dendrimer promotes the amplification of human NK cells in cultures of PBMCs [18]. One of the cellular events leading to the proliferation of NK cells is the specific inhibition of the proliferation of CD4+ T-lymphocytes by the ABP dendrimer, as these cell populations compete for interleukin(IL)-2, a cytokine needed for their proliferation [28]. In the first series of six healthy donors, our results show that after 4 weeks of *ex vivo* cultures of PBMCs, a mean amplification of the total number of NK cells by a factor 105 was achieved in medium supplemented with IL-2 and 20 µM of the ABP dendrimer, whereas a mean amplification by a factor 7.5 was achieved in medium supplemented with IL-2 alone. Later, we produced a prototype batch of 8.9 billion of NK cells (representing 65% of the total number of cells). We started this culture with 360 million of PBMCs from a healthy volunteer (a normal blood sampling obtained from a French-accredited institution), among which 32 million (*i.e.*, 9%) were NK cells (unpublished results). Therefore, the amplification factor was over 275.

The ABP dendrimer is the first chemical compound proposed so far for the *ex vivo* production of NK cells starting with PBMCs from healthy donors.

12.4 ABP Dendrimer as an Anti-inflammatory New Chemical Entity

12.4.1 ABP Dendrimer Promotes Anti-inflammatory Activation of Monocytes

Mononuclear phagocytes, including monocytes and macrophages, are essential in innate immunity as the first line of defense against bacterial and parasitic infections. They also ensure the commitment of the delayed adaptive immune response. Monocytes/macrophages are a heterogeneous population encompassing a large spectrum of phenotypes from pro-inflammatory to anti-inflammatory responses, depending on the stimulus they receive [29, 30]. Indeed, the activation of macrophages can take several aspects. Besides the classical activation pathway delineated earlier in the 1960s [31], an alternative activation mechanism emerged in the mouse model [32]. The classical activation pathway of macrophages is mediated by interferon (IFN)-γ as primer, and then triggering by TNF or bacterial lipopolysaccharide (LPS). These macrophages produce mediators making them effector cells in Th-1 cellular immune responses [33], and are cytotoxic effectors against intracellular pathogens [34]. The "alternative activation" of macrophages describes closely related phenotypes induced by different stimuli such as IL-4, IL-10, and IL-13 [34, 35] or glucocorticoids [34]. Alternative macrophages appear to be involved in immunosuppression and tissue repair [34]. The closely interlinked pathways of the activation of macrophages, and the intricate responses displayed by these cells, explain the still confusing classification of polarized mononuclear phagocytes [30, 36]. Nevertheless, targeting monocytes and macrophages with pharmacological immunomodulators is acknowledged as a promising track for innovative therapies for a wide range of diseases [37].

Once we discovered that the ABP dendrimer can activate human monocytes [17], we further investigated this activation in more details. Using a pan-genomics approach, we studied the transcriptome of human monocytes activated by the ABP dendrimer in comparison with untreated monocytes. We found that the ABP dendrimer induced an anti-inflammatory activation of monocytes. Among over-expressed genes, mannose receptor (MRC1), immuno-modulatory cytokines (IL-10, IL-19, IL-20, IL-24), IL-1 receptor antagonist (IL-1 ra), metalloproteases (MMP1, MMP10), CD23 antigen, and thioredoxine revealed an anti-inflammatory phenotype of human monocytes activated by the ABP dendrimer. Moreover, we observed a decrease in TGF-β, metallothioneins, and IFN-γ-induced genes, which reinforces an anti-inflammatory signature [38].

These results were confirmed by quantitative RT-PCR studies on mRNAs, which are the most indicative of anti-inflammatory activation (MRC1, IL-1 ra, IL-10, CD23). Those mRNAs were shown to be significantly increased in monocytes treated with the ABP dendrimer (compared to untreated ones), whereas mRNAs of inflammatory activation (IL-1β, IL-6, IL-12) were not modified [38].

Finally, the anti-inflammatory phenotype of monocytes activated by the ABP dendrimer was definitely validated by functional experiments. We demonstrated the capacity of these monocytes to inhibit allogeneic mixed lymphocyte reactions (MLR), which is a consequence of an anti-inflammatory activation [38]. Later, we showed that the ABP dendrimer could also modulate the pro-inflammatory activation of human DC [39].

Dozens of PPH dendrimers of different generations (generation 0, 1, and 2), bearing different terminal surface groups such as sym-metrical and asymmetrical azabisphosphonates, azamonophospho-nates [17, 40], azabiscarboxylates, and azabissulfonates [41, 42], have been synthesized and screened regarding the activation of hu-man monocytes. A series of analogs of the ABP dendrimers varying by the density of azabisphosphonate groups has also been prepared and their bioactivity tested [43]. The ABP dendrimer has emerged as the lead compound among these numerous series. More recently, in an unprecedented study comparing the bioactivity of 13 dendrimers representing seven different families, all bearing azabisphosphonate groups at their surfaces, we have shown that the internal scaffold and the three-dimensional shape of the molecules induced thereof are crucial to have bioactive nanodrugs [44].

12.4.2 Chronic Inflammatory Diseases: An Unmet Clinical Need

Chronic inflammatory diseases (CIDs) are medical conditions characterized by persistent inflammation. Patients develop a CID because the immune system has an inappropriate, uncontrolled response to either endogenous (autoimmunity, ageing) or exogenous (environmental factors) stimuli. People with CIDs undergo a great deal of suffering and invalidating disadvantages. CIDs include, among others, rheumatoid arthritis (RA, prevalence between 0.5 and 1%), psoriasis, inflammatory bowel diseases (IBDs, such as ulcerative colitis and Crohn's disease), atherosclerosis, chronic obstructive pulmonary disease (COPD), and neurodegenerative diseases such as multiple sclerosis (MS, prevalence 0.1%) and Alzheimer's disease (AD, prevalence around 1%, strong increase scheduled in the coming decades). Given the pivotal role of pro-inflammatory (upstream in the inflammatory cascade) and inflammatory (downstream in the inflammatory cascade) cytokines in the onset, development, and persistence of CIDs, tremendous efforts have been made to delineate the cytokine network in each CID, including CIDs of the central nervous system (CNS). Regarding the latter, systemically produced pro-inflammatory mediators (such as TNF-α, IL-1β, and IL-6) normally signal to the brain, leading to the activation of microglial cells (the macrophages of the CNS), which in turn signal to neurons to induce adaptive metabolic and behavioral changes. In healthy persons, this is a normal response of the defense system against infection of the CNS [45]. On the contrary, in patients with chronic neurodegeneration, systemic inflammation leads to sustained inflammatory responses in the brain. Release of inflammatory mediators by microglia fuels a vicious circle of inflammation [46]. Moreover, it was shown in rodent models after peripheral administration of LPS that systemic levels of TNF-α gradually subside over a period of several hours (in serum) to days (in liver), whereas amounts of TNF-α in the brain persist for months [47]. Thus, both systemic and tissue-specific inflammation contribute to neurodegeneration in AD, for instance [48].

Depicting and understanding the hierarchical involvement of pro-inflammatory and inflammatory cytokines in CIDs have led to the development of biological therapeutics: monoclonal antibodies (directed against these cytokines or their receptors) or soluble receptors neutralizing these cytokines to treat CIDs [49]. Although these biotherapies have been highly effective, they have also strong drawbacks essentially regarding secondary risks (increase in infections, malignancies, and cardiac failures) and cost (at least €20,000 per patient per year—*i.e.*, several billions euros only in France—for long-term treatments, which only suspend the disease without curing it, sometimes up to €50,000 per patient per year).

Overall, CIDs represent a major medical, scientific, social, and economic challenge for all industrialized countries in which lifespan has continuously increased over the last century, strengthening the global problem raised in developed societies with regard to ageing and healthcare costs.

12.4.3 Proofs of Efficacy of ABP Dendrimer in Mouse Models of CIDs

After showing that the ABP dendrimer skews human monocytes toward an anti-inflammatory activation *ex vivo* [38], we challenged its immunomodulatory and anti-inflammatory properties in rodent models of inflammatory diseases. We have chosen experimental arthritis (relevant to RA) and experimental autoimmune encephalomyelitis (EAE, relevant to MS) in mice, and endotoxin (LPS)-induced uveitis (EIU) in rat as preclinical models.

A model of spontaneous arthritis provoked by the absence of IL-1 receptor antagonist (IL-1 ra) appeared as particularly interesting. Mice knocked-out for IL-1 ra (IL-1 ra-/-) develop arthritis as early as 6 weeks of age. TNF-α is of crucial importance in the physiopathology of this model [50], as in RA. We assayed the effect of the ABP dendrimer in this mouse model. Starting at 8 weeks of age (thus with a developing arthritis, green arrow on the X-axis of the left graph in Fig. 12.2), mice were treated weekly with 10 mg/kg of the ABP dendrimer administered intravenously. A severity clinical score was established from 0 to 3 for each paw. The assay ended after 12 weeks (week 20) due to the necessity of sacrificing untreated mice because of the severity of their disease. On the contrary, inflammation and arthritis were resolved in treated mice (Fig. 12.2) [51]. This dramatic effect of the ABP dendrimer was also observed with 1 mg/kg of dendrimer (not shown). Moreover, we have shown that when the ABP dendrimer is administered orally at 10 mg/kg, the inflammation and arthritis were also resolved in treated mice, with a delay of a few weeks when compared to intravenous administration [52].

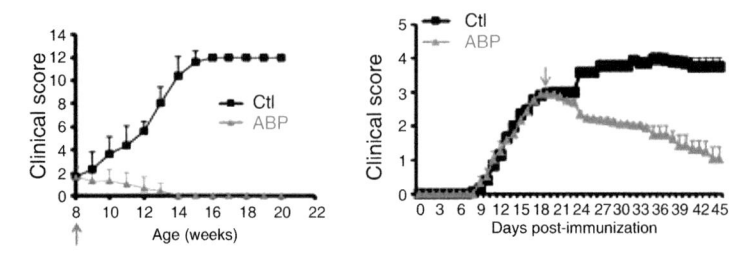

Figure 12.2 Proofs of the efficacy of the ABP dendrimer in two mouse models of CIDs (experimental arthritis on the left, EAE on the right). The graphs give the evolution of the clinical scores of the diseases *versus* time (age of the mice for experimental arthritis, the days post-immunization for EAE, respectively). Clinical scores are evaluated as indicated in Refs. [51] and [53].

During assays testing decreasing doses of the ABP dendrimer (from 10 mg/kg to 1 µg/kg), we followed up the concentration of pro-inflammatory cytokines (IL-1β, IL-6, TNF-α, and IL-17) in the serum of dendrimer-treated IL-1 ra-/- mice, untreated IL-1 ra-/- mice, and healthy controls (Balb/c mice). For these four cytokines, their concentrations in the serum of IL-1 ra-/- mice treated with 1 and 10 mg/kg of the ABP dendrimer decreased to the level of the concentrations in healthy control mice. This indicates that the ABP dendrimer controls the systemic inflammation in this model. We have also shown that the ABP dendrimer is able to mitigate the secretion of matrix metalloproteases, thereby protecting cartilage from degradation [51].

Monocytes can be differentiated *in vitro* into osteoclasts (OC, which are giant multinucleated cells) in the presence of M-CSF and RANK-L. In bone physiology, the role of OC is to degrade the bone matrix then regenerated by osteoblasts. In some pathological contexts, including arthritis, the balance between osteoclastic and osteoblastic activities is tilted toward OC: this causes bone erosion. We have found that the ABP dendrimer inhibits the differentiation of OC in the IL-1 ra-/- mouse model [51]. We have also shown that the ABP dendrimer (at 20 nM and 200 nM) added to the culture inhibits the differentiation of human OC *ex vivo* (Fig. 12.3).

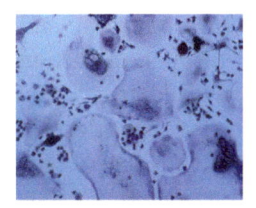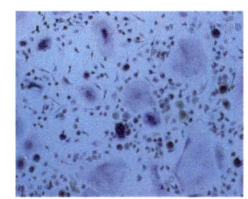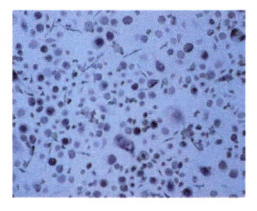

Figure 12.3 Inhibition of the differentiation of human monocytes in OC *ex vivo*. Left: control culture without the ABP dendrimer showing giant multinucleated cells which are OC; central and right: inhibition of the differentiation of OC by 20 nM and 200 nM of the ABP dendrimer, respectively.

This first preclinical *in vivo* study has been positively highlighted by the scientific and business communities [54–57].

EAE is an inflammatory disease of the CNS that shares clinical and immunopathological similarities with MS. The model we have chosen is the classical model of active EAE induced by an immunization against myelin oligodendrocyte protein (MOG) peptide 35–55 in mice [58]. This leads to a chronic, progressive form of EAE resembling MS. Therefore, it is considered a good preclinical model. Disease severity is scored on a clinical scale of 0 to 5 (0 being no detectable sign of EAE, 4 being tetraparalysis, and 5 moribund or death). After MOG immunization, EAE scores for motor functions have been evaluated daily for 45 days for each animal. A preventive protocol and a therapeutic protocol have been set up. In both cases, mice are immunized with the MOG peptide at Day 0. In the preventive protocol, intravenous administration of 10 mg/kg of the ABP dendrimer started at Day 1, and then every 3 days (not shown). In the therapeutic protocol, administration of the ABP dendrimer started once the disease is established at Day 18 (green arrow on the right graph in Fig. 12.2) and was continued under the same conditions as the preventive protocol.

We have shown that the ABP dendrimer inhibits accumulation of antigen-presenting cells (APCs) in the spleen under inflammatory conditions and prevents APC activation; however, the specific molecular targets are not yet known. We have also shown that several cellular mechanisms of action of the ABP dendrimer are operating *in vivo* in the mouse model of EAE: (i) the ABP dendrimer skews the cytokine production by splenocytes from immunized mice from an inflammatory pattern to an anti-inflammatory one; (ii) it redirects myelin-specific CD4 T-cell response toward IL-10 production; and (iii) the latter effect is, at least in part, indirect through the action of the ABP dendrimer on APCs. Taken together, these data strongly suggest that the ABP dendrimer, by down-regulating the activity of APCs, could strongly impact the pathogenic profile of CD4+ T cells interacting with these APCs. Consequently, autoreactive CD4+ T cells produce lesser amount of Th1/Th17 cytokines and are redirected to produce IL-10 [53].

It is noteworthy that the cellular effects of the ABP dendrimer depicted both in experimental arthritis [51] and EAE [53] mouse models strictly correlate to our former observations on human immune cells [28, 38].

EIU is a robust model of acute inflammation. Whereas in arthritis and EAE models the ABP dendrimer was administered systematically, the EIU model gave us the opportunity to administer loco-regionally by the intravitreal route. This study shows that there is a good ocular tolerability of the ABP dendrimer (in non-diseased control animals) that the ABP dendrimer resolves EIU by mediating systemic IL-10 production, likely by targeting the monocyte/macrophage lineage [59]. On the all, we have shown the ABP dendrimer is also a potential drug candidate for inflammatory disorders in ophthalmology.

12.5 Prospects toward "First-in-Man" Clinical Trial

12.5.1 Nanotoxicity

Along with the discussion of their enormous technological and economic potential, a debate about new and specific risks related to nanotechnologies has started. Due to their small size, the properties of nanoparticles (NPs), including dendrimers, not only differ from bulk material of the same composition but also show different interaction patterns with the living organisms. A risk assessment for bulk materials is, therefore, not sufficient to characterize the same material in NP forms. The implications of the special properties of NPs have not yet been fully taken into account by regulators: *e.g.*, size effects are not addressed in the framework of the new European chemicals policy REACH (Registration, Evaluation, Authorization and restriction of CHemicals). NPs raise a number of safety and regulatory issues that governments are now trying to tackle. In 2006, the FDA established the Nanotechnology Task Force to address ways to evaluate nano-products. Since 2009, the European (EMA), American (FDA), and Japanese agencies (PMDA) have worked together to achieve common perspectives for the development of nano-products. Nevertheless, at the international level, the development and manufacturing of nano-products are still regulated by the same ICH guidelines (Q8 for Pharmaceutical development, Q9 for Quality Risk Management, and Q10 for Pharmaceutical Quality System) than classical drugs. The regulatory agencies currently use pre-existing regulatory standards and statutes to regulate nanomedicines [60, 61]. They are fighting to accumulate data and establish testing criteria and agree that further basic research is necessary [60, 62, 63]. Studies on (i) the genotoxic, immunotoxic, hemolytic, carcinogenic, and teratogenic effects of the bioaccumulation and biopersistence of NPs in the human body and (ii) the ecotoxicity of NPs (linked to their manufacturing and potential use in animal health) need a strong involvement of stakeholders—authorities, industrialists, and researchers—to go far beyond the current state of the art.

Regarding their potential applications in the biomedical field, the potential toxicity of dendrimers has questioned the researchers for a long time [64]. Although toxicity studies in non-human primate (NHP) models are not required by regulatory agencies, the use of an NHP model is a crucial step, impossible to circumvent, to evaluate the risks of immunotoxicity induced by therapeutic combinations based on the use of immunomodulatory molecules (assessment of the life-threatening "cytokine storm"). Indeed, the phylogenetic distance between rodents and human represents a limit to adapt to humans the data only gathered in rodent models [65]. Therefore, to mitigate the risk in the preclinical and upcoming clinical developments of the ABP dendrimer, we have assessed the general toxicity and the immunosafety of this drug candidate in *Macaca fascicularis* (cynomolgus monkey). Four monkeys were injected intravenously, once weekly, with 10 mg/kg of the ABP dendrimer during 4 weeks. Each animal was its own control as they had been followed 21 days before the first injection. Then, the toxicity study was set up during the four injections, and 15 days after the last one. Therefore, the whole study was spread over a duration of 56 days. To our knowledge, this was the first time that a dendrimer was administered by a systemic route to NHPs. The animals well tolerated the treatment. All the clinical, biochemical, hematological, and immunological parameters assessed during the study were kept in physiological ranges. Some time-limited mild variations of a few parameters were registered; however, the values went back to normal numbers within 2 or 3 days, and no cumulative effect was noticed during the repeated injections of the ABP dendrimer. The final histopathological analyses of the main thoracic and abdomen organs did not reveal the systemic toxicity of the molecule. The *ex vivo* immunological studies showed that no immunosuppression was induced by the ABP dendrimer during the assay [66].

12.5.2 Perspectives and Hopes

In July 2003, the FDA allowed the first clinical trials of a dendrimer-based pharmaceutical: VivaGel®, a topical microbicide for the prevention of HIV infection in women, developed by the Australian company Starpharma Holdings Ltd. Phase I clinical trials have been successfully completed [67], and now VivaGel is in Phase II clinical trial (search for "SPL7013 and HIV Infections" at www.clinicaltrials.gov). In the European Union (EU), none of dendrimer-based therapeutics is in clinical trial in humans. An observation from which one can conclude that the advent of dendrimer-based nanobiotechnology for human health is a failure [68].

After more than 10 years of a fruitful collaborative project of basic research between chemists and biologists, the ABP dendrimer is now facing the regulatory preclinical requirements regarding the following:

  (i) CMC: Chemical-manufacturing-control
 (ii) ADME-T: Absorption-distribution-metabolism-excretion – toxicity

Acknowledgments

We thank INSERM, CNRS, and the University of Toulouse for institutional funding. We thank the French "Institut National du Cancer" (INCa), the "Etablissement Français du Sang" (EFS), the "Midi-Pyrénées" region, the French "Agence Nationale de la

Recherche" (ANR), the French agency "OSEO", and the French "Fondation pour la Recherche Médicale" (FRM) for having granted several of our projects since 2004.

References

1. Buhleier, E., Wehner, W., and Vögtle, F. (1978). Cascade-chain-like and nonskid-chain-like syntheses of molecular cavity topologies, *Synthesis*, **2**, pp. 155–158.

2. Vögtle, F. and Weber, E. (1974). Octopus molecules, *Angew. Chem. Int. Ed.*, **13**, pp. 814–816.

3. Hyatt, J. A. (1978). Octopus molecules in the cyclotriveratrylene series, *J. Org. Chem.*, **43**, pp. 1808–1811.

4. Menjoge, A. R., Kannan, R. M., and Tomalia, D. A. (2010). Dendrimer-based drug and imaging conjugates: Design considerations for nanomedical applications, *Drug Discov. Today*, **15**, pp. 171–185.

5. Lee, C. C., MacKay, J. A., Fréchet, J. M. J., and Szoka, F. C. (2005). Designing dendrimers for biological applications, *Nat. Biotechnol.*, **23**, pp. 1517–1526.

6. Liu, X. and Peng, L. (2016). Dendrimer nanovectors for SiRNA delivery, *Methods Mol. Biol.*, **1364**, pp. 127–142.

7. Lim, J., Kostiainen, M., Maly, J., da Costa, V. C. P., Annunziata, O., Pavan, G. M., and Simanek, E. E. (2013). Synthesis of large dendrimers with the dimensions of small viruses, *J. Am. Chem. Soc.*, **135**, pp. 4660–4663.

8. Wagner, V., Dullaart, A., Bock, A. K., and Zweck, A. (2006). The emerging nanomedicine landscape, *Nat. Biotechnol.*, **24**, pp. 1211–1217.

9. Mammen, M., Choi, S. K., and Whitesides, G. M. (1998). Polyvalent interactions in biological systems: Implications for design and use of multivalent ligands and inhibitors, *Angew. Chem. Int. Ed.*, **37**, pp. 2754–2794.

10. Varner, C. T., Rosen, T., Martin, J. T., and Kane, R. S. (2015). Recent advances in engineering polyvalent biological interactions, *Biomacromolecules*, **16**, pp. 43–55.

11. Jiang, W., Kim, B. Y. S., Rutka, J. T., and Chan, W. C. W. (2008). Nanoparticle-mediated cellular response is size-dependent, *Nat. Nanotechnol.*, **3**, pp. 145–150.

12. Rolland, O., Turrin, C. O., Caminade, A. M., and Majoral, J. P. (2009). Dendrimer and nanomedicine: Multivalency in action, *New J. Chem.*, **33**, pp. 1809–1824.

13. Espinosa, E., Belmant, C., Sicard, H., Poupot, R., Bonneville, M., and Fournié, J. J. (2001). Y2K+1 state-of-the-art or non-peptide phosphoantigens, a novel category of immunostimulatory molecules, *Microbes Infect.*, **3**, pp. 645–654.

14. Martinet, L., Poupot, R., and Fournié, J. J. (2009). Pitfalls on the roadmap to γδ T cell-based cancer immunotherapies, *Immunol. Lett.*, **124**, pp. 1–8.

15. Constant, P., Davodeau, F., Peyrat, M. A., Poquet, Y., Puzo, G., Bonneville, M., and Fournié, J. J. (1994). Stimulation of human gamma delta T cells by nonpeptidic mycobacterial ligands, *Science*, **264**, pp. 267–270.

16. Belmant, C., Espinosa, E., Halary, F., Tang, Y., Peyrat, M. A., Sicard, H., Kozikowski, A., Buelow, R., Poupot, R., Bonneville, M., and Fournié, J. J. (2000). A chemical basis for selective recognition of nonpeptide antigens by human γδ T cells, *FASEB J.*, **14**, pp. 1669–1670.

17. Poupot, M., Griffe, L., Marchand, P., Maraval, A., Rolland, O., Martinet, L., L'Faqihi-Olive, F. E., Turrin, C. O., Caminade, A. M., Fournié, J. J., Majoral, J. P., and Poupot, R. (2006). Design of phosphorylated dendritic architectures to promote human monocyte activation, *FASEB J.*, **20**, pp. 2339–2351.

18. Griffe, L., Poupot, M., Marchand, P., Maraval, A., Turrin, C. O., Rolland, O., Métivier, P., Bacquet, G., Fournié, J. J., Caminade, A. M., Poupot, R., and Majoral, J. P. (2007). Multiplication of human Natural Killer cells by nanosized phosphonate-capped dendrimers, *Angew. Chem. Int. Ed.*, **46**, pp. 2523–2526.

19. Pont, F., Familiades, J., Déjean, S., Fruchon, S., Cendron, D., Poupot, M., Poupot, R., L'Faqihi-Olive, F., Prade, N., Ycart, B., and Fournié, J. J. (2012). The gene expression profile of phosphoantigen-specific human γδ T lymphocytes is a blend of αβ T cell and NK cell signatures, *Eur. J. Immunol.*, **42**, pp. 228–240.

20. Waggoner, S. N., Reighard, S. D., Gyurova, I. E., Cranert, S. A., Mahl, S. E., Karmele, E. P., McNally, J. P., Moran, M. T., Brooks, T. R., Yaqoob, F., and Rydyznski, C. E. (2015). Roles of natural killer cells in antiviral immunity, *Curr. Opin. Virol.*, **16**, pp. 15–23.

21. Adib-Conquy, M., Scott-Algara, D., Cavaillon, J. M., and Souza-Fonseca-Guimaraes, F. (2014). TLR-mediated activation of NK cells and their role in bacterial/viral immune responses in mammals, *Immunol. Cell. Biol.*, **92**, pp. 256–262.

22. Bogdan, C. (2012). Natural killer cells in experimental and human leishmaniasis, *Front. Cell. Infect. Microbiol.*, **2**, pp. 69.

23. Shekkar, S. and Yang, X. (2015). Natural killer cells in host defense against veterinary pathogens, *Vet. Immunol. Immunopathol.*, **168**, pp. 30–34.

24. Pahl, J. and Cerwenka, A. (2017). Tricking the balance: NK cells in anti-cancer immunity, *Immunobiology*, **222**, pp. 11–20.

25. Rezvani, K. and Rouce, R. H. (2015). The application of natural killer cell immunotherapy for the treatment of cancer, *Front. Immunol.*, **6**, pp. 578.

26. Long, E. O., Sim Kim, H., Liu, D., Peterson, M. E., and Rajagopalan, S. (2013). Controlling natural killer cell responses: Integration of signals for activation and inhibition, *Annu. Rev. Immunol.*, **31**, pp. 227–258.

27. Childs, R. W. and Carlsten, M. (2015). Therapeutic approaches to enhance natural killer cell cytotoxicity against cancer: The force awakens, *Nat. Rev. Drug Discov.*, **14**, pp. 487–498.

28. Portevin, D., Poupot, M., Rolland, O., Turrin, C. O., Fournié, J. J., Majoral, J. P., Caminade, A. M., and Poupot, R. (2009). Regulatory activity of azabisphosphonate-capped dendrimers on human CD4+ T cell proliferation enhances ex-vivo expansion of NK cells from PBMCs for immunotherapy, *J. Transl. Med.*, **7**, pp. 82.

29. Gordon, S., Plüddemann, A., and Martinez-Estrada, F. (2014). Macrophage heterogeneity in tissues: Phenotypic diversity and functions, *Immunol. Rev.*, **262**, pp. 36–55.

30. Sica, A. and Mantovani, A. (2012). Macrophage plasticity and polarization: In vivo veritas, *J. Clin. Invest.*, **122**, pp. 787–795.

31. Mackaness, G. B. (1964). The immunological basis of acquired cellular resistance, *J. Exp. Med.*, **120**, pp. 105–120.

32. Stein, M., Keshav, S., Harris, N., and Gordon, S. (1992). Interleukin 4 potently enhances murine macrophage mannose receptor activity: A marker of alternative immunologic macrophage activation, *J. Exp. Med.*, **176**, pp. 287–292.

33. Mantovani, A., Sica, A., Sozzani, S., Allavena, P., Vecchi, A., and Locati, M. (2004). The chemokine system in diverse forms of macrophage activation and polarization, *Trends Immunol.*, **25**, pp. 677–686.

34. Mosser, D. M. (2003). The many faces of macrophage activation, *J. Leukoc. Biol.* **73**, pp. 209–212.

35. Gordon, S. (2003). Alternative activation of macrophages, *Nat. Rev. Immunol.*, **3**, pp. 23–35.

36. Italiani, P. and Boraschi, D. (2014). From monocytes to M1/M2 macrophages: Phenotypical vs. functional differentiation, *Front. Immunol.*, **5**, pp. 514.

37. Mantovani, A., Vecchi, A., and Allavena, P. (2014). Pharmacological modulation of monocytes and macrophages, *Curr. Opin. Pharmacol.*, **17**, pp. 38–44.

38. Fruchon, S., Poupot, M., Martinet, L., Turrin, C. O., Majoral, J. P., Fournié, J. J., Caminade, A. M., and Poupot, R. (2009). Anti-inflammatory and immuno-suppressive activation of human monocytes by a bio-active dendrimer, *J. Leukoc. Biol.*, **85**, pp. 553–562.

39. Degboé, Y., Fruchon, S., Baron, M., Nigon, D., Turrin, C. O., Caminade, A. M., Poupot, R., Cantagrel, A., and Davignon, J. L. (2014). Modulation of pro-inflammatory activation of monocytes and dendritic cells by aza-bis-phosphonate dendrimer as an experimental therapeutic agent, *Arthritis Res. Ther.*, **16**, pp. R98.

40. Marchand, P., Griffe, L., Poupot, M., Turrin, C. O., Bacquet, G., Fournié, J. J., Majoral, J. P., Poupot, R., and Caminade, A. M. (2009). Dendrimers ended by non-symmetrical azadiphosphonate groups: Synthesis and immunological properties, *Bioorg. Med. Chem. Lett.*, **19**, pp. 3963–3966.

41. Ledall, J., Fruchon, S., Garzoni, M., Pavan, G. M., Caminade, A. M., Turrin, C. O., Blanzat, M., and Poupot, R. (2015). Interaction studies reveal specific recognition of an anti-inflammatory polyphosphorhydrazone dendrimer by human monocytes, *Nanoscale*, **7**, pp. 17672–17684.

42. Rolland, O., Turrin, C. O., Bacquet, G., Poupot, R., Poupot, M., Caminade, A. M., and Majoral, J. P. (2009). Efficient synthesis of phosphorus-containing dendrimers capped with isosteric functions of amino-bis(methylene) phosphonic acids, *Tetrahedron Lett.*, **50**, pp. 2078–2082.

43. Rolland, O., Griffe, L., Poupot, M., Maraval, A., Ouali, A., Coppel, Y., Fournié, J. J., Bacquet, G., Turrin, C. O., Caminade, A. M., Majoral, J. P., and Poupot, R. (2008). Tailored control and optimization of the number of phosphonic acid termini on phosphorus-containing dendrimers for the ex-vivo activation of human monocytes, *Chem. Eur. J.*, **14**, pp. 4836–4850.

44. Caminade, A. M., Fruchon, S., Turrin, C. O., Poupot, M., Ouali, A., Maraval, A., Garzoni, M., Maly, M., Furer, V., Kovalenko, V., Majoral, J. P., Pavan, G. M., and Poupot, R. (2015). The key role of the scaffold on the efficiency of dendrimer nanodrugs, *Nature Commun.*, **6**, pp. 7722.

45. Teeling, J. L. and Perry, V. H. (2009). Systemic infection and inflammation in acute CNS injury and chronic neurodegeneration: Underlying mechanisms, *Neuroscience*, **158**, pp. 1062–1073.

46. van Gool, W. A., van de Beek, D., and Eikelenboom, P. (2010). Systemic infection and delirium: When cytokines and acetylcholine collide, *Lancet*, **375**, pp. 773–775.

47. Qin, L., Wu, X., Block, M. L., Liu, Y., Breese, G. R., Hong, J. S., Knapp, D. J., and Crews, F. T. (2007). Systemic LPS causes chronic neuroinflammation and progressive neurodegeneration, *Glia*, **55**, pp. 453–462.

48. Franck-Cannon, T. C., Alto, L. T., McAlpine, F. E., and Tansey, M. G. (2009). Does neuroinflammation fan the flame in neurodegenerative diseases? *Mol. Neurodegener.*, **4**, pp. 47.

49. Kopf, M., Bachmann, M. F., and Marsland, B. J. (2010). Averting inflammation by targeting the cytokine environment, *Nat. Rev. Drug Discov.*, **9**, pp. 703–718.

50. Horai, R., Nakajima, A., Habiro, K., Kotani, M., Nakae, S., Matsuki, T., Nambu, A., Saijo, S., Kotaki, H., Sudo, K., Okahara, A., Tanioka, H., Ikuse, T., Ishii, N., Schwartzberg, P. L., Abe, R., and Iwakura, Y. (2004). TNF-alpha is crucial for the development of autoimmune arthritis in IL-1 receptor antagonist-deficient mice, *J. Clin. Invest.*, **114**, pp. 1603–1611.

51. Hayder, M., Poupot, M., Baron, M., Nigon, D., Turrin, C. O., Caminade, A. M., Majoral, J. P., Eisenberg, R. A., Fournié, J. J., Cantagrel, A., Poupot, R., and Davignon, J. L. (2011). A phosphorus-based dendrimer targets inflammation and osteoclastogenesis in experimental arthritis, *Sci. Transl. Med.*, **3**, pp. 81ra35.

52. Hayder, M., Poupot, M., Baron, M., Turrin, C. O., Caminade, A. M., Majoral, J. P., Eisenberg, R. A., Fournié, J. J., Cantagrel, A., Poupot, R., and Davignon, J. L. (2012). Frequency and route of administration in the treatment of experimental arthritis by phosphorus-based dendrimer, *Ann. Rheum. Dis.*, **71** (Suppl. 1), pp. A8.

53. Hayder, M., Varilh, M., Turrin, C. O., Saoudi, A., Caminade, A. M., Poupot R., and Liblau, R. S. (2015). Phosphorus-based dendrimer ABP treats neuroinflammation by promoting IL-10-producing CD4+ T cells, *Biomacromolecules*, **16**, pp. 3425–3433.

54. Bosch, X. (2011). Dendrimers to treat rheumatoid arthritis, *ACS Nano*, **5**, pp. 6779–6785.

55. Leah, E. (2011). Experimental arthritis: Dendrimer drug mends monocytes, *Nat. Rev. Rheumatol.*, **7**, pp. 376.

56. Lou, K. J. (2011). Dendrimer throws a blanket on RA, *SciBX*, **4**, doi:10.1038/scibx.2011.561.

57. Wolf, L. K. (2011). Dendrimer treats joint inflammation, *Chem. Eng. News*, **89**, pp. 39.

58. Delarasse, C., Daubas, P., Mars, L. T., Vizler, C., Litzenburger, T., Iglesias, A., Bauer, J., Della Gaspera, B., Schubart, A., Decker, L., Dimitri, D., Roussel, G., Dierich, A., Amor, S., Dautigny, A., Liblau, R., and Pham-Dinh, D. (2003). Myelin/oligodendrocyte glycoprotein-deficient (MOG-deficient) mice reveal lack of immune tolerance to MOG in wild-type mice, *J. Clin. Invest.*, **112**, pp. 544–553.

59. Fruchon, S., Caminade, A. M., Abadie, C., Davignon, J. L., Combette, J. M., Turrin, C. O., and Poupot, R. (2013). An azabisphosphonate-capped poly(phosphorhydrazone) dendrimer for the treatment of endotoxin-induced uveitis, *Molecules*, **18**, pp. 9305–9316.

60. Ehmann, F., Sakai-Kato, K., Duncan, R., Hernán Pérez de la Ossa, D., Pita, R., Vidal, J. M., Kohli, A., Tothfalusi, L., Sanh, A., Tinton, S., Robert, J. L., Silva Lima, B., and Amati, M. P. (2013). Next-generation nanomedicines and nanosimilars: EU regulators' initiatives relating to the development and evaluation of nanomedicines, *Nanomedicine (Lond.)*, **8**, pp. 849–856.

61. Hamburg, M. A. (2012). FDA's approach to regulation of products of nanotechnology, *Science*, **336**, pp. 299–300.

62. FDA Nanotechnology Regulatory Science Research Plan, www.fda.gov/ ScienceResearch/SpecialTopics/Nanotechnology/ucm273325.htm.

63. Nanomedicine Initiative Project, www.pmda.go.jp/english/rs-sb-std/ standards-development/cross-sectional-project/0008.html#r=s&r=s.

64. Jain, K., Kesharwani, P., Gupta, U., and Jain, N. K. (2010). Dendrimer toxicity: Let's meet the challenge, *Int. J. Pharm.*, **394**, pp. 122–142.

65. Mestas, J. and Hughes, C. C. (2004). Of mice and not men: Differences between mouse and human immunology, *J. Immunol.*, **172**, pp. 2731–2738.

66. Fruchon, S., Mouriot, S., Thiollier, T., Grandin, C., Caminade, A. M., Turrin, C. O., Contamin, H., and Poupot, R. (2015). Repeated intravenous injections in non-human primates demonstrate preclinical safety of an anti-inflammatory phosphorus-based dendrimer, *Nanotoxicology*, **9**, pp. 933–941.

67. McGowan, I., Gomez, K., Bruder, K., Febo, I., Chen, B. A., Richardson, B. A., Husnik, M., Livant, E., Price, C., Jacobson, C., and MTN-004 Protocol Team (2011). Phase 1 randomized trial of the vaginal safety and

acceptability of SPL7013 (VivaGel®) in sexually active young women (MTN-004), *AIDS*, **25**, pp. 1057–1064.

68. Svenson, S. (2015). The dendrimer paradox: High medical expectations but poor clinical translation, *Chem. Soc. Rev.*, **44**, pp. 4131–4144.

Chapter 13

Dendrimer Space Concept: A Futuristic Vision in Nanomedicine to Develop New Drugs

Serge Mignani[a] and Jean-Pierre Majoral[b]

[a]Université Paris Descartes, PRES Sorbonne Paris Cité, CNRS UMR 860,
Laboratoire de Chimie et de Biochimie pharmacologiques et toxicologique,
45, rue des Saints Pères, 75006 Paris, France
[b]Laboratoire de Chimie de Coordination du CNRS, 205 route de Narbonne,
31077 Toulouse Cedex 4, France
serge.mignani@parisdescartes.fr

The emergence of nanotechnology has significantly impacted the drug-delivery field with many applications in clinical medicine and pharmaceutical research. In this area, dendrimer nanostructures represent outstanding nanocarriers in nanomedicine, and they have often been referred to as the "Polymers of the 21st century." The main potential advantages of dendrimers in medicinal chemistry can be well defined within a new concept. For this aim, we proposed the dendrimer space concept, per analogy with the chemistry and

Phosphorus Dendrimers in Biology and Nanomedicine: Synthesis, Characterization, and Properties
Edited by Anne-Marie Caminade, Cédric-Olivier Turrin, and Jean-Pierre Majoral
Copyright © 2018 Pan Stanford Publishing Pte. Ltd.
ISBN 978-981-4774-33-8 (Hardcover), 978-1-315-11085-1 (eBook)
www.panstanford.com

biology space concepts, which are extensively used in pharmaceutical industry to develop new drugs. This new concept represents a powerful exploration tool for chemists (*e.g.*, visualization, mapping, and traveling) of both the vast chemical and biological spaces to find new biologically active compounds and then to develop original drugs.

13.1 Introduction

The principal goal of pharmaceutical companies is the discovery and development of novel medicines that satisfy unmet patient needs. Generally speaking, these medicines consist not only in offering new treatments of currently untreated diseases but also in the improvement of treatments of diseases with safer and more efficacious drugs than the existing, including generic drugs [1], biosimilar antibodies, and very recently generics of nanodevice medicines [2]. For several decades, the sector has suffered from major issues such as reduction in the number of new chemical entities (NCEs) and biologics [3] FDA approved, reduction in R&D budgets, and increase in global R&D costs. While we rely heavily on this industry in terms of our healthcare, pharmaceuticals is a business and must make a return on its investment to survive [4].

There is a strong correlation between the lack of productivity of the pharmaceutical industry, as visualized by the number of NCEs approved, and the low clinical success rate. This trend could be related to two main factors, including the quantity of the small-molecule drug candidates and their quality [5]. Consequently, the likelihood of success could be enhanced by increasing the number of clinical candidates that possess an optimal/acceptable physicochemical profile, which plays a crucial role in the attrition of drug candidates [6]. Parameters such as absorption, distribution, metabolism, excretion, and toxicity (named ADMET) can be evaluated using *in vitro* and *in vivo* prediction screens and/or in silico by computational ADMET studies [7]. In addition, understanding the role of physicochemical properties in the attrition of drug candidates and drug development is crucial to developing new active chemical entities [8]. Very recently, an excellent review has been published by

Yusof *et al.* for practical compound prioritization decisions based on the application of multiparameter rules [9].

Importantly, today, traditional Lipinski's criteria/guidelines (called rule of 5, Ro5) are widely used by the medicinal chemistry community to predict not only the oral absorption of compounds, but also overall drug-likeness [10]. Additional parameters determining favorable oral bioavailability are as follows: fully rotatable bonds <5 and polar surface area (PsA) <140Å^2 (blood–brain barrier penetration: <80Å^2) [11]. Ro5 provides suitable information about absorption or permeation, thus helping to reduce the attrition rate at later pre-market stages.

The term "drug-like" corresponds to specific compound properties that confer to these molecules to become successful drug products. Consequently, drug-like characteristics allow to qualify or disqualify compounds for further development phase. For instance, PK, toxicity, and solubility issues need to be addressed in the early development phases in order to decrease the clinical failures due to shifted issues to patients such as poor drug absorption, inadequate dosage regimens, metabolic instability, etc. [12]. The concept of Ro5 represents a good vision of "drug-likeness" and "druggability" predictions and has been extended to proteins and genes for target identification and selection [13], and for difficult targets named "beyond rule of five (called bRo5)" [14]. Other drug-likeness criteria included chemical diversity [15], privileged structures for drug discovery [16], favorable physical and metabolic properties [17], fraction of carbons that is *sp^3* hybridized [18], and the number of aromatic rings [19]. Recently, Hopkins *et al.* described a new quantitative estimation of drug-likeness score (called QED) [20]. This drug-likeness parameter represents a single measure of the distance from Ro5. Based on the chemico-biological space of the 2P2I dataset, Morelli *et al.* calculated the general characteristics of protein–protein interaction inhibitors (PPI) by defining a specific cluster inside the vast chemical space as the "Rules-of-Four" (Ro4) [21]. Generic profile of a PPI inhibitor follows the following criteria: MW > 400 Da, log P > 4, number of rings >4, and number of hydrogen bond acceptors > 4. In an interesting article, Zeneca's Edfeld *et al.* analyzed the druggability (so-called ligandability) of 36 drug-discovery projects for lead discovery success based on fragment screening *versus* HTS approaches [22].

In parallel to the use of quality compound criteria, the optimization guidelines have been used as sequential filters to select compounds [23]. This process consists in comparing the new compounds to a series of criteria: those that fail to meet a criterion are discarded, while those that meet the criterion are progressed forward for comparison against the next criterion in the sequence. One or more "ideal" compounds will emerge from the sequence of filters. Common filters include criteria relating to potency, selectivity, hydrophobicity, solubility, molecular weight (MW), number of aromatic ring [24], ADMET parameters (Caco-2 permeability, intrinsic clearance), cytochrome PE50 interaction, and hERG [25].

13.2 Continuum Chemical Space

One of the foremost challenges in drug discovery is the identification and expansion of chemical areas that contain specific biologically active compounds with adequate physicochemical or topological properties. The estimated number of existing individual molecules below 500 Da in weight—chemical space—that present a possible interest for drug discovery is in excess of 10^{60} [26]. The numbers of commercially available and patent literature compounds are estimated at approximately 10^7 and 10^8, respectively [27]. Thus, the exploration and the multidimensional analysis of novel discrete areas within the vast chemical diversity of this chemical space remain a fundamental challenge shared by academic, pharmaceutical, and agrochemical researchers in the discovery of original classes of active derivatives [28]. Thus, in medicinal chemistry, these molecularly diverse discrete areas are associated with the following specific characteristics/descriptors such as: (1) the biological activities of diverse "target classes," *e.g.*, kinase space, phosphatase space, GPCRs chemical space, protease chemical space, protein–protein interactions, etc. and (2) drug-like chemical space (Ro5 , *vide supra*) lead-like chemical space (Oprea's criteria for lead-likeness, called Ro4) [29], fragment chemical space (criteria for fragments, called the rule-of-three, Ro3) [30], most popular building blocks (called the rule-of-two, Ro2) [31], natural product chemical space [32], and commercial library chemical space (existing and virtual compounds)

[33]. Interestingly, Hajduk *et al.* discussed the potential utility of several strategies based on bioinformatic approaches for predicting protein druggability [34]. Prediction tools of druggability have been developed to prioritize therapeutic targets [35] and to evaluate the druggability of binding site pockets [36]. Also, Oprea highlighted the use of the chemical global positioning system (ChemGPS) as an attractive chemography approach that combines 72 crucial eADMET descriptors to afford scores [37].

Generally, today almost all medicinal chemists ubiquitously agree on the crucial importance of identifying good chemical starting points for lead optimization, library construction, etc. based on Ro2, Ro3, Ro4, and Ro5 (*vide supra*). Interestingly, Oprea *et al.* analyzed and defined 3D descriptor space of biologically active and non-active hit-like cancer compounds such as genotoxic, kinase inhibitors, proteasome inhibitors, and antimitotic agents. These in silico chemoinformatic filters are based on Ro5 and Ro3 [38] or specific chemical structures [39].

One of the utmost important challenges of drug discoverers is to identify and expand chemical areas that contain specific biologically active derivatives with adequate physicochemical or topological properties. Thus, the concept of boundaries of the continuum chemical space, the navigation and the exploration inside this vast space has been outstandingly pointed out by Lipinski [26]. The far-ranging goal is to identify new, discrete chemical regions (called clusters, subfractions,...) in order to find and develop original drugs, especially for challenging targets. The relationship between the continuum of chemical space and several clusters occupied by biological compounds with specific mechanism of action is represented in Fig. 13.1. These different spaces are mapped onto coordinates of chemical descriptors based on physicochemical or topological properties. Thus, for instance, oral drug-like space based on Ro5 parameters can be used. These criteria determine the boundaries of each chemical cluster and are used as early-stage tool filters to select appropriate potential druggable final drugs. The overlapping of the drug-likeness chemical space continuum (Ro5) and the 2D "target classes," including, for instance, PPI space, kinase space, a "poor" druggable target, etc., defined an overlap volume (truncated space) for which all the compounds (virtual or real) within this space are druggable. The anti-overlap area corresponds to the poorly druggable compounds. The same parameters used to define the boundaries of druggable compounds (*e.g.*, Ro5) can be used to define a specific target space, including drugs. By analogy, other cubes can be drawn for drugs destined for other administrative routes such as ocular, inhalation, and transdermal [40]. In addition, several other spaces (*vide supra*) can be defined (clusterized) such as natural product chemical space and commercial library chemical space (existing and virtual compounds), not shown in Fig. 13.1. In summary, an anti-overlap between the drug-like space and chemical space defines the chemical space of a "poor" drug lead's properties, while the overlap between drug-like space and chemical space defines a good chemical property space on which druggable active compounds can be developed. Importantly, once the boundaries of each chemical cluster is defined, and based on guidelines such as Ro3–5, the navigation inside each cluster can be performed using metrics-filters, such as ligand efficiency (LE) or others [41], in order to select the "best" druggable compounds within each cluster.

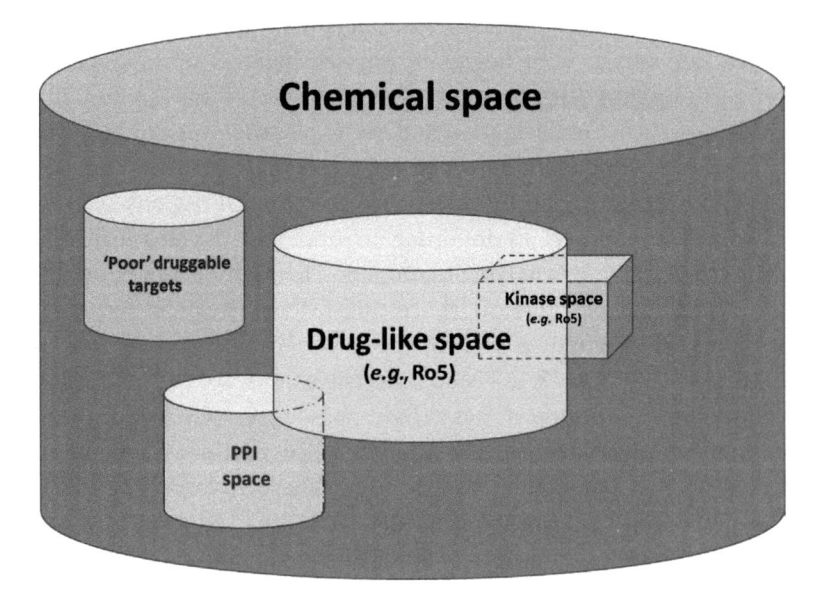

Figure 13.1 Three-dimensional representation of the chemical space, different specific spaces corresponding to targets (PPI, kinases, poor druggable targets, etc.).

Very importantly, helpful simple optimization or selection metrics/indices were implemented in order to navigate inside the different chemical spaces either for the selection of compounds in the existing collections or for the design of compounds to be synthesized. Thus, in order to avoid property inflation (*e.g.*, e-ADMET parameters), molecular mass properties (molecular obesity), and lipophilicity (logP) during the multidimensional approaches of the progression from hit to lead and then to final drug molecule, the concept of LE indice has been emphasized. LE is defined as the Gibbs free energy of binding per non-hydrogen (heavy) atoms. These crucial metrics abolish the concept that only the potency is the appropriate driver for medicinal chemistry optimization. Other metrics were also described such as size-independent ligand efficiency (SILE), lipophilic ligand efficiency (LLE), enthalpic efficiency (EE), and, very recently, drug efficiency (DRUGeff), which is a simple parameter that accounts for all the factors influencing compound concentration at the site of action. A helpful summary and analysis of these different metrics/indices have been mentioned in the Keserü and Hann's review [42].

13.3   Dendrimer Space Concept

In the nanomedicine domain, taking inspiration from various relevant chemical space explorations and from the large number of biomedical applications of dendrimers and dendrons developed by a few in the early 1990s, we introduced the dendrimer space concept as a druggable cluster identified within the vast volume of chemical space [43].

The chemistry of dendrimers was first introduced in 1978 by Fritz Vögtle and coworkers [44]. Numerous biological studies using dendrimers were carried out and highlighted in several review articles [45]. Dendrimers represent a unique class of polymers, with highly branched 3D architectures, whose shape and size can be precisely controlled. They display an exponential number of dendritic branches (hydrophobic and hydrophilic moieties) radiating out from a central core unit. Interior layers (generations, Gn, where n is generally from 1 to 6 and more exceptionally to 12) are made of regularly repeating branching units attached to the core.

The dendrimer diameter increases linearly, while the number of surface groups increases exponentially for each generation.

Dendrimers can be employed as nanocarriers for the delivery of drugs [46]. For this aim, two different approaches have been used: (1) physical encapsulation of drugs in the void spaces of the dendrimers (dendrimer boxes) or electrostatic binding between the drugs and the ionic peripheral groups on the surface of dendrimers; (2) covalent linking of the drug to the dendrimer surface. The last approach is similar to the prodrug approach (Fig. 13.2). This should be extended to other biocompatible nanodevices currently used in the drug-delivery approach such as liposomes, micelles, and polymers.

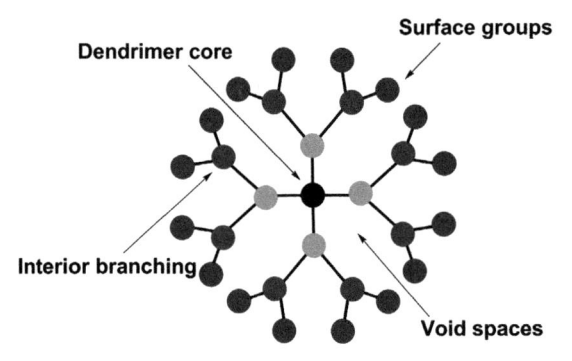

Figure 13.2 Two-dimensional chemical structure of dendrimers as nanocarriers.

Importantly, dendrimers can be used as drugs *per se* in different therapeutic fields. Thus, Majoral and Caminade developed phosphorus dendrimers as anti-cancer [47], anti-prion [48], anti-Alzheimer's [49], anti-coagulant, antidote, and anti-inflammatory [50, 51] (Fig. 13.3). Interestingly, in 2012 Starpharma (Melbourne, Australia) started two important pivotal phase III for the treatment of bacterial vaginosis with VivaGel® [52].

The use of dendrimers offers the following advantages: (1) Encapsulation of poorly soluble drugs into the hydrophobic void spaces within water-soluble dendrimers allows solubilization of the plain drug. In this case, the dendrimers function as unimolecular micelles. (2) Dendrimers having a diameter larger than 5 nm, exceeding the renal threshold, cannot be filtered out of the bloodstream by kidneys, and consequently they circulate for longer. (3) The presence of hydrophilic terminal surface groups on the dendrimers prevents their opsonization or the recognition by macrophages and elimination by the nonspecific reticuloendothelial system (RES). (4) Dendrimers tend to passively extravasate through the leaky vasculature (large pore size: 400–800 nm) of solid tumors. Therefore, a preferential accumulation of dendrimers into tumor tissues, *versus* healthy tissues, is observed due to ineffective lymphatic drainage, which is known as EPR (enhanced permeation and retention) effect [53]. In the case of encapsulated drugs, the drugs can be selectively released in the tumor tissue and diffused throughout the tumor cells (passive targeting).

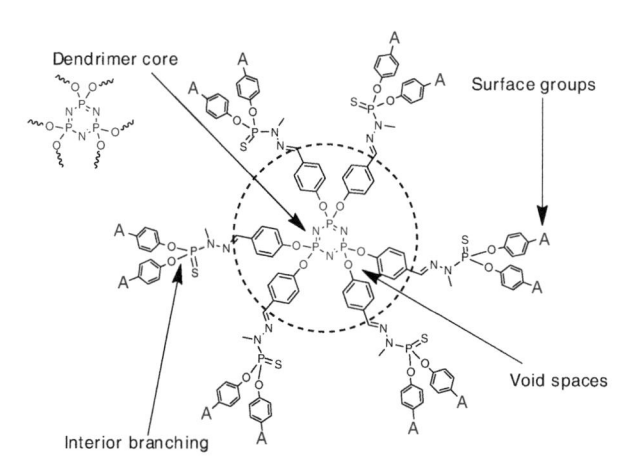

Figure 13.3 Two-dimensional structural units of phosphorus-based dendrimer for pharmaceutical drug carriers or active *per se*.

Taking inspiration from both, the different chemical space exploration/navigation approaches (*vide supra*) and the large number of biomedical applications of dendrimers developed from a handful in the early 1990s, whose one of us (J.-P. Majoral) had highly contributed by opening new areas in medicinal chemistry (*vide supra*), we paved the term of dendrimer space concept as a new druggable cluster, which is included in the vast volume of chemical space (Fig. 13.4) [43]. This new approach affords a new vision of pharmaceutical science research and opens new and promising avenues to find new drug-based dendrimers.

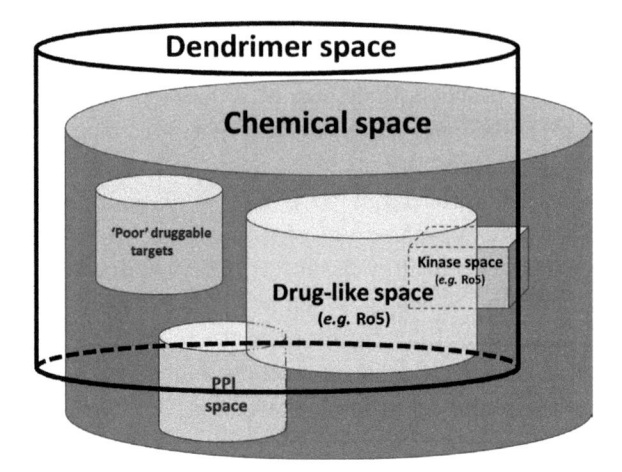

Figure 13.4 Three-dimensional representation of the chemical space, different clusters of chemical space and dendrimer space.

Figure 13.4 depicts the overlapping of the continuum of chemical space (parallelepiped box) and, for instance, diverse discrete areas such as drug-like space (Ro5), the "target classes" PPI space, kinase space, and dendrimer space (block-cylinders). For instance, the overlap volumes between drug-like space and PPI space represent the druggable PPI space (including, for instance, the PPI small-molecule inhibitors), whereas the anti-overlap area corresponds to the current poorly druggable PPI inhibitors/targets, which is a very challenging domain in medicinal chemistry. The dendrimer space covers greater part of the drug-like space (Ro5) and, very interestingly, should cover the poorly druggable PPI space, opening new way to find new drugs.

Notably, the multidimensional limits of drug-dendrimer space are associated with numerous biological and pharmacological applications of both dendrimer-based products (dendrimers as therapeutic compounds *per se*) and dendrimers as drug carriers (covalent conjugation or noncovalent encapsulation of drugs). Clearly, navigating inside the dendrimer space and encompassing both of its characteristics and boundaries, the drug-discovery community will take advantage of the versatile dendrimeric platform for the development of various new biomedical applications in nanoscience. This innovative biomedical approach creates exciting and interesting opportunities for novel nanomedicine developments.

Going into more detail, the development of dendrimer platforms has been directed toward specific organs, tissues, cells, and various biological targets [45]. Very interestingly, multifunctional dendrimers can be used for a wide range of biomedical applications, including intracellular delivery, for instance, of small and large molecules such as cyclic-peptides [54], short hairpin RNA (shRNA) [55], small interfering RNA (siRNA) [56], antibodies [57], and aptamers [58]. These multiple applications in medicinal chemistry are the result of the development of over 100 different dendritic structures with a huge number of functionalities on their surfaces.

Consequently, dendrimers represent also a novel non-viral gene-delivery carrier. Thus, several studies on the transfection efficiency in neuronal cells using dendrimers have been performed. For interesting examples, neuroprotective effect of rat cortical neurons with anti-HIF1-α siRNA complexed with cationic carbosilane dendrimers has been mentioned by Posadas *et al.* [59], and the neuroprotection of rat neurons, astrocytes, microglia, and oligodendrocytes with HMGB1 shRNA-expressing plasmid complexed with cationic arginine-grafted PAMAM dendrimers was portrayed by Kim and colleagues, as well [60].

13.4 Conclusion and Perspectives

For the medicinal chemist, the exploration of dendrimer space is an additional useful way to find and develop the drugs of tomorrow and represents a key concept in drug discovery. Based on several and selected success stories, the boundaries of the dendrimer space can be summarized as the main following dendrimer's propensities: (1) enhance the therapeutic potency, the pharmacokinetic and pharmacodynamic behaviors of the plain drug; (2) reduce toxicity *versus* activity, deliver drugs in designated place of supply; (3) possible use of both active and passive drug targeting; (4) overcome low oral bioavaibility; (5) allow non-classical routes of administration (transdermal, transnasal, ocular delivery system, etc.); and (6) permit the development of a theranostic nanomedicine directed to a personalized medicine. These non-exhaustive dendrimer characteristics defining the dendrimer space will be illustrated with several examples such as classical and non-classical routes of administration of a drug complexed with dendrimers. In the way to use dendrimers in the theranostic approach for nanomedicine, the design of nontoxic, biocompatible, and efficient organic dendritic nanodots for diagnosis will open new avenues in medicine.

This new concept of dendrimer space fully corroborates D. J. Triggle's suggestion: "The chemist is as astronaut searching for biologically useful space in the chemical universe" [61]. Generally speaking, we agree with Antoine de Saint-Exupéry's sentence: "The only things you learn are the things you tame" (The little Prince).

Acknowledgments

Thanks are due to the CNRS and CEFIPRA (Project number 5303-2) for financial support.

References

1. Dunne, S., Shannon, B., Dunne, C., and Cullen, W. (2013). A review of the differences and similarities between generic drugs and their originator counterparts, including economic benefits associated with usage of generic medicines, using Ireland as a case study, *BMC Pharmacol. Toxicol.*, **14**, pp. 1–19.

2. Calo-Fernandez, B. and Martinez-Hurtado, J. L. (2012). Biosimilars: Company strategies to capture value from the biologics market, *Pharmaceuticals.*, **5**, pp. 1393–1408.

3. Davenport, M. (2014). Covering the spread, *CEN*, **10**, pp. 10–13.

4. Jarvis, L. M. (2015). The year in new drugs, *CEN*, **2**, pp. 11–16.

5. Schulze, U., Baedeker, M., Chen, Y. T., and Greber, D. (2014). R&D productivity: On the comeback trail, *Nat. Rev. Drug Disc.*, **13**, pp. 331–332.

6. Borchard, R. T. (2008). Drug design with ADME in mind: Recent paradigm shifts in drug discovery, in: *Towards Drugs of the Future: Key Issues in Lead Finding and Lead Optimization*, Kruse, C. G. and Timmerman, H. (Eds.) (IOS Press, Amsterdam).

7. Kuseru, G. M. and Makara, M. G. (2009). The influence of lead discovery strategies on the properties of drug candidates, *Nat. Rev. Drug Disc.*, **18**, pp. 203–212.

8. Yusof, I. and Segall, D. (2013). Considering the impact drug-like properties have on the chance of success, *Nat. Rev. Drug Disc.*, **18**, pp. 659–666.

9. Tyrchan, C., Blomber, N., Engkvist, O., Kogei, T., and Muresan, S. (2009). Physico property profiles of marketed drugs, clinical candidates, and bioactive compounds, *Bioorg. Med. Chem. Lett.*, **15**, pp. 6943–6947.

10. Yusof, I., Shah, F., Hashimoto, T., Segall, M. D., and Greene, N. (2014). Finding the rules for successful drug optimization, *Drug Discov. Today*, **19**, pp. 680–687.

11. Leeson, P. (2012). Drug discovery: Chemical beauty contest, *Nature*, **481**, pp. 455–456.

12. Veber, R., Johnson S. R., Cheng, H. Y., Smith, B. R., Ward, K. W., and Kopple, K. D. (2002), Molecular properties that influence the oral bioavailability of drug candidates, *J. Med. Chem.*, **45**, pp. 2615–2623.

13. Prentis, R. A. (1988). Pharmaceutical innovation by the seven UK-owned pharmaceutical companies (1964–1985), *Br. J. Clin. Pharmacol.*, **25**, pp. 387–396.

14. Doak, B. C., Zheng, J., Dobritzsch, D., and Kihlberg, J. (2016). How beyond rule of 5 drugs and clinical candidates bind to their targets, *J. Med. Chem.*, **59**, pp. 2312–2327.

15. Schamberger, J., Grimm, M., Steinmeyer, A., and Hillisch, A. (2011). Rendezvous in chemical space? Comparing the small molecule compound libraries of Byer and Schering, *Drug Discov. Today*, **16**, pp. 636–641.

16. Constantino, L. and Barlocco, D. (2006). Privileged structures as leads in medicinal chemistry, *Curr. Med. Chem.*, **13**, pp. 65–85.

17. St Jean, D. T. and Fotsch, C. (2012). Mitigating heterocycles metabolism in drug discovery, *J. Med. Chem.*, **55**, pp. 6002–6020.

18. Tajabadi, F. M., Campitelli, M. R., and Quinn, R. J. (2013). Scaffold flatness: Reversing the trend, *Springer Sci. Rev.*, **1**, pp. 141–151.

19. Ritchie, T. J. and Macdonald, J. F. (2009). The impact of aromatic ring count on compound developability: Are too many aromatic rings a liability in drug design, *Drug Discov. Today*, **14**, pp. 1011–1020.

20. Bickerton, G. R., Paolini, G. V., Besnard, J., Muresan, S., and Hopkins, A. L. (2012). Quantifying the chemical beauty of drugs, *Nat. Chem.*, **4**, pp. 90–98.

21. Morelli, X., Bourgeas, R., and Roche, P. (2011). Chemical and structural lessons from recent successes in protein–protein interaction inhibition (2P2I), *Curr. Opin. Chem.Biol.*, **15**, pp. 475–481.

22. Edfeldt, F. N. B., Folmer, R. H. A., and Breeze, A. L. (2011). Fragment screening to predict druggability (ligandability) and lead discovery success, *Drug Discov. Today*, **16**, pp. 284–287.

23. Segall, M. D. (2012). Multi-parameter optimization: Identifying high-quality compounds with balance of properties, *Curr. Pharm. Des.*, **18**, pp. 1292–1310.

24. Jadhav, P. B., Yadav, A. R., and Gore, M. G. (2015). Concept of drug likeness in pharmaceutical research, *Int. J. Pharm. Bio. Sci.*, **6**, pp. 142–154.

25. Kerns, E. H. and Di, L. (2008). *Drug-Like Properties: Concepts, Structure Design and Methods. From ADME to Toxicity Optimization* (Elsevier, Amsterdam).

26. Lipinski, C. and Hopkins, A. (2004). Navigating chemical space for biology and medicine, *Nature*, **432**, pp. 855–861.

27. Reymond, J.-L. (2010). Chemical space as a source for new drugs, *Med. Chem. Commun.*, **1**, pp. 30–38.

28. Wong, Y.-S. (2012). Exploring chemical space: Recent advances in chemistry, *Methods Mol. Biol.*, **800**, pp. 11–23.

29. Oprea, T. I. (2002). Current trends in lead discovery: Are we looking for the appropriate properties, *J. Compt. Aided Mol. Des.*, **16**, pp. 325–334.

30. Makara, G. M. (2007). On sampling of fragment space, *J. Med. Chem.*, **14**, pp. 3214–3221.

31. Goldberg, F. W., Kettle, J. G., Kogej, T., Perry, M. W. D., and Tomkinson, N. P. (2015). Designing novel building blocks is an overlooked strategy to improve compound quality, *Drug Discov. Today*, **20**, pp. 11–17.

32. Lachance, H., Wetzel, S., Kumar, K., and Wadmann, H. (2012). Charting, navigating, and populating natural product chemical space for drug discovery, *J. Med. Chem.*, **55**, pp. 5989–6001.

33. Van Drie, J. H. (1998). Approaches to virtual library design, *Drug Discov. Today*, **3**, pp. 274–283.

34. Hajduk, P. J. (2005). Druggability indices for protein targets derived from NMR-based screening data, *J. Med. Chem.*, **48**, pp. 2518–2525.

35. Barril, X. (2013). Druggability predictions: Methods, limitations, and applications, *Wiley Interdiscip. Rev. Comput. Mol. Sci.*, **3**, pp. 327–338.

36. Perot, S., Sperandio, O., Miteva, M. A., Camprox, A. C., and Villoutreix, B. O. (2010). Druggable pockets and binding site centric chemical space: A paradigm shift in drug discovery, *Drug Discov. Today,* **15**, pp. 656–667.

37. Oprea, T. I., Zamora, I., and Ungell, A. L. (2002). Pharmacokinetically based mapping device for chemical space navigation, *J. Comb. Chem.*, **4**, pp. 258–266.

38. Lloyd, D. G., Golfis, G., Knox, A. J., Fayne, D., Meegan, M. J., and Oprea, T. I. (2006). Oncology exploration: Charting cancer medicinal chemistry space, *Drug Discov. Today*, **11**, pp. 149–159.

39. Mirza, A., Desai, R., and Reynisson, J. (2009). Known drug space as a metric in exploring the boundaries of drug-like chemical space, *Eur. J. Med. Chem.*, **44**, pp. 5006–5011.

40. Choy, Y. B. and Prausnitz, M. R. (2011). The rule of five for non-oral routes of drug delivery: Ophthalmic, inhalation and transdermal, *Pharm. Res.*, **28**, pp. 943–948.

41. Hopkins, A. L., Keseru, G. M., Leeson, P. D., Rees, D. C., and Reynolds, C. H. (2014). The role of ligand efficiency metrics in drug discovery, *Nat. Rev. Drug Disc.*, **13**, pp. 105–121.

42. Hann, M. M. and Keseru, G. M. (2012). Finding the sweet spot: The role of nature and nurture in medicinal chemistry, *Nat. Rev. Drug Disc.*, **30**, pp. 355–365.

43. Mignani, S., El Kazzouli, S., Bousmina, M., and Majoral, J.-P. (2013). Dendrimer space concept for innovative nanomedicine: A futuristic vision for medicinal chemistry, *Prog. Polym. Sci.*, **38**, pp. 993–1008.

44. Buhleier, E. Wehner, W., and Vogtle, F. (1978). 'Cascade' – and 'nonskid-chain-like' syntheses of molecular cavity topologies, *Synthesis*, **2**, pp. 155–158.

45. (a) Lee, C. C., Mackay, J. A., Frechet, J. M. J., and Szoka, F. C. (2005). Designing dendrimers for biological applications, *Nat. Biotechnol.*, **23**, pp. 1517–1526; (b) Svenson, S. and Tomalia, D. A. (2005). Commentary: Dendrimers in biomedical applications reflections on the field, *Adv. Drug Deliv. Rev.*, **57**, pp. 2106–2129.

46. Kesharwani, P., Jain, K., and Jain, N. K. (2014). Dendrimer as nanocarrier for drug delivery, *Prog. Polym. Sci.*, **39**, pp. 268–307.

47. El Brahmi, N., El Kazzouli, S., Mignani, S., Essassi, E. M., Aubert, G., Laurent, R., Caminade, A. M., Bousmina, M., Cresteil, T., and Majoral, J. P. (2013). Original multivalent copper(II)-conjugated phosphorus dendrimers and corresponding mononuclear copper(II) complexes with antitumoral activities, *Mol. Pharm.*, **10**, pp. 1459–1464.

48. Solassol, J., Crozet, C., Perrier, V., Leclaire, J., Béranger, F., Caminade, A. M., Meunier, B., Dormon, D., Majoral, J. P., and Lehmann, S. (2004). Cationic phosphorous-containing dendrimers reduce prion replication

both in cell cultures and in mice infected with scrapie, *J. Gen. Virol.*, **85**, pp. 1791–1799.

49. Mignani, S., Bryszewska, M., Zablocka, M., Klajnert-Maculewicz, B., Cladera, J., Shcharbin, D., and Majoral, J. P. (2017). Can dendrimer-based nanoparticles fight neurodegenerative diseases? Current situation *versus* other established approaches, *Prog. Polym. Sci.*, **64**, 23–51.

50. Blattes, E., Vercellone, A., Eutamene, H., Turrin, C. O., Theodorou, V., Majoral, J. P., Caminade, A. M., Prandi, J., Nigou, J., and Puzo, G. (2013). Mannodendrimers prevent acute lung inflammation by inhibiting neutrophil recruitment, *Proc. Nat. Acad. Sci. USA*, **110**, pp. 8795–8800.

51. Hayder, M., Poupot, M., Baron, M., Nigon, D., Turrin, C. O., Caminade, A. M., Majoral, J. P., Eisenberg, R. A., Fournié, J. J., Cantagrel, A., Poupot, R., and Davignon, J. L. (2011). Phosphorus-based dendrimer as nanotherapeutics targeting both inflammation and osteoclastogenesis in experimental arthritis, *Sci. Transl. Med.*, **3**, pp. 81ra35.

52. McCarthy, T. D., Karellas, P., Henderson, S. A., Giannis, M., O'Keefe, D. F., Heery, G., Paull, J. R. A., Matthews, B. R., and Holan, G. (2005). Dendrimers as drugs: Discovery and preclinical and clinical development of dendrimer-based microbicides for HIV and STI prevention, *Mol. Pharmacol.*, **2**, pp. 312–318.

53. Anajwala, C. C., Jani, G. K., and Swamy, S. M. V. (2010). Current trends of nanotechnology for cancer therapy, *Int. J. Pharm. Sci. Drug Res.*, **3**, pp. 1043–1056.

54. Spetzler, J. C. and Tam, J. P. (1996). Self-assembly of cyclic peptides on a dendrimer: Multiple cyclic antigen peptides, *Peptide Res.*, **9**, pp. 290–296.

55. Liu, X., Huang, H., Wang, J., Wang, C., Wang, M., Zhang, B., and Pan, C. (2011). Dendrimers-delivered short hairpin RNA targeting hTERT inhibits oral cancer cell growth *in vitro* and *in vivo*, *Biochem. Pharmacol.*, **82**, pp. 17–23.

56. Patil, M. L., Zhang, M., and Minko, T. (2011). Multifunctional triblock nanocarrier (PAMAM-PEG-PLL) for the efficient intracellular siRNA delivery and gene silencing, *ACS Nano.*, **5**, pp. 1877–1887.

57. New, K., Milenic, D. E., Ray, G. L., Kim, Y. S., and Brechbiel, M. W. (2012). Preparation of cystamine core dendrimer and anti-body-dendrimer conjugates for RMI angiography, *Mol. Pharm.*, **9**, pp. 374–381.

58. Lee, I. H., An, S., Yu, M. K., Kwon, H. K., Im, S. H., and Jon, S. (2011). Targeted chemoimmunotherapy using drug-loaded aptamer-dendrimer bioconjugates, *J. Control. Release*, **7**, pp. 435–441.

59. Posadas, I., Lopez-Hernadez, B., Clemente, M. I., Jimenez, J. L., Ortega, P., de la Mata, P. J., Gomez, R., Munoz-Fernandez, M. A., and Cena, V. (2009). Highly efficient transfection of rat cortical neurons using carbosilane dendrimers unveils a neuroprotective role for HIF-1alpha in early chemical hypoxia-mediated neurotoxicity, *Pharmaceut. Res.*, **26**, pp. 1181–1191.

60. Kim, J. B., Choi, J. S., Nam, K., Lee, M., Park, J. S., and Lee, J. K. (2006). Enhanced transfection of primary cortical cultures using arginine-grafted PAMAM dendrimer PAMAM-Arg, *J. Control. Release*, **114**, pp. 110–117.

61. Triggle, J. (2009). The chemist as astronaut: Searching for biologically useful space in the chemical universe, *Biochem. Pharmacol.*, **78**, pp. 217–223.

Chapter 14

DNA-Based Multiplexing Technology for Rapid and Accurate Diagnosis of Pathogens. An Original Contribution of Phosphorus Dendrimers

Jean Pierre Majoral,[a,b] Alice Senescau,[b] Jean Marie François,[b,c] and Richard Fabre[b]

[a]*Laboratoire de Chimie de Coordination, CNRS, 205 Route de Narbonne, BP 44099, 31077 Toulouse Cedex 4, France*
[b]*Dendris SAS, 335 rue du Chêne vert, ZAC de la Bourgade, 31670 Labège, France*
[c]*Laboratoire d'Ingénierie des Systèmes Biologiques & des Procédés, UMR CNRS 5504 & INRA 792, 135 avenue de Rangueil, 31077 Toulouse Cedex 4, France*
jean-pierre.majoral@lcc-toulouse.fr

14.1 Concept and Approach

14.1.1 Current Methods in In Vitro Diagnosis: Assets and Limits

More than a hundred years ago, Pasteur and his followers introduced diagnosis of infectious diseases by cultivating pathogens on petri

Phosphorus Dendrimers in Biology and Nanomedicine: Synthesis, Characterization, and Properties
Edited by Anne-Marie Caminade, Cédric-Olivier Turrin, and Jean-Pierre Majoral
Copyright © 2018 Pan Stanford Publishing Pte. Ltd.
ISBN 978-981-4774-33-8 (Hardcover), 978-1-315-11085-1 (eBook)
www.panstanford.com

dishes. The Pasteur's method or microbiological method involves isolation, cultivation and identification, and additional biochemical tests of the bacteria, virus, fungus, or parasitic pathogen potentially responsible for infections in the biological sample. The diagnosis can take at best 2 days, unless the etiologic agent responsible for the infectious disease has not been identified, which requires additional (time-dependent) tests. Methods based on automatic sewers and mass spectrometry have recently appeared in some reference centers and medical laboratories. This technology is, however, not applicable to non-cultivable microbes and requires well-trained technicians as it needs an expensive and sophisticated mass spectrometer not accessible to most laboratories for medical analysis.

On the other hand, the PCR (polymerase chain reaction) technology, which brings about a molecular approach to diagnosis, is more sensitive and accurate, offers a short time of response, and can be applied to uncultured species.

14.1.2 Emerging Multiplex Technologies in In Vitro Diagnosis

Since the same clinical symptoms diagnosed by a physician can be caused by more than one pathogen, the new paradigm is to consider a syndrome-based approach to diagnosis, which basically aims at identifying all potential pathogens responsible for the syndrome. According to the Infectious Diseases Society of America and FDA [1], syndrome-based diagnosis is a dramatic new way of *in vitro* diagnosis (IVD) since Pasteur. This new approach also coincides with the exponential demand for new IVD techniques that are more informative by providing more data from a single biological sample, while being more precise, fast, and affordable at cost-effective value [2–4]. The syndrome-based approach of IVD requires a multiplexing detection method, leading to the development and commercialization of multiplex PCR technology allowing parallel identification of up to 22 entities [5], but they all require expensive equipment.

Alternatively, there are also initiatives in the USA to use the next-generation sequencing technology to address this syndrome-based diagnosis, which were presented during international conferences and workshops in 2015. However, these technologies, although quite robust and powerful, are only accessible to big hospitals and clinical centers that can install a fully equipped platform with well-trained staff able to master large date sets with adapted bioinformatic tools.

14.2 Dendris Solution Concept Positioning Toward Existing Methods

After the microbiology based on Pasteur's method and PCR, the company Dendris [6] proposed a third-generation of diagnosis enabling the search of a broad range of pathogens, with high sensitivity and specificity. Successful use and reliability of microarray technology is highly dependent on several factors, including surface chemistry parameters and accessibility of cDNA targets to the DNA probes fixed onto the surface. It was shown that functionalization of glass slides with phosphorus dendrimers with aldehyde functions at their periphery [7–9] (Fig. 14.1) allows production of more sensitive and reliable DNA microarrays.

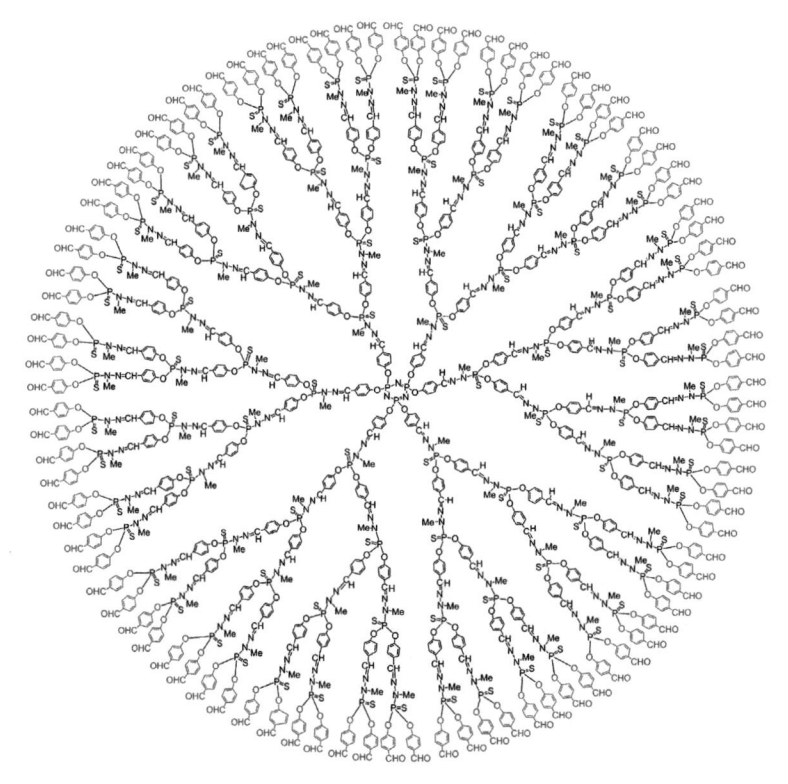

Figure 14.1 Structure of a phosphorus dendrimer of generation 4 bearing 96 terminal aldehyde groups.

Covalent attachment of these spherical reactive chemical structures on amino-silanized glass slides generates a reactive ~50 Å layer onto which amino-modified DNA probes are covalently bound. This new grafting chemistry leads to the formation of uniform and homogenous spots. Moreover, probe concentration before spotting could be reduced from 0.2 to 0.02 mg/ml with PCR products and from 20 to 5 µM with 70mer oligonucleotides without affecting signal intensities after hybridization with Cy3- and Cy5-labeled targets. The process of coating of the dendrimers on silanized glass slide as well as the DNA probes printing (grafting of amino oligonucleotides as well as hybridization with complementary oligonucleotides) is illustrated in Fig. 14.2.

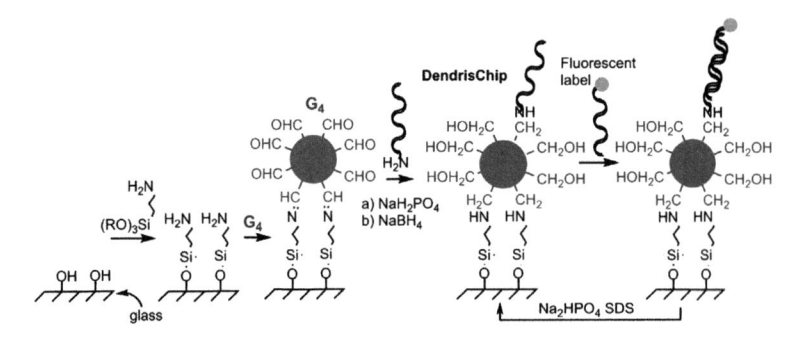

Figure 14.2 Functionalization of glass slides with phosphorus dendrimers bearing aldehyde functions at their periphery (see its structure in Fig. 14.1) to afford a DendrisChip.

The functionalization of the glass slide with phosphorus dendrimers benefits from three advantages: (i) an increase in the density of probes per unit surface and thus in the number of binding sites; (ii) a greater accessibility of the target to the probes with hybridization in 3D and not 2D like many other activated surfaces; (iii) a greater spacer from the glass surface reducing the unspecific interaction. Figure 14.3 focusses on the advantages of DendrisChip compared to other competitors. The interaction between probe and target is 10 to 100 times higher than with the others.

Based on these results, Dendris has developed an affordable and easy-to-use multiplex diagnosis, for syndrome-based diseases and biomarkers validation. The kit is intended for hospitals and medical laboratories with a user-friendly IVD device. In a single test, it provides a rapid and accurate diagnosis, thus improving and accelerating the medical decision-making. The IVD solution shall lead to a new standard, which could reduce public health costs (Table 14.1). Rapid diagnosis delay will establish a faster curative action and determine the best treatment to prescribe in the context of personalized medicine.

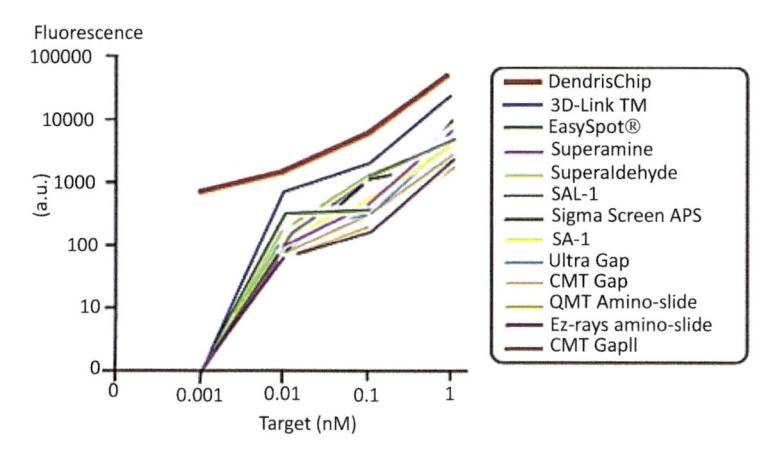

Figure 14.3 The advantages of DendrisChip compared to other potential competitors.

Table 14.1 Comparative analysis of criteria from the different technologies used in IVD

	Pasteur's method	Mass spectrometry	PCR	PCR + DendriChip
Multiplex	No	No	Yes, max 3	Yes, max 20
Time of response	48 h	24 h	3 h	5 h
Non-cultivable species	No	No	Yes	Yes
Reagents cost and equipment	€5 per species	€5.25 per species	€20 per species	€50 per min 15 species or €3.3 per species
Automatization	No	Semi	Yes	Yes
Man power cost	High	Medium	Low	Low

The β-tester prototype available today from Dendris is depicted in Fig. 14.4. It includes a dedicated scanner (Dendriscan) to read the DendrisChip. In addition, it contains a simple SoftDiag for data analysis, which is based on an algorithmic method. Results of this diagnosis method are illustrated in Fig. 14.5.

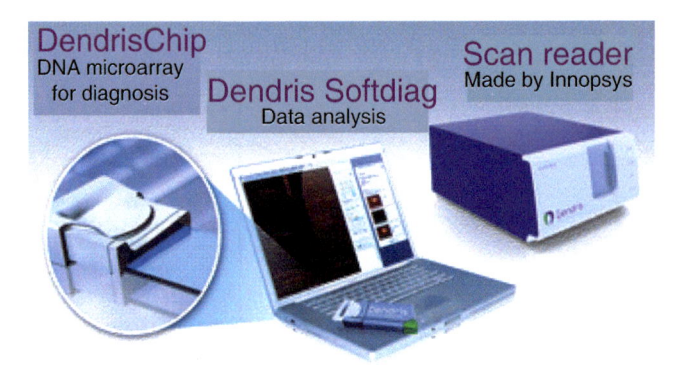

Figure 14.4 β-tester prototype proposed by Dendris.

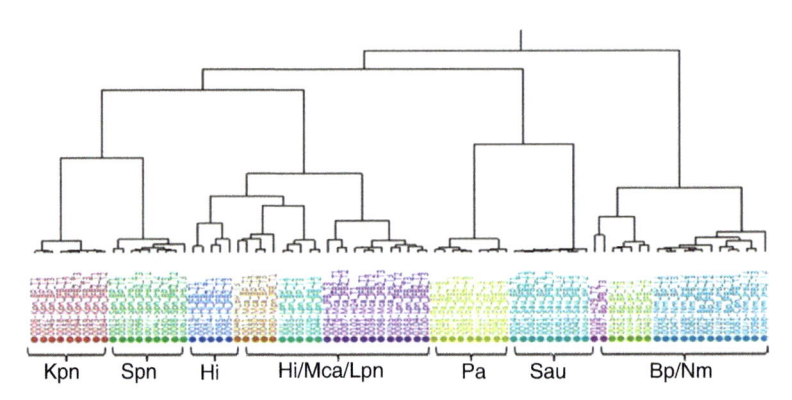

Figure 14.5 Classification tree from 81 tests deduced from DendrisChip analysis. Abbreviations: Kpn: *Klebsiella pneumoniae*; Spn: *Streptococcus pneumoniae*; Hi: *Hemophilis influenza*; Sau: *Staphylococcus aureus*; Lpn: *Legionella Pneumophila*; Pa: *Pseudomonas aeruginosa*; BP: *Bordetella pertussis*; Nm: *Neisseria meningitis*; Mca: *Moraxella catarrhalis*.

The statistical method allows classification of most of the bacteria species used in the training. The collusion of three species in almost the same group (Hi/Mca/Lpn) was actually due to their wrong assignation of species confirmed by sequencing analysis. Thus, the DendrisChip provides an accurate diagnostic and also allows questioning about identification assessed by microbial methods.

14.3 Applications of DendrisChips

14.3.1 Respiratory Diseases

The Dendris solution to IVD in respiratory infection is fully compliant with medical practice. Respiratory tract infection is the most widespread infectious disease and is caused by a wide range of microorganisms, which are difficult to clinically distinguish due to similarities in symptoms. Dendris is developing a symptom approach based on their proprietary DendrisChips technology, which can rapidly discriminate 11 bacteria (Fig. 14.6) responsible for this infection. This method shall not solely complete traditional diagnostic assays but overcome limitations of the current assays in providing a rapid, accurate, and more informative diagnosis, which could reduce the use of antibiotic therapies.

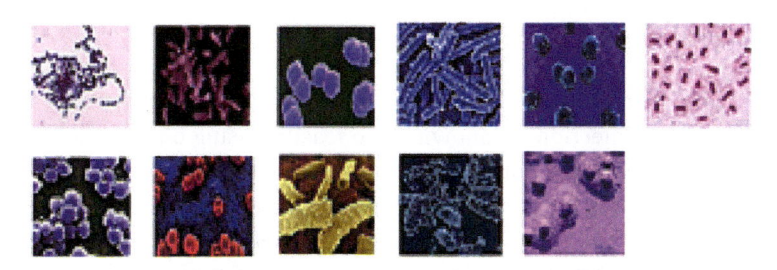

Figure 14.6 Types of bacteria discriminated by the DendrisChip. From left to right, first row: *Streptococcus pneumoniae*; *Pseudomonas aeruginosa*; *Moraxella catarrhalis*; *Legionella pneumophila*; *Chlamydia pneumoniae*; *Haemophilus influenza*. Second row: *Staphylococcus aureus*; *Neisseria meningitidis*; *Bordetella pertussis*; *Klebsiella pneumoniae*; *Mycoplasma influenza*.

In numerous cases, the DendrisChip confirmed the presence of a pathogen suspected but not confirmed by culture in several examples and revealed more information thanks to its ability to detect co-infections (Table 14.2).

Table 14.2 Examples of cases where the chip gave additional information, which could help clinicians to adapt a treatment

Specimens	Patients	Context	Culture	DendrisChipRD
Sputum	A 7-year-old child	Permanent bronchial overload + cerebellar syndrome	No pathogen	Nm, Spn
NPS	A 81-year-old woman	9 days after hospitalization for a bronchial surinfection (antibiotherapy + O_2)	Few Hi	Hi, Pa
Throat	A 36-year-old woman	Spn suspected: dysphagia + erythema on forearm and thorax	Sau	Sau, Spn

Nm: *Neisseria meningitidis*; Spn: *Streptococcus pneumoniae*; Hi: *Haemophilis influenzae*; Pa: *Pseudomonas aeruginosa*; Sau: *Staphylococcus aureus* (NPS: Nasopharingal swabs).

The symptom-based diagnosis of 11 bacteria responsible for respiratory infections is shown to be feasible using our technology and provides a diagnostic value in less than 6 h. The diagnosis is obtained thanks to the implementation of a unique statistical learning method that shall become even more accurate due to its ability of self-training by increasing the number of samples from clinical laboratories.

In addition, another practical reason for choosing these solutions is depicted in Fig. 14.7. A doctor, when receiving a patient suffering from an infectious disease, commonly seeks for the responsible bacteria as it is the cause of more than 80% of the disease leading to the identification of delivering the appropriate medication, whereas for the virus, there is no appropriate treatment[1] in most cases.

---

[1]A viral identification 3-1 leads only to a symptomatic treatment except for the flu-like virus, which usually occurs in an epidemic and seasonal context where the clinician is warned. Thus, direct assay by immunoblots are useful and enough to establish the viral infection with eventually hospitalization.

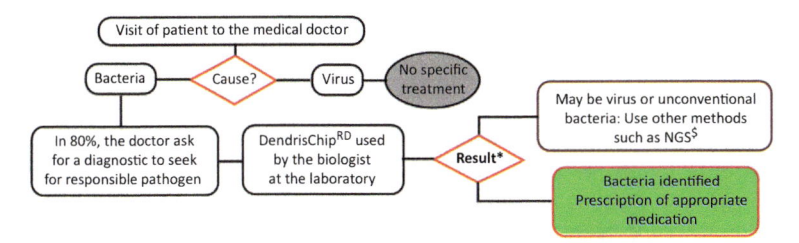

Figure 14.7 The current feasibility of the DendrisChip according to the medical practice for the respiratory infectious diseases. (*: the results can be obtained in less than 5 h; $: NGS: next generation sequencing technology)

14.3.2   Sexual Diagnosis

Another DendrisChip is dedicated to the identification of the 10 pathogens commonly implicated in sexual diseases (Fig. 14.8).

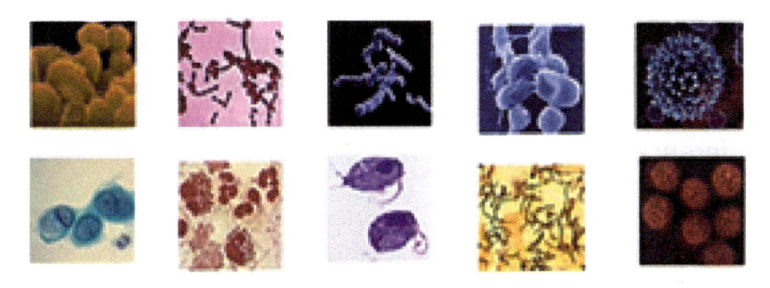

Figure 14.8 Pathogens commonly implicated in sexual diseases. From left to right, first row: *Mycoplasma genitalium*; *Haemophilus ducreyi*; *Steptococcus agalactiae*; *Candida albicans*; HSV 1 & 2 (herpes simplex virus). Second row: *Chlamydia trachomatis*; *Neisseria gonorrhoeae*; *Trichomonas vaginalis*; *Treponema pallidum*; HPV 16 & 18 (human papillomavirus).

14.3.3   Other Main Applications of DendrisChips

Three other main applications can be pointed out: Food safety project allows to detect in multiplex mode several bacteria: *Staphylococcus aureus, Listeria monocytogenes, Yersinia enterolytica, Bacillus cereus, Salmonella* spp., *Shigella* spp., *Escherichia coli*, while an Oncograde project is based on breast cancer recurrence prognosis. The last one concerns the detection of *legionella* species [10].

14.4 Conclusion

Today, more than 70% of clinical decisions are based on IVD tests. IVD helps physicians to provide the therapeutic and good management of patients' health. With this decisive role in healthcare, IVD innovation is foreseen to better contribute to health savings and meanwhile is a very important economic sector. That is why many companies keep on investing an important part of their revenue (10 to 12%) in IVD R&D. To address the clinical needs in combination with greater health concerns of patients, the most suitable solutions in IVD should meet these features: (i) multiplex rather than simplex (*i.e.,* identify pathogen through a syndrome approach rather than actual mode of single identification by phenotypic or genotypic method), (ii) high sensitivity, (iii) high specificity, (iv) acceptable costs of the whole process (reagents, instrument, and workforce), and (v) non-invasive way.

The solution proposed by Dendris based on the use of phosphorus dendrimers fits perfectly with all requirements summarized above.

References

1. Infectious Diseases Society of America. (2011). IDSA Public Policy: An unmet medical need: Rapid molecular diagnostics tests for respiratory tract infections, *Clin. Infect. Diseases*, **52**, pp. S384–S395.

2. World Alliance Against Antibiotic Resistance, June 2014, http://biomarqueursinfos.fr/rencontres/waaar

3. Dohouhaki, P. and Blondeau, J. M. (2012). Advances in laboratory diagnostic technologies in clinical microbiology and what this means for clinical practice? *Clin. Pract.*, **9**, pp. 347–352.

4. Donatin, E. and Drancourt, M. (2012). DNA microarrays for the diagnostic of infectious diseases, *Médecines et Maladies Infectieuses*, **42**, pp. 453–459.

5. Pillet, S., Lardeux, M., Dina, J., Grattard, F., Verhoeven, P., Le Goff, J., Vabret, A., and Pozzetto, B. (2013). Comparative evaluation of six commercialized multiplex PCR kits for diagnosis of respiratory infections, *PlosOne*, **8**, e72174.

6. www.dendris.fr

7. Trevisiol, E., Le Berre-Anton, V., Leclaire, J., Pratviel, G., Caminade, A. M., Majoral, J. P., Francois, J. M., and Meunier, B. (2003). Dendrislides, DendriChips: A simple chemical functionalization of glass slides with phosphorus dendrimers as an effective means for the preparation of biochips, *New J. Chem.*, **27**, pp. 1713–1719.

8. Le Berre, V., Trevisiol, E., Dagkessamanskaia, A., Sokol, S., Caminade, A. M., Majoral, J. P., Meunier, B., and Francois, J. (2003). Dendrimeric coating of glass slides for sensitive DNA microarrays analysis, *Nucleic Acids Res.*, **31**, pp. 8.

9. Trevisiol, E., Leclaire, J., Pratviel, G., Caminade, A. M., François, J., Majoral J. P., and Meunier, B. (2003). Solid support carrying functionalized dendrimer, useful for immobilization or synthesis of *e.g.* nucleic acids or proteins, particularly as biochips for studying interactions, WO 2003091304.

10. Senescau, A., François, J. M., Bernier, M., and Fabre, R. (2014). Biopuce pour la détection et identification de bactéries du genre legionella, kit et procédé d'utilisation. French Patent N° 2995614.

Index

PGMO 05/02/2018